VEDÂNTA PHILOSOPHY: LECTURES ON JNÂNA YOGA. PART I.

VEDÂNTA PHILOSOPHY: JNÂNA YOGA. PART II. SEVEN LECTURES (2 BOOKS IN ONE)

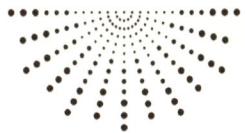

SWÂMI VIVEKÂNANDA

ALICIA EDITIONS

CONTENTS

VEDÂNTA PHILOSOPHY: LECTURES ON JNÂNA YOGA. PART I.

Preface	3
I. The Song of the Sannyasin.	5
II. The Necessity of Religion.	9
III. The Real Nature of Man.	20
IV. Mâyâ and Illusion.	36
V. Mâyâ and the Evolution of the Conception of God.	52
VI. Mâyâ and Freedom.	64
VII. The Absolute and Manifestation.	75
VIII. Unity in Diversity.	88
IX. God in Everything.	101
X. Realization.	111
XI. The Freedom of the Soul.	130
XII. Practical Vedânta. Part I.	143
XIII. Practical Vedânta. Part II.	158
XIV. Practical Vedânta. Part III.	175
XV. Practical Vedânta. Part IV.	187
XVI. Vedânta in All Its Phases.	203
XVII. Vedânta.	222

VEDÂNTA PHILOSOPHY: JNÂNA YOGA. PART II. SEVEN LECTURES

Editor's Preface	259
I. The Sânkhya Cosmology.	265
II. Prakriti and Purusha.	275
III. Sânkhya and Advaita.	286
IV. The Free Soul.	297
V. One Existence Appearing as Many.	309
VI. Unity of the Self.	318
VII. The Highest Ideal of Jnâna Yoga.	325

VEDÂNTA PHILOSOPHY: LECTURES ON JNÂNA YOGA.
PART I.

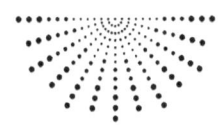

PREFACE

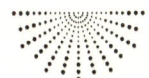

Vedânta Philosophy regards the religious tendencies of mankind as being of four main divisions, the dividing lines not being necessarily sharply defined, for more than one of these tendencies may be found in one individual. Broadly speaking, there is a large class of men who seek to express their religious ideas through ethical work, through constant effort to help and uplift their fellow-men. Then there are others of a strongly devotional character, who find in love and worship the satisfaction of their religious needs. Others again, of more mystical nature, prefer to realize their ideals through concentration and meditation. Lastly, there is a class of men of strongly analytical natures who must have the sanction of logic and reason for every belief and who therefore take the path of philosophy and discrimination.

The books by Swâmi Vivekânanda already published have been intended to meet the inquiries of the first three classes of men. The present work is adapted for the last class, the philosophers. *Jnâna Yoga* is, as its name implies, the yoga, or method, of realizing our divine nature through wisdom (Jnâna). Wisdom is not knowledge in its ordinary sense, although it includes it. It is that higher knowledge which is self-illumination.

This is equally the goal of every *yoga*, or method, the difference lying only in the path chosen for reaching that goal.

The present volume consists chiefly of lectures which were delivered in London, England. Two were given in India, and are consequently new both in England and in this country. The lectures deal with the teachings of the Upanishads, which contain the essence of Vedânta. Some of these Upanishads are among the most ancient of the Hindu Scriptures, and show a wonderful insight into the great truths underlying all religious aspiration. It is because Vedânta is a religion of principles, not of external authority, that the late Professor Max Müller said of it: "Vedânta has room for almost every religion; nay, it embraces them all."

I. THE SONG OF THE SANNYASIN.

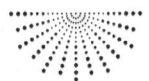

Wake up the note! The song that had its birth
    Far off, where worldly taint could never reach;
In mountain caves, and glades of forest deep,
Whose calm no sigh for lust or wealth or fame
Could ever dare to break; where rolled the stream
Of knowledge, truth, and bliss that follows both.
Sing high that note, Sannyâsin bold! Say—

                              "Om tat sat, Om!"

Strike off thy fetters! Bonds that bind thee down,
Of shining gold, or darker, baser ore;
Love, hate—good, bad—and all the dual throng.
Know slave is slave, caressed or whipped, not free;
For fetters tho' of gold, are not less strong to bind.
Then off with them Sannyâsin bold! Say—

                              "Om tat sat, Om!"

Let darkness go; the will-o'-the-wisp that leads

With blinking light to pile more gloom on gloom.
This thirst for life, for ever quench; it drags,
From birth to death and death to birth, the soul.
He conquers all who conquers self. Know this
And never yield, Sannyâsin bold! Say—

"Om tat sat, Om!"

"Who sows must reap," they say, "and cause must bring
The sure effect; good, good; bad, bad; and none
Escape the law. But whoso wears a form
Must wear the chain." Too true, but far beyond
Both name and form is Atman, ever free.
Know thou art That, Sannyâsin bold! Say!

"Om tat sat, Om!"

They know not truth, who dream such vacant dreams
As father, mother, children, wife and friend.
The sexless Self! Whose father He? Whose child?
Whose friend, whose foe is He who is but One?
The Self is all in all, naught else exists; And thou art
That, Sannyâsin bold! Say!

"Om tat sat, Om!"

There is but One—The Free—The Knower—Self!
Without a name, without a form or stain;
In Him is Mâyâ dreaming all this dream.
The Witness, He appears as nature, soul.
Know thou art That, Sannyâsin! Say—

"Om tat sat, Om!"

Where seekest thou? That freedom, friend, this world
Nor that, can give. In books and temples vain

Thy search. Thine only is the hand that holds
The rope that drags thee on. Then, cease lament,
Let go thy hold, Sannyâsin bold! Say—

"Om tat sat, Om!"

Say—"Peace to all; from me no danger be
To aught that lives; in those that dwell on high,
In those that lowly creep, I am the Self in all!
All life, both here and there, do I renounce,
And heav'ns, earths and hells; all hopes and fears."
Thus cut thy bonds, Sannyâsin bold! Say—

"Om tat sat, Om!"

Heed then no more how body lives or goes,
Its task is done. Let Karma float it down,
Let one put garlands on, another kick
This frame; say naught. No praise or blame can be
Where praiser, praised—and blamer, blamed—are one.
Thus be thou calm, Sannyâsin bold! Say—

"Om tat sat, Om!"

Truth never comes where lust and fame and greed
Of gain reside. No man who thinks of woman
As his wife can ever perfect be;
Nor he who owns the least of things, nor he
Whom anger chains, can pass thro' Mâyâ's gates.
So, give these up, Sannyâsin bold! Say—

"Om tat sat, Om!"

Have thou no home. What home can hold thee, friend?
The sky thy roof, the grass thy bed; and food
What chance may bring, well cooked or ill, judge not.

No food or drink can taint that noble self
Which knows itself. Like rolling river, be
Thou ever free, Sannyâsin bold! Say—

                                      "Om tat sat, Om!"

Few only know the truth. The rest will hate
And laugh at thee, great one; but pay no heed.
Go thou, the free, from place to place, and help
Them out of darkness, Mâyâ's veil. Without
The fear of pain or search for pleasure, go
Beyond them both Sannyâsin bold! Say—

                                      "Om tat sat, Om!"

Thus day to day, till Karma's powers spent
Release the soul for ever. No more is birth
Nor I, nor thou, nor god, nor man.
The "I" Has all become, the all is "I," and bliss.
Know thou art That, Sannyâsin bold! Say—

                                      "Om tat sat, Om!"

II. THE NECESSITY OF RELIGION.

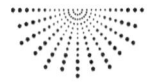

Of all the forces that have worked and are still working, to mould the destinies of the human race, none, certainly, is more potent than that, the manifestation of which we call religion. All social organizations have as a background, somewhere, the workings of that peculiar force, and the greatest cohesive impulse ever brought into play amongst human units has been derived from this power of religion. It is obvious to all of us, that in very many cases the bonds of religion have proved stronger than the bonds of race, of climate, or even of descent. It is a well known fact that persons worshipping the same God, believing in the same religion, have stood by each other, with much greater strength and constancy than people of merely the same descent, or even than brothers. Various attempts have been made to trace the beginnings of religion. In all the ancient religions which have come down to us at the present day we find one claim made—that they are all supernatural; that their genesis is not, as it were, in the human brain, but that they have originated somewhere outside of it.

Two theories have gained some acceptance amongst modern scholars. One is the spirit theory of religion, the other the evolution of the Infinite. One party maintains that ancestor worship is the beginning of religious ideas; the other that religion originates in the personification of the powers of nature. Man wants to keep up the memory of his dead relatives, and thinks they are living even when the body has been dissolved, and he wants to place food for them and, in a certain sense, to worship them. Out of that came the growth we call religion. Studying the ancient religions of the Egyptians, Babylonians, Chinese, and many other races in America and elsewhere, we find very clear traces of this ancestor worship being the beginning of religion. With the ancient Egyptians the first idea of the soul was that of a double. This physical man contained in it another being very similar to it, and when a man died this double went out of the body and yet lived on. But the life of the double lasted only as long as the dead body remained intact, and that is why we find among the Egyptians so much solicitude to keep the body intact. That is why they built those huge pyramids in which they preserved bodies. For, if any portion of the external body was hurt, just so would the double be hurt. This is clearly ancestor worship. With the ancient Babylonians we find the same idea of the double, but with a variation. The double lost all sense of love; it frightened the living to give it food and drink, and to help it in various ways. It even lost all affection for its own children, its own wife or daughter. Among the ancient Hindûs, also, we find traces of this ancestor worship. Among the Chinese the basis of their religion may also be said to be clearly ancestor worship, and it still permeates the length and breadth of that vast country. In fact the only religion that can really be said to flourish in China is that of ancestor worship. Thus it seems on the one hand a very good position is made out for those who hold to the theory of ancestor worship as the beginning of religion.

On the other hand there are scholars who go back to ancient Âryan literature. Although in India we find proofs of ancestor worship everywhere, yet in the oldest records there is no trace of it whatsoever. In the Rig Veda Samhita, the most ancient record of the Âryan race, we do not find any trace of it at all. Modern scholars think it is the worship of nature that they find there.

The human mind seems to struggle to get a peep behind the

scenes. The dawn, the evening, the hurricane, the stupendous and gigantic forces of nature, its beauties, these have exercised the human mind, and it aspires to go beyond, to understand something about them. In the struggle they endow these phenomena with personal attributes, giving them souls and bodies, sometimes beautiful, sometimes transcendent. Every attempt ends by these phenomena becoming abstractions whether personalized or not. So also it is found with the ancient Greeks; their whole mythology is simply this abstracted nature worship. So also with the ancient Germans, the Scandinavians, and all the other Âryan races. Thus, on this side too a very strong case has been made out that religion has its origin in the personification of the powers of nature.

These two views, though they seem to be contradictory, can be reconciled on a third basis, which to my mind is the real germ of religion, and that I propose to call the struggle to transcend the limitations of the senses. Either man goes to seek for the spirits of his ancestors, or the spirits of the dead, or he wants to get a glimpse of what there is after the body is dissolved, or he desires to understand the power working behind the stupendous phenomena of nature. Whichever of these is the case, one thing is certain, that he is trying to transcend the limitations of the senses. He cannot remain satisfied with his senses; he wants to go beyond them. The explanation need not be mysterious. To me it seems very natural that the first glimpse of religion should come through dreams. The first idea of immortality man must get through dreams. Is not the dream state a most wonderful state? We know that children and untutored minds find very little difference between dreaming and their waking state. What can be more natural than that they find, as natural logic, that even during the sleep state, when the body is apparently dead, the mind goes on with all its intricate workings? What wonder that men will at once come to the conclusion that when this body is dissolved for ever the same working will go on? This, to my mind, would be a more natural explanation of the supernatural, and through this dream idea the human mind rises to higher and higher concepts. Of course in time the vast majority of mankind found out that these dreams were not verified by their awakened states, and that during the dream state it is not that man has a fresh existence, but simply that he recapitulates the experiences of the awakened state.

But by this time the search had begun, and the search was inward, and they continued to inquire more deeply into the different stages of the mind, and discovered higher states than either the waking or dreaming. This state of things we find in all the organized religions of the world, called either a state of ecstasy, or inspiration. In all the organized religions, their founders, prophets and messengers are declared to have gone into states of mind which were neither waking nor sleeping, but states in which they came face to face with a new series of facts, those relating to what is called the spiritual kingdom.

They realized things there in a much more intense sense than we realize facts around us in our waking state. This we find in all the existing religions. Take, for instance, the religions of the Brâhmans. The Vedas are said to be written by Rishis. These Rishis were sages who realized certain facts. The exact definition of the Sanskrit word is "The Seers of the Mantrams"—of the thoughts conveyed in the Vedic Hymns. These men declared that they had realized—*sensed*, if that word can be used with regard to the supersensuous—certain facts, and these facts they proceeded to put on record. We find the same thing declared among both the Jews and the Christians.

Some exception may be taken in the case of the Buddhists as represented by the Southern sect. It may be asked—if the Buddhists do not believe in any God, or a soul, how can their religion be derived from this supersensuous state of existence?

The answer to this is, that even the Buddhists find an eternal moral law, and that moral law was not reasoned out in our sense of the word, but Buddha found it, discovered it, in a supersensuous state. Those of you who have studied the life of Buddha, even as shortly given in that beautiful poem "The Light of Asia," may remember that Buddha is represented as sitting under the Bo-tree until he had reached the supersensuous state of mind. All his teachings came from this, and not from intellectual cogitations.

Thus, here is a tremendous statement made by all religions, that this human mind, at certain moments, transcends not only the limitations of the senses, but also the power of reasoning. It then comes face to face with facts which it could never have sensed, could never have reasoned out. These facts are the basis of all the religions of the world. Of course we have the right to challenge these facts, to put them to the test of reason, nevertheless, all the existing religions of the world claim for the human mind this peculiar power of transcending the limits of the senses, and the limits of reason; and this power they put forward as a statement of fact.

Apart from the consideration of the question how far these facts claimed by religions are true, we find one characteristic common to them all. They are all abstractions as contrasted with the concrete discoveries of physics, for instance; and in all the highly organized religions they take the purest form of Unit Abstraction, either in the form of an Abstracted Presence, as an Omnipresent Being, as an Abstract Personality, called God, as a Moral Law, or in the form of an Abstract Essence underlying every existence. In modern times, too, the attempts made to preach religions without appealing to the supersensuous state of the mind, have had to take up the old abstractions of the Ancients, and put different names to them as "Moral Law," the "Ideal Unity," and so forth, thus showing that these abstractions are not in the senses. None of us have yet seen an Ideal Human Being, and yet we are told to believe in an Ideal Human Being.

None of us have yet seen an ideally perfect man, and yet without that ideal we cannot progress. Thus, this one fact stands out from all these different religions, that there is an Ideal Unit Abstraction, and this is either put before us in the form of a Person, or as an Impersonal Being, or as Law, or a Presence, or an Essence. We are always struggling to raise ourselves up to that ideal. Every human being whosoever and wheresoever he may be, has an ideal of infinite power. Every human being has an ideal of infinite pleasure. Most of the works that we find around us, the activities displayed everywhere, are due to the struggle for this infinite power, or this infinite pleasure. But a few quickly discover that although they are struggling for infinite power, it is not through the senses that it can be reached.

They find out very soon that that infinite pleasure is not to be got through the senses, or, in other words, the senses are too limited, and the body is too limited to express the Infinite. To manifest the Infinite through the finite is impossible, and, sooner or later, man learns to give up the attempt to express the Infinite through the finite. This giving up, this renunciation of the attempt, is the background of ethics. Renunciation is the very basis upon which ethics stand. There never was an ethical code preached which had not renunciation for its basis.

Ethics always says: "Not I, but thou." Its motto is, "Not self, but non-self." The vain ideas of individualism to which man clings when he is trying to find that Infinite Power, or that Infinite Pleasure through the senses, have to be given up, say the laws of ethics. You have to put *yourself* last, and *others* before you.

The senses say, "Myself first." Ethics says, "I must hold myself last." Thus, all codes of ethics are based upon this renunciation; destruction, not construction, of the individual on the material plane. That Infinite will never find expression upon the material plane, nor is it possible or thinkable.

So, man had to give up the plane of matter, and rise to other spheres to seek a deeper expression of that Infinite. In this way the various ethical laws are being moulded, but all have that one central idea, eternal self-abnegation. Perfect self-annihilation is the ideal of ethics. People are startled if they are asked not to think of their individualities. Everybody seems so very much afraid of losing what he calls his individuality. At the same time, the same men would declare the highest ideals of ethics to be right; never for a moment thinking that the scope, the goal, the idea of all ethics is destruction of the individual, and not the building up of the individual.

Utilitarian standards cannot explain the ethical relations of men; for, in the first place we cannot derive any ethical laws from considerations of utility. Without this supernatural sanction, as it is called, or the perception of the super-conscious, as I prefer to term it, there can be no ethics. Without this struggle towards the Infinite there can be no ideal. Any system that wants to bind men down within the limits of their own societies would not be able to find an explanation for the ethical laws of mankind. The Utilitarian wants us to give up all this struggle after the Infinite, all this going to the Supersensuous, as impracticable and absurd, and, in the same breath, asks us to take up ethics, and do good to society. Why should we do good? Doing good is a secondary consideration. We must have an ideal. Ethics itself is not the end, but the means to the end. If the end is not there why should we be ethical? Why should I do good to other men, and not injure them? If happiness be the goal of mankind, why should I not make myself happy and other's unhappy? What prevents me? In the second place, the basis of utility is too narrow. All these forms and methods are derived from society as it exists, but what right has the Utilitarian to assume that society is eternal? Society did not exist ages ago, possibly will not exist ages hence. Most probably it is one of the passing stages through which we are going towards a higher evolution, and any law that is derived from society alone cannot be eternal, cannot cover the whole ground of man's nature. At best, therefore, Utilitarian theories can only work under present social conditions. Beyond that, they have no value. But a morality, an ethical code derived from religion and spirituality, has the whole of infinite man for its scope. It takes up the individual but its relations are to the Infinite, and it takes up society also—because society is nothing but numbers of these individuals grouped together— and applying to the individual and *his* eternal relations, it must necessarily apply to the whole of society, in whatever condition it may be at any given time. Thus we see that there is always the necessity of spiritual religion for mankind. Man cannot always think of matter, however pleasurable it may be.

It has been said that too much attention to things spiritual disturbs our practical relations in this world. As long ago as the days of the Chinese sage Confucius it was said: "Let us take care of this world, and then, when we have finished with this world, we will take care of other worlds." It is all very well that we should take care of this world and let the other go, but though too much attention to the spiritual may hurt a little our practical relations, yet too much attention to the so-called practical hurts us here and hereafter. It makes us materialistic. For man is not to regard *Nature* as his goal, but something higher than Nature.

Man is man so long as he is struggling to rise above Nature, and this nature is both internal and external. Not only does nature comprise the laws that govern the particles of matter outside us and in our bodies, but there is the more subtle nature inside us, which is, in fact, the motive power which is governing the external and the internal nature. It is good and very grand to conquer external nature, but grander still to conquer the internal nature of man. It is grand and good to know the laws that govern the stars and planets; it is infinitely grander and better to know the laws that govern the passions, the feelings, the will of mankind. This conquering of the inner man, understanding the secrets of the subtle workings that are within the human mind, and knowing its wonderful secrets, belong entirely to religion. Human nature—the ordinary human nature, I mean—wants to see big material facts. Ordinary mankind cannot understand anything that is subtle. Well has it been said that mobs would run after a lion that could kill a thousand lambs, and never for a moment think that it is death unto the lambs, although it may be a momentary triumph for the lion, because in that the mob finds the greatest manifestation of physical strength. Thus with the ordinary run of mankind, they understand and find pleasure in everything that is external; but in every society there is a section whose pleasures are not in the senses, but beyond, and who now and then catch glimpses of something higher than matter, and want to struggle thither. And if we read the histories of nations between the lines we shall always find that the rise of a nation comes with an increase in the number of such men in society; and the fall begins when this pursuit after the Infinite, however vain utilitarians may call it, has ceased.

That is to say, the mainspring of the strength of every race lies in the spirituality manifested in religion, and the death of that race will begin the day that spirituality wanes and materialism begins.

Thus, apart from the solid facts and truths that we may learn from religion, apart from the comforts that we may gain therefrom, religion itself, as a science, as a study, is the greatest and healthiest exercise that the human mind can have. This pursuit of the Infinite, this struggle to grasp the Infinite, this effort to get beyond the limitations of the senses, out of matter, as it were, and to evolve the spiritual man, instead of filling the mind with low, narrow and little ideals; this striving day and night to make the Infinite one with our being—this struggle itself is the grandest and most glorious that man can make. Some persons find the greatest pleasure in eating. We have no right to say they should not. Others find the greatest pleasure in possessing certain things. We have no right to say they should not. But they also have no right to say "no" to the man who finds his highest pleasure in spiritual thought. The lower the organization the more is the pleasure in the senses. Very few men can eat a meal with the same gusto that a dog, or a wolf can.

But all the pleasures of the dog or the wolf have gone, as it were, into the senses, into that eating. The lower types of humanity in all nations find more pleasure in the senses, while the cultured and the educated find more in thought, in philosophy, in the arts and sciences. Spiritual thought is a still higher plane. The subject being infinite, that plane is the highest, and the pleasure there is the highest for those who appreciate it. So, even on the utilitarian ground—that man is to seek for pleasure—he should cultivate religious thought, for that is the highest pleasure that exists. Thus religion as a study, seems to me to be absolutely necessary. We can see it in its effects. It is the greatest motive power that moves the human mind. No other ideal can put into us the same mass of energy as the spiritual. So far as human history goes, it is obvious to all of us that this has been the case, and its powers are not dead. I do not deny that men on simply utilitarian grounds can be very good and moral. There have been many great men in this world perfectly sound and moral and good simply on utilitarian grounds, but the world-movers, men who bring, as it were, a mass of magnetism into the world, whose spirit works in hundreds and in thousands, whose life produces a halo around them wherever they go, igniting others with a spiritual fire—such men we always find had that spiritual background. The motive power of their energy came from religion. Religion is the greatest motive power to release that infinite energy which is the birthright and nature of every man. Nothing can compare with religion there. In building up character, in making for everything that is good and great, in bringing peace to others, and peace to one's own self, religion is the highest motive power, and religion ought to be studied therefore from that standpoint. Religion must be studied on a broader basis than formerly. All narrow, limited, fighting ideas of religion have to go. All sect ideas and tribal or national ideas of religion must be given up. Each tribe or nation having its own particular God, and thinking that every other is wrong, is superstition that should belong to the past. All such ideas must be abandoned.

As the human mind broadens, so its spiritual steps must broaden. The time has already come when a man cannot record a thought without it reaching to all corners of the earth; by merely physical means we have come into touch with the whole world—so the future religions of the world have to become as universal, as wide.

The religious ideals of the future must embrace all that exists in the world that is good and great, and, at the same time, have infinite scope for future development. All that was good in the past must be preserved and kept; and yet the doors must be open for future addition to this already existing store. Religions must also be inclusive. Religions must not look down with contempt upon people who have not the particular ideal of God which governs their special sect. In my life I have seen a great many spiritual men, a great many sensible persons, who did not believe in God at all. That is to say, not in our sense of the word. Perhaps they understood God better than we can ever do. The Personal idea of God or the Impersonal, the Infinite, the Moral Law, or the Ideal Man—these all have to come under the definition of religion. And when religions have become thus broadened, their power for good will have increased a hundred times beyond the present. Religions, having tremendous power in them, have often done more injury to the world than good, simply on account of their narrowness, and limitations.

Even at the present time we find many sects and societies, with almost the same ideas, fighting each other, because the one does not want to set forth those ideas in precisely the same way as the others. Therefore religions will have to broaden. Religious ideas will have to become universal, vast and infinite, and then alone we shall have the fullest play of religion, for the power of religion has only just begun in the world. It is sometimes said that religions are dying out, that spiritual ideas are dying out of the world. To me it seems that they have just begun. The power of religion, broadened and purified, is going to penetrate every part of human life. So long as religion was in the hands of a chosen few, or of a body of priests, it was in the temples, it was in the churches, it was in books, in dogmas, in ceremonials, forms and rituals. When men have come to the real, universal, spiritual concept, then, and then alone, religion will become real and living; it will come into our very nature, live in every movement of the human being, it will penetrate every pore of society, and be infinitely more a power for good than it has ever been before.

What is needed is a fellow-feeling between the different types of religion, seeing that they all stand or fall together; a fellow-feeling which springs from mutual esteem and mutual respect, and not the condescending, patronizing, niggardly expression of goodwill unfortunately in vogue at the present time with many. And above all, this is needed, between types of religious expression coming from the study of mental phenomena—unfortunately even now laying exclusive claim to the name of religion—and those expressions of religion whose heads are penetrating more and more into the secrets of heaven, though their feet are clinging to earth—the so-called materialistic sciences.

To bring about this harmony both will have to make concessions, sometimes very large, nay, more, sometimes painful; but after all, each will find itself better for the sacrifice and more advanced in truth. And in the end, the knowledge which has its basis in changes in time, and that which is founded on changes in space will both meet and become one, where there is neither space nor time, where the mind cannot reach, nor the senses—the Absolute, the Infinite. the "One without a second."

III. THE REAL NATURE OF MAN.

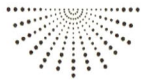

Great is the tenacity with which man clings to the senses, yet however substantial he may think the external world in which he lives and moves, there come times in the lives of individuals and of races when, involuntarily they ask, "Is this real?" To the person who never finds a moment to question the credentials of his senses, whose every moment is occupied with some sort of sense-enjoyment—even to him death comes, and he also is compelled to ask: "Is this real?" Religion begins with this question and ends with the answer. Even in the remote past where recorded history cannot help us, in the mysterious light of mythology, back in the dim twilight of civilization, we find the same question was asked "What becomes of this? What is real?"

One of the most poetical of the Upanishads, the Katha Upanishad, begins with the inquiry: "When a man dies there is a contention. One party declares that he has gone forever, the other insists that he is still living. Which is true?" Various answers have been given. The whole sphere of metaphysics, philosophy and religion is really filled with various answers to this question. Attempts at the same time have been made to suppress it, to put a stop to this unrest of mind, which asks, "What beyond? What is real?"

But so long as death remains all these attempts at suppression will uniformly prove to be unsuccessful. We may very easily talk about seeing nothing beyond and keeping all our hopes and aspirations confined to the present moment. We may struggle hard, and perhaps everything outside may help to keep us limited within the narrow bonds of the senses. The whole world may combine to prevent us from broadening out beyond the present; yet, so long as there is death the question must come again and again, "Is death the end of everything, of all these things to which we are clinging as if they were the most real of all realities, the most substantial of all substances?" The world vanishes in a moment and is gone. Standing on the brink of a precipice beyond which is the infinite yawning chasm, every mind, however hardened, is bound to recoil, and ask, "Is this real?" The hopes of a lifetime, built little by little with all the energies of a great mind, vanish in one second. Are they real? This question will have to be answered. Time will never lessen its power. As time rolls on it adds value to itself. Then there is the desire to be happy; we run after everything to make ourselves happy, we run after the senses, go on madly careering into the external world. The young man, with whom life is successful, if you ask him, declares that it is real; he thinks it is all quite real. Perhaps the same man, growing old, and with fortune ever eluding him, will declare that it is fate. He finds at last that his desires cannot be fulfilled. Wherever he goes there is an adamantine wall beyond which he cannot pass. Every sense-activity results in a reaction. Everything is evanescent. Enjoyment, misery, luxury, wealth, power and poverty, even life itself are all evanescent.

Two positions remain to mankind. One is to believe with the Nihilists that all is nothing. We know nothing. We can never know anything either about the future, the past, or even of the present. For we must remember that he who denies the past and the future and wants to stick to the present is simply a madman. One may as well deny the father and mother and assert the child. It would be equally logical. To deny the past and future, the present must inevitably be denied also. This is one position, that of the Nihilists. I have never seen a man who could really become a Nihilist for one minute. It is very easy to talk.

Then there is the other position, to seek for an explanation, to seek for the real, to discover in the midst of this eternally changing and evanescent world whatever is real. In this body which is an aggregation of molecules of matter, is there anything which is real? And this has been the search throughout the history of the human mind. In the very oldest times we often find glimpses of light coming into men's minds. We find man even then going a step beyond this body finding something which is not this external body, but which although very much like it, is not it, being much more complete, much more perfect, which remains even when this body is dissolved. We read in the hymns of the Rig Veda addressed to the God of Fire who is burning a dead body, "Carry him, Fire, in your arms gently, give him a perfect body, a bright body, carry him where the fathers live, where there is no more sorrow, where there is no more death." The same idea you will find present in every religion, and we get another idea with it. It is a curious fact that all religions, without one exception, hold that man is a degeneration of what he was, whether they clothe this in mythological words, or in the clear language of philosophy, or in the beautiful expressions of poetry. This is the one fact that comes out of every scripture and of every mythology, that the man that is, is a degeneration of what he was. This is the kernel of truth behind the story of Adam's fall in the Jewish scripture. This is again and again repeated in the scriptures of the Hindûs; the dream of a period which they call the age of truth, when no man died unless he wished to die; when he could keep his body as long as he liked and his mind was pure and strong. There was no death at that time, and no evil and no misery; and the present age is a corruption of that state of perfection. Side by side with this we find the story of the deluge everywhere. That story itself is a proof that this present age is held to be a corruption of the former by every religion. It went on becoming more and more corrupt until the deluge swept away a large portion of mankind and again the ascending series began. It is going up slowly again to reach once more that early state of purity. You are all aware of the story of the deluge in the Old Testament. The same story was current among the ancient Babylonians, the Egyptians, the Chinese and the Hindûs. Manu, a great ancient sage, was praying on the banks of the Ganges when a little minnow came to him for protection and he put it into a pot of water he had before him. "What do you want?" asked Manu. The little minnow declared he was pursued by a bigger fish and wanted protection. Manu carried the little fish to his home, and in the morning it had become as big as the pot, and said, "I cannot live in this pot any longer." Manu put him in a tank, and the next day he was as big as the tank and declared he could not live there any more. So Manu had to take him to a river, and in the morning the fish filled the river. Then Manu put him in the ocean, and he declared, "Manu, I am the creator of the Universe, I have taken this form to come and warn you that I will deluge the world. You build an ark, and in it put a pair of every kind of animal, and let your family enter the ark and there will come out of the deluge my horn. Fasten the ark to it, and when the deluge subsides come down and people the earth." So the world was deluged, and Manu saved his own family and a pair of every kind of animal and seeds of every plant, and when it subsided he came and peopled the world and we are all called "man" because we are progeny of Manu.[1] Now human language is the attempt to express the truth that is within. A little baby whose language itself consists of imperceptible, indistinct sounds, I am fully persuaded is attempting to express the highest philosophy, only the baby has not got the organs to express it, nor the means. The difference in the language between the highest philosophers and the utterances of babies is one of degree and not of kind. What you call the most correct, systematic, mathematical language of the present time and the hazy, mystical, mythological languages of the ancients, differ only in degree. All of them have a grand idea behind, which is, as it were, struggling to express itself, and many times behind these ancient mythologies are nuggets of truth, and many times, I am sorry to say, behind the fine, polished phrases of the modern, is arrant trash. So we need not throw overboard everything because it is clothed in mythology, because it does not fit in with the notions of Mr. So-and-So, or Mrs. So-and-So of modern times. If they laugh at religion because most religions declared that men must believe these things, because such and such a prophet has said them, they ought to laugh more at these moderns. In modern times if a man quotes a Moses, or a Buddha, or a Christ, he is laughed at; but let him give the name of a Huxley, a Tyndall, or a Darwin, and it is swallowed without salt. "Huxley has said it," that is enough for many. We are free from superstitions indeed! That was a religious superstition, and this is a scientific superstition; only in and through that superstition came life-giving lines of spirituality; in and through this modern superstition come lust and greed. That superstition was worship of God, and this superstition is worship of filthy lucre, of fame or power. That is the difference.

To turn back to our mythology, behind all these stories we find one idea standing supreme—that man is a degeneration of what he was. Coming to the present times, modern research seems to repudiate this position absolutely. Evolutionists seem to entirely contradict this assertion. According to them man is the evolution of the mollusc, and therefore what this mythology states cannot be true. There is in India, however, a mythology which is able to reconcile both these positions. The Indian mythology has a theory of cycles, that all progression is in the form of waves. Every wave is attended by a fall, and that by a rise the next moment, that by a fall in the next, and again another rise. The motion is in cycles. Certainly it is true even on the grounds of modern research, that man cannot be simply an evolution. Every evolution presupposes an involution. The modern scientific man will tell you that you can only get the amount of energy out of a machine which you put into it before. Something cannot be produced out of nothing. If man is an evolution of the mollusc, then the perfect man, the Buddha man, the Christ man, was involved in the mollusc. If it is not so, whence come these gigantic personalities? Something cannot come out of nothing. Thus we are in the position of reconciling the scriptures with modern light. That energy which manifests itself slowly through various stages until it becomes the perfect man cannot come out of nothing. It existed somewhere, and if the mollusc, or the protoplasm, is the first point to which you can trace it, that protoplasm, somehow or other, must have contained the energy. There is a great modern discussion going on as to whether this aggregate of materials we call the body is the cause of manifestation of the force we call the soul and thought, etc., or whether it is the thought that manifests this body. The religions of the world of course hold that the force called thought manifests the body, and not the reverse.

There are schools of modern people who hold that what we call thought is simply the outcome of the adjustment of the parts of the machine which we call body. Taking the second position, that the soul or the mass of the thought, or however you may call it, is the outcome of this machine, the outcome of the chemical and physical combinations of matter making up the body and brain, the question remains unanswered. What makes the body? What force combines all these molecules into the body form? What force is there which takes up material from the mass of matter around and forms my body one way, another body another way, and so on? What makes these infinite distinctions? To say that the force called soul is the outcome of the combinations of the molecules of the body is putting the cart before the horse. How did the combinations come: where was the force to make them? If you say some other force was the cause of these combinations and that soul was the outcome of that matter, and that soul—which combined a certain mass of matter— was itself the result of the combinations, it is no answer. That theory ought to be taken which explains most of the facts, if not all, and without contradicting other existing theories. The force which takes up the matter and forms the body is the same which manifests through that body, and this is more logical. To say therefore that the thought-forces manifested by the body are the outcome of the arrangement of molecules and have no existence at all, has no meaning, neither can force evolve out of matter. It is rather more possible to demonstrate that what we call matter does not exist at all. It

is only a certain state of force. Solidity, hardness, or anything, can be proved to be the result of motion. Increase of vibration will make things solid. A mass of air vibrated at a tremendous rate would become as solid as a table. A thread of a spider's web moved at almost infinite velocity would be as strong as an iron chain, would cut through an oak tree, such force would be given to it by motion. Looking at it that way it would be rather easier to prove that what we call matter and so on does not exist. But the other way cannot be proved.

What is this force which is manifesting itself through the body? It is obvious to all of us, whatever that force be, that it is taking particles up, as it were, and manipulating forms out of them—the human body. None other comes here to manipulate bodies for you and me. I never saw anybody eat food for me. I have to assimilate it, manufacture blood and bones and everything out of that food. What is this mysterious force? Ideas about the future and about the past seem to be terrifying to man. To many they seem to be mere speculation. We will take the present theme. What is this force now which is working through us? We have seen how in old times in all the ancient scriptures this power, this manifestation of power, was thought to be a bright substance having a body like this body, and which remains even after this body falls. Later on, however, we find a higher idea coming even—that this body does not represent the force. Whatsoever has form must be the result of combinations of particles and requires something else behind it to move it. If this body requires something which is not the body to manipulate it, the bright body, by the same necessity, will also require something other than itself to manipulate it. So that something was called the soul, the Âtman, in Sanskrit. It was the Âtman which through the bright body, as it were, worked on the gross body outside. The bright body is considered as the receptacle of the mind, and the Âtman is beyond that. It is not the mind even, it operates the mind, and through the mind the body. You have an Âtman, I have another, each one of us has a separate Âtman, and a separate fine body, and through that we work on the gross external body. Questions were then asked about this Âtman, about its nature. What is this Âtman, this soul of man which is neither a body nor a mind? Great discussions followed. Speculations came, various shades of philosophic inquiry came into existence, and I will try to place before you some of the conclusions that have been reached about this Âtman. The different philosophies seem to agree that this Âtman, whatever it be, has neither form nor shape, and that which has neither form nor shape must be omnipresent. Time begins with mind, space also is in the mind. Causation cannot stand without time. Without the idea of succession there cannot be any idea of causation. Time, space, and causation, therefore, are in the mind, and as this Âtman is beyond the mind and formless it must be beyond time, beyond space, and beyond causation. Now if it is beyond time, space and causation, it must be infinite. Then comes the highest speculation in our philosophy. The infinite cannot be two. If the soul be infinite there can be only one soul, and all these ideas of various souls—you having one soul, and I having another, and so forth—are not real. The real man therefore is one and infinite, the omnipresent spirit. And the apparent man is only a limitation of that real man. In that sense all these mythologies are true, that the apparent man, however great he may be, is only a dim reflection of the real man which is beyond. The real man, the spirit, being beyond cause and effect, not bound by time and space, must therefore be free. He was never bound, and could not be bound. The apparent man, the reflection, is limited by time, space and causation, and he is therefore bound. Or in the language of some of our philosophers, he appears to be bound, but really is not. This is the reality in our souls, this omnipresence, this spiritual nature, this infinity, which we are already. Every soul is infinite, therefore there is no question of birth and death. Some children were being examined. The examiner put them rather hard questions, and among them was this question: "Why does not the earth fall?" He wanted to evoke answers about gravitation and so forth. Most of the children could not answer at all; a few answered that it was gravitation or something. One bright little girl answered it by putting another question: "Where should it fall?" The question is nonsense. Where should the earth fall? There is no falling or rising for the earth. In infinite space there is no up or down; that is only in the relative. Where is going or coming for the infinite? Whence should it come and whither should it go? When people refuse to think of the past, or future, or what is going to become of them—when they give up the ideas of body, because being limited, the body comes and goes—

then they have risen to a higher ideal. The body is not the real man, neither is the mind, for the mind waxes and wanes. It is the spirit beyond which alone can live forever. The body and mind are continually changing. These are the names of series of changeful phenomena, rivers where every particle of water is in a constant state of flux; yet we recognize the series as the same river. Every particle in this body is continually changing; no one has the same body for several minutes together. Yet a sort of impression left in the mind makes us call it the same. So with the mind, one moment happy, another moment unhappy; one moment strong, another weak. An ever-changing whirlpool. That cannot be the spirit, for spirit is infinite. Change can only be in the limited. To say that the infinite changes in any way is absurd; it cannot be. You can move and I can move as bodies; every particle in this universe is in a constant state of flux, but taking the universe as a unit, as one whole, it cannot move, it cannot change. Motion is always a relative thing. I move only in relation to something else. Any particle in this universe can change in relation to any other particle, but the whole universe as one—in relation to what will that move? There is nothing beside it. So this infinite unit is unchangeable, immovable, absolute, and this is the Real Man. Our reality, therefore, consists in the Universal, and not in the limited. These are old delusions, however comfortable they are, to think that we are little limited beings, constantly changing. People are frightened when they are told that they are Universal Being, everywhere present. Through everything you work, through every foot you move, through every lip you talk, through every breath you breathe. People are frightened when they are told this. They will again and again ask you if they are not going to lose their individuality. What is any man's individuality? I should be glad to see it.

A little baby has no moustache; when he grows older he has a moustache and beard. His individuality is lost if it is in the body. If I lose one eye, or if I lose one of my hands my individuality will be lost if it is in the body. A drunkard should not give up drinking because he would lose his individuality. A thief need not be a good man because he would therefore lose his individuality. No man ought to change his habits for fear of this. There is no individuality except in the Infinite. That is the only condition which does not change. Everything else is in a constant state of flux. Neither can individuality be in memory. Suppose I receive a blow on the head and forget all about my past; then I have lost all my individuality; I am gone. I do not remember two or three years of my childhood, and if memory and existence are one, then whatever I forget is gone. That part of my life which I do not remember I did not live. That is a very narrow idea of individuality. We are not individuals yet. We are struggling towards individuality and that is the Infinite; that is the real nature of man. He alone lives whose life is in the whole universe, and the more we concentrate our lives on little limited things the faster are we going towards death. That moment alone we have lived when our lives were in the universe, in others; and all those minutes which we concentrated upon this little life was death, simply death, and that is why the fear of death comes. The fear of death can only be conquered when man realizes that so long as there is one life in this universe he is living. When he can say: "I am in everything, in every body; I am in all lives, I am the universe, this whole universe is my body. How can I die so long as one particle remains? Who says I will die?" then alone comes the state of fearlessness. To talk of immortality in little constantly changing things is ridiculous. Says an old Sanskrit philosopher: It is only the spirit that is the individual because it is infinite; no infinity can be divided; infinity cannot be broken into pieces. It is the same one, undivided unit forever, and this is the individual man, the Real Man. The apparent man is merely a struggle to express, to manifest this individuality, which is beyond, and that evolution is not in the spirit. These changes which are going on, the wicked becoming good, the animal becoming man, take it whatever way you like, are not in the spirit. Evolution of nature and manifestation of spirit. Suppose here is a screen hiding you from me, and there is a small hole in the screen, and through that I can just see some of the faces before me, just a few faces. Now suppose this hole begins to grow larger and larger. As the hole goes on becoming larger and larger, more and more of the scene before me reveals itself, and when the hole has become identified with the screen I stand face to face with you. You did not change at all in this case, you were where you always were. It was the hole that was evolving and you were manifesting yourself. So it is with the spirit. You are already free and perfect. No perfection is going to be attained. You are that already—free and perfect. What are all these ideas of religion and God and searching for the hereafter? Why does man go to look for a God? Why in every nation, in every state of society did man want a perfect ideal somewhere, either in man, in God, or anywhere else? Because that idea is in you. It is your own heart beating and you did not know, you were mistaking it for something external. It is the God within your own self that is impelling you to seek for Him, to realize Him, and after long search here and there, in temples and in churches, in earths, in heavens, and in all various ways, at last you come back, complete the circle from where you started, back to your own soul and find that He for whom you have been seeking all over the world, for whom you have been weeping and praying in churches and temples, on whom you were looking as the mystery of all mysteries shrouded behind the clouds, He nearest of the near, your own Self, the reality of your own life, your body and your soul. That is your own nature, the real nature of man. Assert it, manifest it. You are pure already. You are not to become perfect, you are that already. This whole of nature is like that screen which was hiding the reality beyond. Every good thought that you think or act upon is simply tearing the veil, as it were, and the purity, the Infinity, the God behind, manifests itself. This is the whole history of man. Finer and finer becomes the veil, more and more of the light behind shines by its own nature, for it is its nature to shine. It cannot be known; in vain we try to know it. Were it knowable, it would not be what it is, for it is the Eternal Subject: knowledge is a limitation, knowledge is objectifying. He is the eternal subject of everything, the eternal witness in this universe, your own Self. Knowledge is, as it were, a lower step, a degeneration. We are that Eternal Subject already; how to know it? That is the real nature of every man and he is struggling to express it in various ways; else why are there so many ethical codes? Where is the explanation of all ethics? One idea stands out as the centre in all ethics, expressed in various forms; doing good to others. The guiding motive of mankind is charity towards men, charity towards all animals. But these are all various expressions of that eternal truth that "I am the universe; this universe is one." Else where is the reason? Why shall I do good to my fellow men? Why should I do good to others? What compels me? It is this sympathy, this feeling the sameness everywhere. The hardest hearts feel sympathy to other beings sometimes. Even the man who gets frightened if he is told that this assumed individuality is really a delusion, that it is ignoble to try to cling to this apparent individuality, that very man will tell you that extreme self-abnegation is the centre of all morality; and what is perfect self-abnegation? What remains? Self-abnegation means the abnegation of this apparent self, the abnegation of all selfishness. This idea of "me" and "mine"—*ahankâra* and *mama*—is the result of past superstition, and the more this present self rolls away, the more the Real Self becomes manifest in its full glory. This is real self-abnegation, the centre, the basis, the gist of all moral teaching, and whether men know it or not, the whole world is slowly going towards that, practising that more or less. Only the vast majority of mankind do it unconsciously. Let them do it consciously. Let them make the sacrifice knowing that this is not the real self; this is nothing but a limitation. One glimpse of that Infinite Reality which is behind, one spark of that Infinite Fire that is the All, represents the present man, but that Infinite is his true nature.

What is the utility, the effect, the result of this knowledge? In these days we have to measure everything by utility. That is to say generally, by how many pounds, shillings and pence it represents. What right has a person to ask that truth should be judged by the standard of utility or money? Suppose there is no utility, will it be less truth? Utility is not the test of truth. Nevertheless, there is the highest utility in this. Happiness, we see, is what every one is seeking for, but the majority seek it in things which are evanescent, and which are not real. No happiness was ever found in the senses. There never was a person who found happiness in the senses, or in enjoyments of the senses. Happiness is only found in the spirit. Therefore the highest utility to mankind is to find this happiness in the spirit. The next point is, that ignorance is the great mother of all misery, and this is the fundamental ignorance, to think that the Infinite weeps and cries that he is finite, and this is the basis of all ignorance, that we, the immortal, the ever pure, the perfect spirit, think that we are little minds, that we are little bodies; this is the mother of all selfishness. As soon as I am a little body I want to preserve it, to protect it, to keep it nice, at the expense of other bodies; you and I have become separate. As soon as this idea of separation comes, it opens the door to all mischief and leads to all misery. This is the utility, that if a very small fractional part of the human beings living to-day can put aside this idea of selfishness and narrowness and littleness, this earth will become a paradise to-morrow, but with machines and improvements of material knowledge it will never come.

These only increase misery, as oil poured on fire increases the flame all the more. Without the knowledge of spirit, every bit of material knowledge is only adding fuel to fire, only giving into the hands of selfish man one more instrument to take what belongs to others, to live upon the life of others, instead of giving up his life for others.

Is it practical, is another question. Can it be practised in modern society. *Truth does not pay homage to any society, modern or ancient. Society has to pay homage to Truth, or die.* Societies and all beings are moulded upon truth, and truth has not to adjust itself to society. If such noble truth as unselfishness cannot be practised in society, better give up society and go into forests. That is the daring man. There are two sorts of courage. One is the courage to jump at the mouth of a cannon.

Tigers, in that case, have been braver than men and wolves also. But there is also the courage of spiritual boldness. An invading Emperor went to India. His teacher told him to go and see some of those sages of India. After a long search he found a very old man sitting on a block of stone. The Emperor talked with him a little and became very much pleased with the conversation of the man. He asked the sage to go with him to his country. "No, I am quite satisfied with my forest here." Said the Emperor, "I will give you money, position, wealth. I am the Emperor of the world." "No," replied the man, "I don't care for those things." The Emperor replied, "If you do not go I will kill you." The man smiled serenely. "That is the most foolish thing you ever said, Emperor. You cannot kill me. Me the sun cannot dry, neither fire can burn, neither instrument kill, for I am the birthless, the deathless, the omnipotent, omnipresent spirit, ever living." That is another boldness. In the Mutiny of 1857 there was a great Swâmi, a very great soul. A Mahommedan mutineer stabbed him and nearly killed him. The Hindu mutineers brought the Mahommedan to the Swâmi and offered to kill him. But the Swâmi turned and said: "Yet, brother, thou art He, thou art He!" and expired. That is another bravery. What is it to talk of the bravery of your muscles, of the superiority of your Western institutions, if you cannot make a truth square with your society, if you cannot build up a society into which the highest truth will fit? What is this boastful talk about your grandeur and greatness, if you above all things stand up and say, "This kind of courage is not practical." Is nothing practical, but pounds, shillings, and pence? If so, why the boast of your society? *That society is the greatest where the highest truths become practical.* That is my opinion, and if society is not fit for the highest truths, make it fit. Make it if you can, and the sooner you do so, the better. Stand up, men and women, in the spirit, dare to believe in the truth, dare to practise the truth. The world requires a few hundred bold men and women. It is very hard to be bold. In that animal boldness, the tigers can do better. Wolves have it naturally. Even the ants are better than all other animals. What use to talk of this physical boldness! Practice that boldness which does not quake before death, which welcomes death, which stands there and knows it is the spirit and in the whole universe, no arms can kill it, not all the lightnings can kill it. Not all the fire in the universe can burn it. It dares know the truth and show the truth in life.

This is the free man, this is the real soul. "This Âtman is first to be heard, then thought about, and then meditated upon."

There is a great tendency in modern times to talk too much of works and decry all thought. Doing is very good, but even that comes from thinking. Little manifestations of energy which have originated in thought are escaping through the muscles and are called work. Where there is no thought, there will be no work. Fill the brain, therefore, with high thoughts, highest ideals, place them day and night before you, and out of that will come great work. Talk not about impurity, but tell the mind we are pure. We have hypnotized ourselves into this thought that we are little, that we are born and that we are going to die, and into living in a constant state of fear.

There was a lioness, heavy with young, going about in search of prey, and there was a flock of sheep, and the lioness jumped upon the flock. She died in the attempt and a little baby lion was born, motherless. It was taken care of by the sheep and the sheep brought it up and it grew with the sheep, lived on grass like the sheep, bleated like the sheep, and although it became a big full-grown lion, to all intents and purposes it thought it was a sheep. In course of time another big lion came in search of prey, and what was its astonishment to find that in the midst of this flock was this lion flying like the sheep at the approach of danger. He tried to get near to teach it that it was not a sheep, but a lion, but at the very approach of the other lion the sheep fled, and with it the sheep-lion. But the other lion was rather kind, he watched, and one day found the big sheep-lion sleeping. He jumped on it and said, "You are a lion." "I am a sheep," cried the other lion. He would not believe, but bleated.

The lion dragged him towards a lake and said, "Look there, there is my reflection and yours." Then came the comparison. He looked at this lion and then at his own reflection, and in a moment came the idea that he was a lion. The lion roared, the bleating was gone. You are the lions, you are souls, pure, infinite and perfect. The might of the universe is in you. "Why weepest thou, my friend? There is neither birth nor death for thee. Why weepest thou? There is no disease nor misery for thee, but thou art like the infinite sky, clouds of various colors come over it, play for a moment, then vanish. It is the same eternal blue." Why do we see wickedness? There was a stump of a tree in the dark at night. A thief came that way and said, "That is a policeman." A young man waiting for his beloved came that way and thought that was his sweetheart. A child who had been told ghost stories came out and began to shriek that it was a ghost. But it was the stump of a tree. We see the world as we are. Put on the table a bag of gold and let a baby be here. Let a thief come and take the gold. Would the baby know it was stolen? That which we have inside we see outside. The baby has no thief inside and sees no thief outside. So with all knowledge. Do not talk of the wickedness of the world and all its sins. Weep that you are bound to see wickedness yet. Weep that you are bound to see sin everywhere, and if you want to help the world do not condemn it. Do not weaken it all the more. For what is sin and what is misery, and what are all these, but the results of weakness? The world has been made weaker and weaker every day by such teachings. Men are taught from childhood that they are weak and are sinners. Teach them that they are all glorious children of immortality, even those who are the weakest in manifestation. Let positive, strong, helpful thought, enter into their brains from very childhood and not weakening and paralyzing thought. Lay yourselves open to those thoughts. Tell your own minds "I am He, I am He." Let it ring day and night in your minds like a song, and at the point of death declare: "I am He." That is the truth, the infinite strength of the world is yours. Drive out the superstition that has covered your minds. Let us be brave. Know the truth and practise the truth. The goal may be distant, but awake, arise, and stop not till that goal is reached.

---

1. Sanskrit root *man*, to think.

IV. MÂYÂ AND ILLUSION.

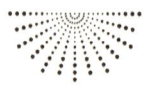

Almost all of you have heard of the word *Mâyâ*. Generally it is used, though I am afraid very wrongly, to denote illusion, or delusion, or some such thing, but as the theory of *Mâyâ* forms, as it were, one of the pillars upon which the Vedânta rests, it is necessary that it should be properly understood, and I ask a little patience of you, for there is great danger of being misunderstood in expounding the theory of *mâyâ*. The oldest idea of *mâyâ* that we can find in Vedic literature is where this word is used in the sense of delusion, but then the real theory had not been reached. We find such passages as "Indra through his *mâyâ* assumed various forms." Here it is true the word *mâyâ* means something like magic. So we find various other passages, always taking the same meaning. The word *mâyâ* then drops out of sight altogether. In the meanwhile the idea is developing. Later the question is raised, why cannot we know the secret of the Universe, and the answer given is very significant. "Because we talk in vain, and because we are satisfied with the things of the senses, and because we are running after desires; therefore we, as it were, cover this reality with a mist." Here the word *mâyâ* is not used at all, but we get one idea, that the cause of our ignorance is a kind of mist that has come between us and the truth. Much later on, in one of the latest Upanishads, we find the word *mâyâ*, reappearing, but by this time a good deal of transformation has been worked upon it, a mass of new meaning has by this time attached itself to the word. Theories have been propounded and repeated; others have been taken up, until at last the idea of *mâyâ* has become a fixed quantity. We read in the *Svetasvatara* Upanishad "Know nature to be *mâyâ* and the mind, the ruler of this *mâyâ* is the Lord Himself." Coming to our philosophers, we find that this word *mâyâ* has been manipulated in various fashions, until we come to the great Sankarâcharya. The theory of *mâyâ* was manipulated a little by the Buddhists, too, but in their hands it became very much like what is called Idealism, and that is the meaning that is now generally given to the word *mâyâ*. When the Hindu says the world is *mâyâ*, at once people get the idea that the world is an illusion. This interpretation has some basis, as coming through the Buddhistic philosophers, because there was one section of them who did not believe in the external world at all. But the *mâyâ* of the Vedânta, in its last developed form, is neither idealism nor realism, nor is it theory. It is a simple statement of facts—what we are, and what we see around us. As I have told you before, the minds of the people from whom the Vedas came were intent upon following principles, discovering principles. They had no time to work upon details, or to wait for them; they wanted to go deep into the heart of things. Something beyond was calling them, as it were, and they could not wait. We find that, scattered all through the Upanishads and other books the details of subjects which we now call modern sciences, are often very erroneous, but, at the same time, their principles are correct. For instance, the idea of ether, which is one of the latest theories of modern science, is to be found in our ancient literature in forms much more developed than is the modern scientific theory of ether to-day; but it was in principle; when they tried to demonstrate the workings of that principle, they made many mistakes. The theory of the all-pervading life principle, of which all life in this universe is but a differing manifestation, was understood in Vedic times; it is found in the *Brahmanas*. There is a long hymn in the *Samhita* in praise of *Prâna*, of which all life is but a manifestation. By the bye, it may interest some of you to know that there are in the Vedic philosophy theories about the origin of life on this earth very similar to those which have been advanced by some modern European scientists. You, of course, all know that there is a theory that life came from other planets. It is a settled doctrine with some Vedic philosophers that life comes in this way from the moon.

Coming to the principles, we find these Vedic thinkers very courageous and wonderfully bold in propounding large and generalized theories. The answer which they gave as a solution of the mystery of this Universe from the external world was a general one. The detailed workings of modern science do not bring the question one step nearer to solution, because the principles have failed. If the theory of ether failed in ancient times to give a solution of the mystery of the Universe, working out the details of that ether theory will not bring us much nearer to the truth. If the theory of all-pervading life failed as a theory of this Universe, it would not mean anything more if worked out in detail, for the details do not change the principle of the Universe. What I mean is, that in their inquiry into the principle, the Hindu thinkers were as bold, and in some cases much bolder, than the moderns. They made some of the grandest generalizations that have yet been reached, and some still remain in India as theories, which modern science has yet to get even as theories. For instance, they not only arrived at the ether theory, but went beyond and classified mind also, as a still more rarefied ether. Beyond that they found a still more rarefied ether. Yet there is no solution, it does not answer the problem. No amount of knowledge of the external world would answer the problem. We find here we were just beginning to know a little; wait a few thousand years and we shall get the solution. "No," says the Vedantist, for he has proved beyond all doubt that the mind is limited; that it cannot go beyond certain limits; we cannot go beyond time, space and the law of causation. As no man can jump out of his own self, so no man can go beyond the limits that have been put upon us by the laws of time and space. Every attempt to solve the law of causation, time and space, will be futile, because the very attempt would have to be made by taking for granted the existence of these three. It cannot be. What form does the statement of the existence of the world take then? "This world has no existence." What is meant thereby? That it has no existence-absolute. It exists only as relative to my mind, to yours, and to the minds of everybody else. We see this world with the five senses. If we had another sense, we would see in it something else. If we had still another sense, it would appear as something yet different. It has, therefore, no real existence; that unchangeable, immovable, infinite existence it has not. Nor can it be called non-existence, seeing that it exists, and we have to work in and through it. It is a mixture of existence and non-existence.

Coming from abstractions to the common everyday details of our lives, we find that our whole life is a mixture of this contradiction of existence and nonexistence. There is this contradiction in knowledge. It seems that man can know everything, if he only wants to know; but before he has gone more than a few steps he finds an adamantine wall which he cannot move. All his work is in a circle, and he cannot go beyond that circle. The problems which are nearest and dearest to him, are impelling him and calling on him day and night for a solution, but he cannot solve them, because he cannot go beyond his intellect. And yet the desire is implanted strongly in him. Still we know that the only good is to be obtained by controlling and checking these impulses. With every breath, every impulse of our heart asks us to be selfish. At the same time, there is some power beyond us which says that it is unselfishness alone which is good. Every child is a born optimist; he is dreaming golden dreams. In youth he becomes still more optimistic. It is hard for a young man to believe that there is such a thing as death, such a thing as defeat or degradation. Old age comes, and life is a mass of ruin. Dreams have vanished into air, and the old man has become a pessimist. Thus we are going on, from one extreme to the other, buffeted by Nature, without hope, without limit, without knowing the bounds, without knowing where we are going. It reminds me of a celebrated song written in the *Lalita Vistara*, in the biography of Buddha. Buddha was born, says the book, as the saviour of mankind, but he forgot himself in the luxuries of his palace, and some angels came to sing a song to rouse him up, and the burden of the whole song is, we are floating down this river, continually changing, with no stop and no rest. So are all our lives, going on and on without knowing any rest. What are we to do? The man who has enough to eat and drink is an optimist, and he avoids all mention of misery, for it frightens him. Tell not to him the sorrows and the sufferings of the world; go to him and tell that it is all good.

"Yes, I am safe," says he; "look at me, I have a nice house to live in. I do not care for cold; therefore do not bring these horrid pictures before me." But, on the other hand, there are others dying of cold and hunger. Go and teach them that it is all good and they will refuse to believe you. There may be a man who has suffered tremendously in this life, and he will not hear of anything joyful, of anything beautiful, of anything that is good.

"Frighten everybody," says he; "why should it be that anybody should laugh while I am weeping? I must make them all weep with me, for I am miserable; that is my only consolation." Thus we are going on, between optimism and pessimism. Then there is the tremendous fact of death. The whole world is going to death; everything is dying. All our progress, our vanities, our reforms, our luxuries, our knowledge have that one end— death. That is all that is certain. Cities come and go, empires rise and fall, planets break into pieces and crumble into dust, to be blown about by the atmospheres of other planets. Thus it is going on from time without beginning. What is the goal? Death is the goal of everything. Death is the goal of life, of beauty, of power, of wealth, of virtue, too. Saints die and sinners die, kings die and beggars die. They are all going to death, and yet this tremendous clinging on to life exists. Somehow, we do not know why, we have to cling on to life; we cannot give it up. And this is *mâyâ!*

The mother is nursing a child with great care; all her soul, her life, is in that child. The child grows, becomes a man, and perchance becomes a blackguard and a brute, kicks her and beats her every day; and yet the mother clings on to the child, and when her reason awakes, she covers it up with the idea of love. She little thinks it is not love, it is something which has got hold of her nerves, she cannot shake it off; however she may try, she cannot shake off the bondage she has—and this is *mâyâ!* We are all after the golden fleece. Every one of us thinks that this will be ours, but very few of them are in the world. Every reasonable man sees that the chance of getting it is perhaps one in twenty millions, yet every one must struggle for it, and the majority never get anything. And this is *mâyâ!* Death is stalking day and night over this earth of ours, but at the same time we always believe that we shall live eternally. A question was once asked of King Yudhisthira, "What is the most wonderful thing on this earth?" And the King replied, "Every day people are dying around us, and yet men think they will never die." And this is *mâyâ!* This tremendous contradiction, pleasure succeeding pain, and pain pleasure, seems quite natural to us. A reformer arises and wants to remedy the evils that are existing in a certain nation; and before they have been remedied a thousand other evils have arisen in another place. It is an old house that is falling; patch it up in one place, the ruin extends to another corner. In India our reformers cry and preach against the evils which enforced widowhood brings to Indian women. In the West non-marriage is the great evil. Help the unmarried on one side; they are suffering. Help the widows on the other; they are suffering. Like the old rheumatism in the body, drive it from the head and it goes to the body, drive it from there and it goes to the feet. Some people become richer than others; learning, and wealth, and culture become their exclusive possession. Reformers cry that these treasures should not be in the hands of a select few; that they should be distributed, that all ought to share them. More happiness might possibly be brought to the masses in the sense of physical happiness, but, perhaps, as culture comes, this physical happiness vanishes. Which way shall we go, for the knowledge of happiness brings the knowledge of unhappiness? The least bit of material prosperity that we enjoy is elsewhere causing the same amount of misery. This is the state of things. The young, perhaps, do not see it clearly, but those who have lived long enough and those who have struggled enough will understand it. And this is *mâyâ!* These things are going on day and night, and to find a solution of this problem would be impossible. Why should it be thus? This is an impossible question to answer, because the question cannot be logically formulated. There is neither how nor why in this. We must grasp it before we can answer it; we must know what it is before we can answer. But we cannot make it steady one moment, it eludes our grasp every minute. We are like blind machines. We struggle to find a solution of a problem that incessantly changes; we have to do this, we cannot help ourselves. And this too is *mâyâ!* I stand up and lecture to you, and you sit and listen; we cannot help it. And you will go home, and some of you may have learned a little, while, perhaps, others will think this man has talked nonsense. I will go home thinking I have been lecturing. And this is *mâyâ!*

Mâyâ, is a statement of the facts of this Universe, of how it is going on. People generally get frightened when these things are told to them. Bold we must be. Hiding facts is not the way to find a remedy. As the hare, you all know, hunted down by dogs, puts its head down and thinks itself safe, so, when we run into optimism or pessimism, we are doing just like the hare, but that is not a remedy. On all sides there are objections and these objections, you may remark, are generally from people who possess more of the good things of life, or of enjoyments. In this country (England) it is very difficult to become a pessimist. Every one tells me how wonderfully the world is going on, how progressive, but what he himself is, is his own world. Old questions arise; Christianity must be the only true religion of the world, because Christian nations are prosperous. But that assertion contradicts itself, because the prosperity of the Christian nations depends on the misfortune of non-Christian nations. There must be some to prey upon. Suppose the whole world were to become Christian, then the Christian nations would become poor, because there would be no non-Christian nations for them to prey upon. Thus the argument would kill itself. Animals are living upon the plants, men upon animals, and worst of all upon each other, the strong upon the weak; this is going on everywhere, and this is *mâyâ!* What solution do you apply to this? We hear every day of such and such explanations, and are told that in the long run it will be all good. Suppose it be possible—which is very much to be doubted—but let us take it for granted, why should there be this diabolical way of doing good? Why cannot good be done through good instead of through these diabolical methods? The descendants of the human beings of to-day will be happy; but why must there be all this suffering so now? This is *mâyâ*; there is no solution to it.

Again, we often hear that it is one of the features of evolution that it eliminates evil, and this evil being continually eliminated from the world, at last there will remain only good and good alone. That is very nice to hear, and it panders to our vanities, at least with those of us who have enough of this world's goods, who have not a hard struggle to face every day, and are not being crushed under the wheels of this so-called evolution. It is very good and comforting, indeed, to such fortunate ones.

The common herds may suffer, but they do not care; let them die, they are of no consequence. Very good, yet this argument is fallacious from beginning to end. It takes for granted, in the first place, that manifested good and evil in this world are certain quantities. In the second place, it makes a still worse assumption, that the amount of good is an increasing quantity, and the amount of evil is a decreasing quantity. So, if evil is being eliminated in this way by what they call evolution, there will come a time when this evil will be eliminated and what remains will be all good. Very easy to say, but can it be proved that evil is a lessening quantity? Is it not increasing all the time? Take the man who lives in a forest, who does not know even how to cultivate the mind, cannot read a book, has not heard of such a thing as writing. Run a bayonet through that man and take it out, and soon he is all right again, while we, who are more cultured, get scratched in the streets and die. Machines are making things cheap, making for progress and evolution, but are crushing down millions, that one may become rich, making one richer than others, and thousands at the same time poorer and poorer, making slaves of whole masses of human beings.

That way it is going on. The animal man has enjoyments only in the senses. If he does not get enough to eat, he is miserable, or if something happens to his body, he is miserable. In the senses, both his misery and his happiness begin and end. As soon as this man progresses, as soon as the horizon of his happiness increases, his horizon of unhappiness increases proportionately. The man in the forest does not know what it is to be jealous, to be in the Law Courts, to pay taxes regularly, what it is to be blamed by society, to be watched day and night by the most tremendous tyranny that human diabolism ever invented, prying into the secrets of every human heart. He does not know how man becomes a thousand times more diabolical than any other animal, with all his vain knowledge, and with all his pride. Thus it is that, as we emerge out of the senses we develop higher powers of enjoyment, and, at the same time, we have to develop higher powers of suffering, too. The nerves, on the other hand, are becoming finer and capable of suffering more. Often, in every society, we find that the ignorant, common man, if he is abused, does not feel much, but he feels a good thrashing. But the gentleman cannot hear a single word of abuse, he has become so finely nerved. Misery has increased with his susceptibility to happiness. This does not go much to prove the philosopher's case. As we increase our power to be happy, we are always increasing our power to suffer, and in my humble opinion, if we advance in our power to become happy in arithmetical progression, we shall progress, on the other hand, in the power to become miserable in geometrical progression. We who are progressing know that the more we progress the more avenues are opened to pain as well as to pleasure. And this is *mâyâ!*

Thus we find that *mâyâ* is not a theory for the explanation of the world; it is simply a statement of facts as they exist. The very basis of our being is contradiction, everywhere we have to move through this tremendous contradiction, that wherever there is good there must also be evil, and wherever there is evil there must be some good, wherever there is life death must follow it as its shadow, and every one who smiles will have to weep, and whoever weeps must smile also. Nor can this state of things be remedied. We may verily imagine that there will be a place where there will be only good, and no evil, that there will be places where we shall only smile and never weep. Such a thing is impossible in the very nature of things, for the conditions will be the same. Wherever there is the power of producing a smile in us, there lurks the power of producing tears in our eyes. Wherever there is the power of producing happiness in us, there lurks somewhere the power of making us miserable.

Thus the Vedânta philosophy is neither optimistic nor pessimistic. It voices both these views and takes things as they are; it admits that this world is a mixture of good and evil, happiness and misery; and that to increase the one, of necessity must increase the other. There will never be a good world, because the very idea is a contradiction in terms; nor can there be a bad world. The great secret revealed by this analysis is this, that good and bad ire not two cut-and-dried, separate existences. There is not one thing in this world of ours which you can label as good, and good alone, and there is not one thing in the universe which you can label as bad, and bad alone. The very same phenomenon which is appearing to be good now, may appear to be bad to-morrow. The same thing which is producing misery in one, may produce happiness in another. The fire that burns the child may cook a good meal for a starving man. The same nerves that carry the sensations of misery carry also the sensations of happiness. The only way to stop evil, therefore, is to stop the good also; there is no other way that is sure. To stop death, we shall have to stop life also. Life without death, and happiness without misery, are contradictions, and neither can be found alone, because each of them is but a different manifestation of the same thing. What I thought to be good yesterday, I do not think to be good now. In all my life, when I look back upon it, and see what were my ideals at different times, I find this to be so. At one time my ideal was to drive a strong pair of horses. I do not hold that ideal now. At another time, when I was a little child, I thought if I could make a certain kind of sweetmeat I should be perfectly happy. At another time I imagined that I should be entirely satisfied if I had a wife and children and plenty of money. To-day, I laugh at all these ideals as mere childish nonsense. The Vedânta says, there must come a time when we look back and laugh at these ideals of ours which make us afraid of giving up our individuality. Each one wants to keep this body and not give it up, and our idea is that if we can keep the body for an indefinite time we shall be very happy, but there will come a time when we shall laugh at that too. Now, if such be the state of things, we are in a state of helpless contradiction, neither existence, nor non-existence, but a mixture of them both; neither misery, nor happiness, but a mixture of them both. What, then, is the use of Vedânta, and all other philosophies and religions? And, above all, what is the use of doing good work? This is the question that comes to the mind. If this be the truth, that whenever you try to do good the same evil remains, and whenever you try to create happiness there will always be mountains high of misery, people will always ask you—what is the use of doing right? The answer is, in the first place, that we must work in the way of lessening misery, for that is the only way of making ourselves happy. Every one of us finds it out sooner or later in our lives. The bright ones find it out a little earlier, and the dull ones a little later. The dull ones pay very dearly for the discovery and the bright ones less dearly. In the second place, apart from that, although we know there never will come a time when this universe will be full of happiness and without misery, still this is the work to be done; although misery increases, we must do our part at the same time. Both these forces will make the universe live until there will come a time when we shall awake from our dreams and give up this building of mud-pies, which we are doing all the time, for it is true that it is only a building of mud-pies. That one lesson we shall have to learn. It will take a long, long time to learn it.

Attempts have been made in Germany to build a system of philosophy on the basis that the Infinite has become the finite. Such attempts are made even in England now, and the analysis of the position of these philosophers is this, that the Infinite is trying to express Itself in this universe. The mistake is that they imagine there will come a time when the Infinite will succeed in expressing itself. In that case the absolute state would be a lower one than the manifested, because in the manifested state, the Absolute expresses itself, and we are to help this expression more and more, until the Infinite pours itself out on this side as the finite. This is all very nice, and we have used the words infinite and manifestation and expression, and so on, but philosophers naturally ask for a logical, fundamental basis for the statement that the finite can fully express the Infinite.

The Absolute and the Infinite can become this universe only by limitation. Everything here, therefore, must be limited, everything that comes out of the senses, or through the mind, or through the intellect, must of necessity be limited, and for the limited to be the unlimited is simply absurd, and can never be.

The Vedânta, on the other hand, says that it is true that the Absolute, or the Infinite, is trying to express itself in the finite, but there will come a time when it will find that it is impossible, and it will then have to beat a retreat, and this beating a retreat is the real beginning of religion. It is very hard for modern people to talk of renunciation. I stand, as it was said of me in America, as a man coming out of a world that has been dead and buried these five thousand years, and talking of renunciation. So says, perhaps, the English philosopher. Yet it is true that that is the only path to religion —renounce and give up. Struggle hard and try your best to find any other way. What did Christ say? "He that loseth his life for my sake, shall find it." Again and again did he preach renunciation as the only way to be perfect. There comes a time when the mind awakes from this long and dreary dream, and longs for some satisfying reality. It finds the truth of the statement: "Desires are never satisfied by the enjoyment of desires they only increase the more, as butter poured upon the fire increases the flame the more." This is true of all sense enjoyments, of all intellectual enjoyments, and of all the enjoyments of which the human soul is capable. They are all without real value, they are within *mâyâ*, within this net-work beyond which we cannot go. We may run therein through infinite time and find no end, and whenever we struggle to get a little bit of enjoyment, a mass of misery will be on our back. How awful is this state of things! And when I think of all this, I cannot but think that this theory of *mâyâ*, this statement that it is all *mâyâ*, is the best and only explanation. What an amount of misery there is in this world, and if you travel among various nations you will find that one nation has attempted to cure its evils by one means, and another by another. Evil has been taken up by the various races, and attempts have been made in various ways to check it, yet no nation has succeeded. If it has been minimized in one point, a mass of evil has been crowded into another point. Thus it goes. The Hindus, to produce a little chastity in the race, have sanctioned child-marriage, which in the long run has degraded the race. At the same time, I cannot deny that this child-marriage makes the race more chaste. What would you have? If you want the nation to be more chaste, you weaken men and women physically by child-marriage. On the other hand, are you in England any safer? No, because chastity is the life of a nation. Do you not find in history that the first death-sign of a nation has been unchastity? When that has entered, the end of the race is in sight. Where shall we get a solution of these miseries then? If parents select husbands and wives for their children, will this evil be prevented? The daughters of India are more practical than sentimental. Very little of poetry remains in their lives. Again, if people select their own husbands and wives, that does not seem to bring much happiness, if the records of the divorce court are to be trusted. The Indian woman is very happy; there is scarcely a case of quarrelling between husband and wife. On the other hand, in the United States, where the greatest liberty obtains, the number of unhappy homes and marriages is very large. Unhappiness is here, there and everywhere. What does it show? That, after all, not much happiness has been gained by all these ideals. We all struggle for happiness, and before we get a little on one side on the other side there begins unhappiness.

Shall we not work to do good then? Yes, with more zest than ever, but what this knowledge will do for us is to break down our fanaticism. The Englishman will no more become a fanatic to curse the Hindu. He will have learned to respect the customs of different nations. There will be less fanaticism and more real work; fanatics cannot work, they waste three-fourths of their energy. It is the level-headed, calm, practical man who works.

Mere ranting fanatics do not do much. So the power to work will increase from this idea. Knowing that this is the state of things, there will be more patience. The sight of misery or of evil will not be able to throw us off our balance and make us run after shadows. Therefore, patience will come to us, knowing that the world will have to go on in this way. Say, for instance, that all men will have become good, then the animals will have become men, and will have to go through the same state, and so the plants. But only one thing is certain; the mighty river is rushing towards the ocean, and there are bits of straw and paper in the stream, which are trying to get back, but we are sure that the time will come when each one of these pieces will be drawn into that boundless ocean. So, in this life, with all its miseries and sorrows, its joys and smiles and tears, one thing is certain, that all things are rushing towards their goal and it is only a question of time when you and I, and plants and animals, and every particle of life that exists must go into the Infinite Ocean of perfection, must attain unto freedom, unto God.

Let me repeat, once more, because the mistake is constantly being made, that the Vedantic position is neither pessimism nor optimism. It does not say that this world is all evil or all good. It says that our evil is of no less value than our good, and our good of no more value than our evil. They are all bound together. This is the world, and knowing this you work with patience. What for? Why should we work? If this is the state of things what shall we do? Why not become agnostics? The modern agnostics also know that there is no solution of this problem, no getting out of this evil, or this *mâyâ*, as we should say in our language; therefore, they tell us to be satisfied and enjoy life. Here, again, is a mistake, a tremendous mistake, a most illogical mistake. And it is this. What do you mean by life? Do you mean only the life of the senses? In this, every one of us differs only slightly from the brutes. I am sure that no one is present here whose life is only in the senses. Then this present life means something more than that. Our feelings and thoughts and aspirations are all part and parcel of our life, and is not the struggle towards the great ideal, towards perfection, one of the most important components of what we call life? According to the agnostics, we must enjoy life as it is. But this life means, above all, this tremendous search after the ideal; the backbone of life is going towards perfection. We must have that, and, therefore, we cannot be agnostics, or take the world as it appears. The agnostic position takes this life minus this latter component, to be all that exists, and this he claims cannot be known, wherefore he must give up the search. This is what is called *Mâyâ*, this Nature, this Universe. This according to the Vedantist is Nature.

All religions are more or less attempts to get beyond nature, the crudest, or the most developed, expressed through mythology, or symbology, or through the abstractions of philosophy, through stories of gods, or angels, or demons; through stories of saints, or seers, or great men, or prophets, all have that one object, all are trying to get beyond these limitations, to find something better and higher. In one word, they are all struggling towards freedom. Man feels, consciously or unconsciously, that he is bound; that he is not what he wants to be. It was taught to him at the very moment he began to look around; that very instant he learned that he was bound, and he also found that there was something in him which wanted to fly beyond, where the body could not follow, something which was as yet chained down by this limitation. Even in the lowest of religious ideas, where departed ancestors, and other spirits, mostly violent and cruel, lurking about the houses of their friends, fond of bloodshed and strong drink—even there we find that one common factor, that of freedom. The man who wants to worship the gods, sees in them above all things greater freedom than in himself. If a door is closed, he imagines that the gods can get through walls and so on; the walls have no limitations for them. This one idea of liberty is increasing, until it comes to the ideal of a Personal God, of which the central concept is that God is a Being beyond the limitation of Nature, of *mâyâ*. I hear, as it were, a voice before me, I feel as if this question were being discussed by those ancient sages of India, in some of those forest retreats, and in one of them even the oldest and the holiest fail to reach the solution, but a young boy is standing up in the midst of them and declaring: "Hear ye children of immortality, hear ye who live in the highest places, I have found the way. There is a way out beyond the darkness by knowing Him who is beyond this darkness."

This *mâyâ* is everywhere, it is terrible; to work through *mâyâ* is impossible. If a man says I will sit beside this great river and I will ford the river when all the water has run down into the ocean, that man would be as likely to succeed as the man who says he will work till this world has become all good, and then he will enjoy this world. Great Ganges herself might sooner run dry than the world become all good! The way is not with *mâyâ* but against *mâyâ*. This is another fact to learn. We are not born helpers of Nature, but competitors with Nature. We are the bondmasters, and we are trying to bind ourselves down. Why is this house here? Nature did not give it. Nature says go and live in the forest. Man says I will build a house and fight with Nature, and he does. The whole history of humanity is a continuous fight against the so-called laws of Nature, and man gains in the end. Coming to the internal world, there, too, the same fight is going on, this fight between the animal man and the spiritual man, between light and darkness, and here, too, man becomes victorious. He, as it were, cuts his way out of Nature to his idea of freedom. We have seen so far, then, that here is a statement of *mâyâ*, and beyond this *mâyâ* the Vedantic philosophers find something which is not bound by *mâyâ*, and if we can get where that stands, certainly we shall be beyond *mâyâ*. This, in some form or other, is the common property of all religions, and is what is called Theism. But with the Vedânta, it is the beginning of religion and not the end. The idea of a personal God, the Ruler and Creator of this Universe, as He has been styled, the Ruler of *mâyâ*, or Nature, is not the end of these Vedantic ideas, it is only the beginning, and the idea grows and grows until the Vedantist finds that He who was standing outside was he himself, and was in reality inside. It was the very one who is free, who through limitation thought he was bound.

V. MÂYÂ AND THE EVOLUTION OF THE CONCEPTION OF GOD.

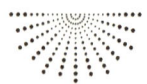

We have seen how the idea of *Mâyâ*, which forms; as it were, one of the basic doctrines of the Advaita Vedânta, is, in its germ, found even in the Samhitas, and that in reality all the ideas which are developed in the Upanishads are to be found already in the Samhitas in some form or other. Most of you are by this time perfectly acquainted with the idea of *Mâyâ*, and know that it is sometimes very erroneously explained as illusion, so that when the universe is said to be *Mâyâ*, that also would have to be explained as being illusion. The translation of the word is neither happy nor correct. *Mâyâ* is not a theory, it is simply a statement of facts about the universe as it exists, and to understand *Mâyâ* we must go back to the Samhitas and begin with the conception in the germ. We have seen how the ideas of the *Devas* came. At the same time these *Devas* were at first only powerful beings, nothing more. Most of you are horrified when reading the old scriptures, whether of the Greeks, the Hebrews, the Persians, or others, to find that the ancient gods sometimes did things which, to us, are very repugnant, but when reading these books, we entirely forget that we are persons of the nineteenth century, and these gods were beings existing thousands of years ago, and we also forget that the people who worshipped these gods found nothing incongruous in their characters, found nothing to frighten them in depicting their gods as they did, because they were very much like them themselves. I may also remark that this is the one great lesson we have to learn throughout our lives. In judging others we always judge them by our own ideals. That is not as it should be. Every one must be judged according to his own ideal, and not by that of any one else. In all our dealings with our fellow-beings we constantly labor under this mistake, and I am of the opinion that the vast majority of our quarrels with our fellow-beings arise simply from this one cause, that we are always trying to judge other gods by our own, other ideals by our ideals, and others' motives from our motives. Under certain circumstances I might do a certain thing, and when I see another person taking the same course I think he has also the same motive actuating him, little dreaming that although the effect may be the same, yet many thousands of causes may produce the same effect. He may have performed the action with quite a different motive from what would impel me to do the same thing. So in judging of those ancient religions we must not take the ordinary standpoint to which we incline in our judgment of others, but must throw ourselves, as it were, into the position of thought in those early times.

The idea of the cruel and ruthless Jehovah in the Old Testament has frightened many—but why? What right have they to assume that the Jehovah of the ancient Jews must represent the conventional idea of God of the present day? And at the same time we must not forget that there will come men after us who will laugh at our ideas of religion and God in the same way that we laugh at those of the ancients. Yet through all these various conceptions runs the golden thread of unity, and it is the purpose of the Vedânta to unfold this thread. "I am the thread that runs through all these various ideas, each one of which is like one pearl," says the Lord Krishna; and it is the duty of Vedânta to establish this connecting thread, however incongruous, hideous, horrible, or disgusting may seem these ideas when judged according to the conceptions of to-day. When these ideas had the setting of past times they were harmonious, they were not more hideous than our present ideas. It is only when we try to take them out of these settings and apply them to our own present circumstances that the hideousness becomes obvious. It is all dead and gone and past. Just as the old Jew has developed into the keen, modern, sharp Jew, and the ancient Âryan into the intellectual Hindû, similarly Jehovah has grown, and *Devas* have grown. The great mistake is in recognizing the evolution of the worshippers, while we do not acknowledge the evolution of the God. He is not credited with the advance that his devotees have made.

That is to say, you and I, as representing ideas, have grown; these gods also, as representing ideas, have grown. This may seem somewhat curious to you—how can God grow? He cannot. He is unchangeable, but man's ideas about God are constantly changing and expanding. In the same sense the real man never grows. We will see later on how the real man behind each one of these manifestations is immovable, unchangeable, pure, and always perfect; and in the same way the idea that we form of God is a mere manifestation, our own creation. Behind that is the real God who never changes, the ever pure, the immutable. But the manifestations are always changing, revealing the reality behind more and more. When it reveals more of the fact behind, it is called progression; when it hides more of the fact behind, it is called retrogression. Thus, as we grow, so the gods grow. From the common-sense point of view, just as we reveal ourselves as we evolve, so the gods reveal themselves.

We shall now be in a position to understand the theory of *Mâyâ*. In stating all the religions of the world one question they propose to discuss is this: Why is there disharmony in the universe? Why is there evil in the universe? We do not find this question in the very primitive inception of religious ideas because the world did not appear incongruous to the primitive man. Circumstances around him were not inharmonious; there was no clash of opinions; no antagonism of good and evil. There was merely the fight in his own heart between something which said yea, and something which said nay. The primitive man was a man of impulse. He did what occurred to him, and tried to bring out into his muscles whatever thought came into his mind. He never stopped to judge, and seldom tried to check his impulses. So with the gods, they also were creatures of impulse. Indra comes and shatters the forces of the demons. Jehovah is pleased with one person and displeased with another, for what reason no one knows or asks; for the habit of inquiry had not then arisen, and whatever he did was regarded as right. There was no idea of good or evil. The *Devas* did many wicked things in our sense of the word; again and again Indra and other gods committed very wicked deeds, but to the worshippers of Indra the ideas of wickedness and evil did not occur, so they did not question.

With the advance of ethical ideas came the fight. There arose a certain sense in man; different languages and nations called it by different names, and it acted as a checking power; for the impulses of the human heart are the voice of God, or the result of past education, but whatever it is called the effect is the same. There is one impulse in our minds which says: "do." Behind it rises another voice which says: "do not." There is one set of ideas in our mind which is always struggling to get outside through the channels of the senses, and behind that, although it may be thin and weak, an infinitely small voice which says do not go outside. The two beautiful Sanskrit words for these phenomena are *pravritti* and *nivritti*, "circling forward" and "circling inward." It is the circling forward which usually governs our actions. Religion begins with the circling inward. Religion begins with this "do not." Spirituality begins with this "do not." When the "do not" is not there, religion has not begun. And this "do not" came, causing men's ideas to grow despite the brutal fighting gods which they had made.

A little love awoke in the hearts of mankind. It was very small indeed, and even now it is not much greater. It was at first confined to the tribe, embracing perhaps members of the same tribe; these gods loved their tribes and each god was a tribal god, the protector of that tribe. And sometimes the members of those tribes would think of themselves as the descendants of that god, just as the clans in different nations think that they are the common descendants of some one who was the founder of the clan. There were in ancient times, and are even now, some people claiming to be descendants not only of these gods, but also of the Sun and Moon. You read in the ancient Sanskrit books of the great heroic emperors of the solar dynasty. They were first worshippers of the Moon and Sun, and gradually came to think of themselves as descendants of the god of the Sun, of the Moon, and so forth. So when these tribal ideas began to grow there came a little love, some slight idea of duties towards each other, a little social organization, and immediately began the idea, how can we live together without bearing and forbearing? How can one man live with another man—even one—without having some time or other to check his impulses, restrain himself, forbear from doing things which his mind would prompt him to do. It is impossible. Thus comes the idea of restraint. The whole social fabric is based upon that idea of restraint, and we all know that the man or woman who has not learned the great lesson of bearing and forbearing, leads a most miserable life.

Now when these ideas of religion came, a glimpse of something higher, more ethical, dawned upon the intellect of mankind. The old gods were found to be incongruous, these boisterous, fighting, drinking, beef-eating gods of the ancients, whose delight was in the smell of burning flesh and libations of strong liquor. Sometimes Indra drank so much that he fell upon the ground and began to talk unintelligently. These gods could no longer be tolerated. The notion had arisen of inquiring into motives, and the gods had to come in for their share of inquiry. What is the reason for such an action of such and such a god?—and the reason was wanting. Therefore men gave up these gods, or rather they developed higher ideas concerning them; they collected together and discarded all the actions and qualities of the gods which they could not harmonize, and they kept those which they could understand and harmonize, and combining these, labelled them with one name, *Deva-deva*, the "God of gods of the universe. The god to be worshipped was no more a simple symbol of power; something more was required than power. He was an ethical god; he loved mankind, did good to mankind. But the idea of god still remained. They increased his ethical significance, and increased also his power. He became the most ethical being in the Universe, as well as almost almighty.

But all this patchwork would not do. As the explanation assumed greater proportion, the difficulty which it sought to solve did the same. If the qualities of the god increased in arithmetical progression, the difficulty and doubt increased in geometrical progression. The difficulty of Jehovah was very little beside the difficulty of the god of the universe, and this question remains to the present day. Why, under the reign of an almighty and all loving God of the Universe, should such diabolical things be allowed to remain? Why so much more misery than happiness? and so much more wickedness than good? We may shut our eyes to all these things, but the fact still remains, this world is a hideous world. At best it is the hell of Tantalus and nothing else. Here we are with strong impulses, and stronger cravings for sense enjoyments and nothing outside to satisfy them. There rises a wave which impels us forward in spite of our own will, and as soon as we move one step comes a blow. We are all doomed to live here and die here like Tantalus. Ideals come into our head, far beyond the limit of our sense ideals, but when we seek to express them, we never can see them fulfilled. On the other hand, we are crushed into atoms by the surging mass around us. Yet if I give up all ideality and merely struggle through this world, my existence is that of a brute, and I degenerate and degrade myself. Neither way is happiness. Unhappiness is the fate of those who are content to live in this world born as they are. A thousandfold unhappiness is the fate of those who dare to stand forth for truth and for higher things, and who dare to ask for something higher than mere brute existence here. These are the facts; there is no explanation. There cannot be any explanation, but Vedânta shows the way out. You must bear in mind that I must tell you facts in this course which will frighten you sometimes, but remember what I say, think of it, digest it, and it will be yours, it will raise you high, and make you capable of understanding and living in truth.

Now this is a statement of fact, not a theory, that this world is a Tantalus' hell, that we do not know anything about this Universe, yet at the same time we cannot say that we do not know. I cannot say that this chain exists, when I think of it I do not know. It may be an entire delusion in my brain. I may be dreaming all the time. I am dreaming that I am talking to you, and that you are listening to me. No one can prove that it is not a dream. My brain itself may be a dream, and as to that, no one has ever seen his own brain yet. We all take that for granted. So it is with everything. My own body I take for granted. At the same time I cannot say I do not know. This standing between knowledge and ignorance, this mystic twilight, the mingling of truth and falsehood, where they meet no one knows. We are walking in the midst of a dream, half sleeping, half waking, passing all our lives in a haze, this is the fate of every one of us. This is the fate of all sense knowledge. This is the fate of all philosophy, of all boasted science, of all boasted human knowledge. This is the Universe.

What you call matter, or spirit, or mind, or anything else you may like to call them, any nickname you may choose to give them, the fact remains the same, we cannot say they are; we cannot say they are not. We cannot say they are one, we cannot

say they are many. This eternal play of light and darkness, indiscriminate, indistinguishable, inseparable is always there. A fact, yet at the same time, not a fact, awake, and at the same time, asleep. This is a statement of facts, and this is what is called *Mâyâ*. We are born in this *Mâyâ*, we live in it, we think in it, we dream in it. We are philosophers in it, we are spiritual men in it, nay, we are devils in this *Mâyâ*, and we are gods in this *Mâyâ*. Stretch your ideas as far as you can, make them higher and higher, call it infinite or by any other name you please, even that idea is within this *Mâyâ*. It cannot be otherwise, and the whole of human knowledge is generalization of this *Mâyâ*, trying to know it as it really is. This is the work of *Nâma-Rûpa*— name and form. Everything that has form, everything that calls up an idea in your mind, is within *Mâyâ*, for, everything that is bound by what the German philosophers call the laws of time, space, and causation, is within *Mâyâ*.

Let us go back a little to those earlier ideas of God, and see what became of them. We perceive at once that with such a state of things the idea of some being who is eternally loving us— the word love in our sense—eternally unselfish and almighty, ruling this universe, cannot be. It requires the boldness of the poet to withstand this idea of the personal God. Where is your just, merciful God? the poet asks. Does he not see millions and millions of his children perish, either in the form of men, or of animals; for who can live one moment here without killing others? Can you draw a breath without destroying thousands of lives? You live because millions die. Every moment of your life, every breath that you breathe, is death to thousands, every movement that you make is death unto millions. Every morsel that you eat is death unto millions. Why should they die? There is an old sophism, "But they are very low existences." Supposing they are; it is a question. Who knows whether the ant is greater than man, or the man than the ant? Who can prove one way or the other? Man can build a house or invent a machine, therefore the man is greater! The same argument will apply, because the ant cannot build a house nor make a machine, therefore he is greater. There is no more reason for one than for the other.

Apart from that question, even taking it for granted that these are very low beings, still why should they die? If they are low they ought to live the more. Why not? Because they live more in the senses, they feel pleasure and pain a thousandfold more than you or I can. Which of you can eat a dinner with the same gusto as a dog or a wolf? Because our energies are not in the senses, they are in the intellect, the spirit. But in the dog the whole soul is in the senses, and they become mad, enthusiastic, enjoy things which we human beings can never dream of, and the pain is commensurate with the pleasure.

Pleasure and pain are meted out in equal measure. If the pleasures felt by animals are so much keener than those felt by man, it follows absolutely that the animals' sense of pain is as keen, if not keener than that in men; and they have to die. So the fact is that the pain and misery men would feel in dying is intensified a thousandfold in animals, and yet we have to kill them, without troubling about their misery. This is *Mâyâ*, and if we suppose there is a personal God like a human being, who made all, these so-called explanations and theories which try to prove that out of evil comes good are not sufficient. Let twenty thousand good things come, why should they come from evil? On that principle I might cut the throats of others because I want the full pleasure of my five senses. That is no reason. Why should good come through evil? The question remains to be answered, and it cannot be answered; and philosophy in India was compelled to admit this.

The Vedânta is the boldest system of religion. It stopped nowhere, and it had one advantage. There was no body of priests seeking to suppress every man who tried to tell the truth. There was always absolute religious freedom. In India the bondage of superstition was a social one; here society is very free. Social matters in India have not been free, but religious opinion has. In England a man may dress as he likes, or eat what he likes—no one says nay, or objects; but if he misses attending his church then Mrs. Grundy is down on him. He has to look a thousand times at what society says, and then think of the truth. In India, on the other hand, if a man dines with another who does not belong to his own caste, down comes society with all its terrible power, and crushes him then and there. If he wants to dress a little differently from the way in which his ancestor dressed ages ago he is done for. I have heard of a man who was outcasted because he went several miles to see the first railway train. Well, we will presume that that was not true!

On the other hand, in religion, we find Atheists, and Materialists, and Buddhists, and creeds and opinions, and speculations of every phase and variety; some of a most startling character. Men going about preaching and gaining adherents, and at the very gates of the temple full of all the gods, the Brahmins—to their credit be it said—allow even the Materialist to stand on the steps of their temples and denounce their gods.

Buddha died at a ripe old age. I remember a friend of mine, a great American scientist, who was fond of reading his life. He did not like the death of Buddha, because he was not crucified. What a false idea! For a man to be great he must be murdered! Such ideas never prevailed in India. This great Buddha travelled all over India denouncing all gods, and even their God, the Governor of the Universe, and he died at a ripe old age. Eighty-five years he lived, until he had converted half the country.

There were the *Chârvâkas*, who preached the most horrible things; the most rank, undisguised materialism, such as in the nineteenth century they dare not preach openly. These *Chârvâkas* were allowed to preach from temple to temple, and city to city, that religion was all nonsense, that it was priestcraft, that the Vedas were the words and writings of fools, rogues and demons, and that there was neither God nor an eternal soul. If there were a soul why did it not come back after death, drawn by love of wife and children? Their idea was that if there was a soul it must still love after death, and want nice things to eat and nice dresses. Yet no one hurt these *Chârvâkas*.

Thus India has always had this magnificent idea of religious freedom—for you must always remember that freedom is the first condition of growth. What you do not make free will never grow. The whole of that idea that you can make others grow, and help their growth, can direct and guide them, always retaining for yourself the freedom of the teacher, is nonsense a dangerous lie, which has retarded the growth of millions and millions of human beings in this world. Let men have the light of liberty. That is the only condition of growth.

We, in India, allowed liberty in spiritual matters, and we have a tremendous spiritual power in religious thought, even to-day. You grant the same liberty in social matters, and so have a splendid social organization. We have not given any freedom to the expansion of social matters, and ours is a cramped society. You have never given any freedom in religious matters. With fire and sword you have enforced your beliefs, and the result is that religion is a stunted, degenerate growth in the European mind. In India we have to take off the shackles from society; in Europe the chains must be taken from the feet of spiritual progress. Then will come a wonderful growth and development of men. If we discover that there is one unity running behind all these developments, either spiritual, moral or social, we shall find that religion in the full sense of the word must come into society, must come into our every day lives. In the light of Vedânta you will understand that all your sciences are but manifestations of religion, and so is everything that exists in this world.

We see then that through freedom these sciences were built, and in them we have two sets of opinions growing slowly in the teaching of the Vedânta, the one about which I have just told you, that of the materialists, the denouncers, and the other the positive, the constructive. This again is a most curious fact; in every society you find it. Supposing there is an evil in society. You will find immediately one group rising up and beginning to denounce it in vindictive fashion. This sometimes degenerates into fanaticism. You always find fanatics in every society, and women frequently join in these outcries, because they are impulsive in their nature. Every fanatic who gets up and denounces something secures a following. It is very easy to break down; a maniac can break anything he likes, but it would be hard for him to build anything in this world.

So there is this set of denouncers in every country, present in some form or other, and they think they will mend this world by the sheer power of denunciation and of exposing evil; they do some good, according to their light, but much more harm, because things are not done in a day. Social institutions are not made in a day, and to change means removing the cause. Suppose there is evil here; denouncing it will not do anything, but you must go to work at the root. First find out the cause, then remove it, and the effect will be removed also. All this outcry will not produce any effect, unless indeed it produces misfortune.

There were others who had sympathy in their hearts and who understood the idea that we must go deep into the cause, and these were the great saints. One fact you must remember, that all the great teachers of the world have declared that they came not to destroy but to fulfil. Many times this has not been understood, and their forbearance has been thought to be an unworthy compromise with existing popular opinions. Even now, you occasionally hear that these prophets and great teachers were rather cowardly, dared not say and do what they thought was right; but it was not so. Fanatics little understand the infinite power of love in the hearts of these great sages.

They looked upon the inhabitants of this world as their children. They were the real fathers, the real gods, filled with infinite sympathy and patience for everyone, they were ready to bear and forbear. They knew how human society should grow, and patiently, slowly, surely, went on applying their remedies, not by denouncing and not by frightening people, but by gently and kindly leading them step by step. Such were the writers of the Upanishads. They knew full well how the old ideas of God were not reconcilable with the advanced ethical ideas of the time; they knew perfectly well that truth was not on that side of the question, but on the other side; they knew full well that what the Buddhists and the other atheists were preaching contained a good deal of truth, nay, great nuggets of truth, but, at the same time, they understood that those who wish to sever the thread that binds the beads, who want to build a new society upon the air, will entirely fail.

We never build anew, we simply change places, we cannot have anything new, we only change the positions of things. The seed grows into the tree, and patiently, gently, we must direct the energies towards truth, and fulfil the truth that exists, not try to make new truths. Thus, instead of denouncing these old ideas of God as unfit for modern times, these ancient sages began to seek out the reality that was in them, and the result was the Vedânta Philosophy, and out of the old deities, out of the monotheistic God, Ruler of the Universe, they found yet higher and higher ideas in what is called the Impersonal Absolute; they found One-ness throughout the Universe. "He who sees in this world of manifoldness that One running through all; in this world of death, he who finds that one Infinite Life; and in this world of insentience and ignorance, he who finds that one Light and Knowledge, unto him belongs eternal peace. Unto none else, unto none else."

VI. MÂYÂ AND FREEDOM.

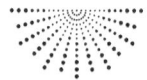

"Trailing clouds of glory we come," says the poet. Not all of us come trailing clouds of glory however, some of us come also trailing black fogs behind us; there can be no question about that. But every one of us is sent into this world as on to the battlefield to fight. We must come here weeping to fight our way, as well as we can, to make a path through this infinite ocean of life without leaving any track; forward we go, long ages behind us, and immense the expanse beyond. So on we go, till death comes, takes us off the field, victorious or defeated, we do not know, and this is *Mâyâ*.

Hope is dominant in the heart of childhood. The whole is a golden vision to the opening eyes of the child; his will he thinks is supreme. As he moves onward, at every step nature stands as an adamantine wall barring his further progress. He may hurl himself against it again and again, striving to break through.

Through his life the farther he goes, the farther recedes the ideal until death comes, and there is release perhaps, and this is *Mâyâ*.

A man of science rises, he is thirsting after knowledge. No sacrifice is too great, no struggle too hopeless for him. He moves onward discovering secret after secret of Nature, searching out the secrets from the innermost heart of Nature, and what for? What is it all for?

Why should we give him glory? Why should he acquire fame? Does not Nature know infinitely more than any human being can know, and Nature is dull, insentient. Why should it be glory to imitate the dull, the insentient? Nature can hurl a thunderbolt of any magnitude to any distance. If a man can do one small part as much we praise him, laud him up to the skies, and why? Why should we praise him for imitating Nature, imitating death, imitating dulness, imitating insentience? The force of gravitation can pull to pieces the biggest mass that ever existed; yet it is insentient. What glory is in imitating the insentient? Yet we are all struggling after that, and this is *Mâyâ*.

The senses drag the human soul out. Man is asking for pleasure, for happiness where it can never be found; for countless ages every one of us is taught that this is futile and vain, there is no happiness here. But we cannot learn; it is impossible for us to learn, except through our own experience. We try them, and a blow comes; do we learn then? Not even then. Like moths hurling themselves against the flame we are hurling ourselves again and again into sense pleasures, hoping to find satisfaction there. We return again and again with freshened energy; thus we go on till crippled, cheated, we die, and this is *Mâyâ*.

So with our intellect, in our desire to solve the mysteries of the universe, we cannot stop our questioning, we must know; and cannot believe that there is no knowledge to be gained. A few steps, and there arises the wall of beginningless and endless time which we cannot surmount. A few steps and there appears a wall of boundless space which cannot be surmounted, and the whole is irrevocably bound in by the walls of cause and effect. We cannot go beyond them. Yet we struggle; we have to struggle; and this is *Mâyâ*.

With every breath, with every pulsation of the heart, with every one of our movements, we think we are free, and the very same moment we are shown that we are not. Bound slaves, Nature's bondslaves, in body, in mind, in all our thoughts, in all our feelings, and this is *Mâyâ*.

There was never a mother who did not think her child a genius, the most extraordinary child that was ever born; she dotes upon her child. Her whole soul is in that child. It grows up, perhaps becomes a drunkard, a brute, ill-treats the mother, and the more he ill-treats her the more her love increases. The world lauds it as the unselfish love of the mother, little dreaming that the mother is a born slave, she cannot help herself. She would throw it off a thousand times, but cannot. So she covers it with a mass of flowers, calls it wonderful love, and this is *Mâyâ*.

So are we all in this world, and the legend tells how once Nârada said to Krishna, "Lord, show me *Mâyâ*." A few days passed away, and Krishna asked Nârada to make a trip with him towards a desert, and after walking for several miles Krishna said, "Nârada, I am thirsty; can you fetch some water to me?" I will go at once, sir, and get you water." So Nârada went. At a little distance from the place there was a village; he entered the village in search of some water, and knocked at a door, the door opened and a most beautiful young girl appeared. At the sight of her he immediately forgot that his master was waiting, thirsty, perhaps dying for want of water. He forgot everything, and began to talk with the girl. All that day he did not return to his master. The next day he was again at the house talking to the girl. That talk ripened into love, he asked the father for the daughter, and they were married, and lived there and had children. Thus twelve years passed. His father-in-law died, he inherited his property, and lived, as he seemed to think, a very happy life with his wife and children, his fields and his cattle, his lands and his house. Then came a flood. One night the river rose until it overflowed its banks and flooded the whole of the village. Houses began to fall, men and animals were swept away and drowned, and everything was floating in the rush of the stream. Nârada had to escape. With one hand he had hold of his wife, with the other two of his children, another child was on his shoulders, and he was trying to ford this tremendous flood.

After a few steps the current was too strong, and the child on his shoulders fell and was borne away. A cry of despair came from Nârada. In trying to save that child he lost his grasp upon one of the others he was holding, and it also was lost. At last his wife, to whom he had clung with all his might and main to save her life, was also torn away by the current, and weeping and wailing he was thrown on the bank, where he fell upon the ground with bitter lamentations. Behind him there came a gentle voice: "My child, where is the water? You went to fetch a pitcher of water, and I am waiting for you; you have been gone about half an hour." "Half an hour!" Twelve whole years had passed through his mind, and all these scenes had passed by in that half an hour—and this is *Mâyâ*. In one shape or another we are all in it. It is a most difficult and intricate state of things to understand. What does it show? Something very terrible, which has been preached in every country, taught everywhere and only believed by a few, because until we get the experiences ourselves we cannot believe in it. After all, it is all futile.

Time, the avenger of everything, comes, and nothing is left. He swallows up the sin and the sinner, the king and the peasant, the beautiful and the ugly; he leaves none. Everything is rushing towards that one goal, destruction. Our knowledge, our arts, our sciences, everything is rushing towards that one inevitable goal of all, destruction. None can stem the tide, none can hold it back for a minute. We may try to forget it, just as we hear of persons in a plague-stricken city becoming paralyzed, trying to create oblivion by drinking and dancing, and other vain devices. So we are all trying hard to forget it, trying to create oblivion with all sorts of sense pleasures. And this is *Mâyâ*.

Two ways of living have been proposed. There is one method very common, which every one knows, and that is to say, "It may be very true, but do not think of it. 'Make hay while the sun shines,' as the proverb says. It is all true; it is a fact; but do not mind it. Seize the few pleasures you have, do what little you can, do not think of this negative side of the picture, always look towards the hopeful, the positive side." There is some truth in this, but there is also danger. The truth is that it is a good motive power; hope and a positive ideal are very good motive powers for our lives, but there is a certain danger in them. The danger lies in our giving up the struggle in despair, as is the case with every one who preaches: "Take the world as it is; sit down calmly, as comfortably as you can, and be contented with all these miseries, and when you receive blows, say they are not blows but flowers, and when you are driven about like a slave, say that you are free, just tell lies day and night to others and to your own souls, because that is the only way to live." This is what is called practical wisdom, and never was it more before the world than in this nineteenth century, because never were blows hitting harder than at the present time, never was competition keener, never were men so cruel to their fellow-men as now, and therefore is this consolation offered. It is strongest at the present time, and it fails, it always fails. We cannot hide carrion with roses; it is impossible. It would not avail long; one day the roses would vanish, and the carrion would become worse than ever before. So with all our lives; we may try to cover our old and festering sores with cloth of gold, but there will come a day when the cloth of gold is removed, and the sore in all its ugliness is revealed. Is there no hope? True it is that we are all slaves of *Mâyâ*, we are all born in *Mâyâ*, we live in *Mâyâ*.

Is there then no way out, no hope? That we are all miserable, that this world is really a prison, that even our so-called trailing beauty is but a prison-house, and that even our intellects and minds are prison-houses, has been known for ages upon ages. There has not been a man, there has not been a human soul, who has not felt it some time or other, however he may talk. And the old people feel it most, because in them is the accumulated experience of a whole life, because they cannot be easily cheated by the lies of Nature; *Mâyâ's* lies cannot cheat them much. What of them? Is there no way out? We find that with all this, with this terrible fact before us, in the midst of all this sorrow and suffering, even in this world, where life and death are synonymous, even here there is a voice that is going through all ages, through all countries, and through every heart.

"This my *Mâyâ* is divine, made up of qualities, and very difficult to cross. Yet those that come unto Me, I cause them to cross this river of life." "Come unto Me, all ye that labor and are heavy laden, and I will give you rest." This is the voice that is leading us forward. Man has heard it, and is hearing it all through the ages. This voice comes to men when everything seems to be lost, and hope is flying away, when man's dependence on his own strength has been crushed down, when everything seems to melt away between his fingers, and life is a hopeless ruin.

Then he hears it. This is called Religion.

On the one side, therefore, is the bold assertion, the most hopeful assertion, to realize that this is all nonsense, that this is *Mâyâ*, but that beyond *Mâyâ* there is a way out. On the other hand our practical men tell us "Don't you bother your heads about such nonsense as religion and metaphysics. Live here; this is a very bad world indeed, but make the best of it." Which put in plain language means—live a hypocritical, lying life, a life of continuous fraud, covering all sores the best way you can. Go on, patch after patch, until everything is lost, and you are a mass of patchwork. This is what is called practical life.

Those that are satisfied with this patchwork will never come to Religion. Religion begins with a tremendous dissatisfaction with the present state of things, with our own lives, a hatred, an intense hatred, for this patching up of life, an unbounded disgust for fraud and lies. He alone can be religious who dares stand up and say as the mighty Buddha once said under the Bo-tree, when this idea of practicality appeared also before him and he saw that it was nonsense, and yet could not find a way out. The temptation came to give up his search, to give up the search after truth, to go back to the world and live the old life of fraud, calling things by wrong names, telling lies to oneself and to everybody—once came this temptation, but he, the giant, conquered it, and said: "Death is better than a vegetating ignorant life; it is better to die on the battlefield than to live a life of defeat." That is the basis of Religion. When a man takes that stand he is in the way to find the truth, he is on the way to God. That determination must be the first impulse towards becoming religious. I will hew out a way for myself. I will know the truth, or give up my life in the attempt. For on this side it is nothing, it is gone, it is vanishing every hour. The beautiful, hopeful young person of to-day is the veteran of to-morrow. Hopes and joys and pleasures will die like blossoms with to-morrow's frost. That is this side; on the other side there are the delights of conquest, victories over all the ills of life, victories over life itself, the conquering of the universe. On that side men can stand. Those who dare, therefore, to struggle for victory, for truth, for religion, are in the right way, and this is what the Vedas preach. "Be not in despair; the way is very difficult; it is, as it were, walking on the blade of a razor. Yet, despair not, awake, arise, and find the ideal, the goal."

Now all the various manifestations of religion, in whatever shape and form they have come to mankind, have this one common central basis. It is the preaching of freedom, the way out of this world. They never came to reconcile the world and religion, but to cut the Gordian knot, to establish religion in its own ideal, and not to compromise with the world. That is what every religion preaches, and the duty of the Vedânta is to harmonize all these aspirations, to make manifest the common ground between all the religions of the world, the highest as well as the lowest. What we call the most arrant superstition and the highest philosophy really have a common aim in that they both are trying to show the way out of the same difficulty, and in most cases this way is through the help of some one who is outside this universe, some one who is not himself bound by the laws of nature, in one word some one who is free. In spite of all the difficulties and differences of opinion about the nature of the one free agent, whether he is God, whether he is a personal God, whether he is a sentient being like man, whether he is a conscious being, whether masculine, feminine, or neuter—and the discussions have been endless—the fundamental idea is the same. In spite of the almost helpless contradictions of the different systems, we find the golden thread of unity running through them all, and in this philosophy, this golden thread has been traced, revealed little by little to our view, and the first step to this revelation is this common ground, that all are advancing towards freedom.

One curious fact is present in the midst of all our sorrows and joys, our difficulties and struggles, we are surely journeying towards freedom. The question was practically what is this universe? From what does it arise? Into what does it go? And the answer was, in Freedom it rises, in Freedom it rests, and into Freedom it melts away. This curious fact you cannot relinquish, your actions, your very lives will be lost without it, this idea of freedom, that we are free. Every moment nature is proving us to be slaves, and not free. Yet, simultaneously rises the other idea that still we are free. At every step we are knocked down as it were, by *Mâyâ*, and shown that we are bound, yet at the same moment, together with this blow, together with this feeling that we are bound, comes the other feeling that we are free. Some inner voice tells us that we are free. But if we attempt to realize this freedom, to make it manifest, we find the difficulties almost insuperable. Yet, in spite of that, it insists on asserting itself inwardly, "I am free, I am free." And if you study all the various religions of the world you will find this idea expressed. Not only Religion—do not take this word in the narrow sense—but the whole life of society, is the assertion of that one principle of freedom. All movements are the assertion of that one freedom. That voice has been heard by every one, whether he knows it or not; that voice which declares, "Come to me all ye that are weary and heavy laden." It may not be in the same language, or the same form of speech, but in some form or other, that voice calling for freedom has been with us. Yes, we are born here on account of that voice; every one of our movements is for that. We are all rushing towards freedom, we are all following that voice, whether we know it or not: like the flute player who attracted the children of the village; we are all following the music of the flute without knowing it.

Why are we ethical but that we must follow that voice? Not only the human soul, but all from the lowest atom to the highest man, have heard the voice and are rushing to meet it; and in the struggle are combining with each other, or pushing each other out of the way. Thus come competition, joys, struggles, life, pleasure and death, and the whole Universe is nothing but the result of this mad struggle to reach the voice. That is what we are doing. This is the manifestation of Nature.

What happens then? The scene begins to shift. As soon as you know the voice and understand what it is, the whole scene changes. The very world which was the ghastly battlefield of *Mâyâ* is changed into something else, into something more beautiful, better. We need not curse nature, we need not say that the world is horrible, we need not say it is all vain, we need not weep or wail. As soon as we understand the voice we see the reason why this struggle should be here, this fight, this competition, this difficulty, this cruelty, these little pleasures and joys—that they are in the nature of things, because we are going towards the voice, to attain which we are called, whether we know it or not. All human life, all Nature, therefore, is struggling to manifest this freedom; the sun is moving towards the goal, so is the earth circling round the sun, so is the moon circling round the earth. For that goal the planet is moving, and the breeze is blowing. "For that goal the sun is shining and so is the moon, for that goal the wind is blowing and thunder is crashing, for that goal death is stalking about." They are all struggling towards that. The saint is going that way; he cannot help it; it is no glory to him. So is the sinner. The most charitable man is going straight towards that voice, he cannot stop; the most hopeless miser is going towards the same destination; the greatest worker of good hears the same voice within, he cannot resist it, he must go towards the voice. So with the most arrant idler. One stumbles more than another, and he who stumbles more we call weak, he who stumbles less we call good. Good and bad are never two different things, they are one and the same; the difference is not one of kind, but of degree.

Now, if the manifestation of this power of freedom is really governing the whole universe—applying that to religion, our special study—we find this idea has been the one assertion throughout. Take the lowest form of religion, where there is a departed ancestor, or certain powerful and cruel gods, and they are worshipped; what is the very idea of the god or departed ancestor? That he is superior to Nature, not bound by this *Mâyâ*. The idea of Nature here is very small, of course.

The worshipper, an ignorant man, of crude ideas, cannot pass through the wall of a room, cannot jump up into the skies, or fly through the air, and his idea of Nature is one of bondage to superior powers; hence the gods whom he worships can pass through walls, or the air, or change shape. What is meant by that, philosophically? That the assertion of freedom is there, that the gods whom he worships are superior to Nature as he knows it. So with those who worship still higher beings; it is the same assertion. As the view of Nature expands, the view of the soul as superior to Nature also expands, and at last we come to what we call Monotheism—that there is *Mâyâ*, (this Nature,) and that there is some Being who is superior to the whole of this *Mâyâ*, and this is the hope.

Vedânta begins where monotheistic ideas first appear, but the Vedânta philosophy wants further explanation. This explanation—that there is a Being beyond all these manifestations of *Mâyâ*, who is superior to, and independent of *Mâyâ*, and who is attracting us towards Himself, and that we are all going towards Him—is very good, says the Vedânta, but yet the perception is not clear, the vision is dim and hazy, although it does not directly contradict reason. Just as in your hymn it is said, "Nearer my God to Thee," the same hymn would be very good to the Vedântin, only he would change a word, and make it, "Nearer my God to me." The idea that the goal is far off, far beyond Nature, attracting us all towards it, has to be brought down nearer and nearer, without degrading or degenerating it, until it comes closer and closer, and the God of Heaven becomes the God in Nature, till the God in Nature becomes the God who is Nature, and the God who is Nature becomes the God within this temple of the body, and the God dwelling in the temple of the body, becomes the temple itself, becomes the soul of man, and there it reaches the last words it can teach. He whom the sages have been seeking in all these places is in our own hearts. The voice that you heard was right, says the Vedânta, but the direction you gave to the voice was wrong.

That ideal of freedom that you perceived was correct, but you projected it outside yourself, and that was your mistake. Bring it nearer and nearer, until you will find that it was all the time within you, that it is the Self of your own self. That freedom is your own nature, and this *Mâyâ* never found you. Nature never had power over you. Like a frightened child you were dreaming that it was throttling you, and the release from this fear is the goal; not only to see it intellectually, but to perceive it, actualize it, much more definitely than we perceive this world. Then we shall know that we are free. Then, and then alone, will all difficulties vanish, then will all the perplexities of the heart be smoothed away, all crookedness made straight, then will vanish the delusion of manifoldness and nature; and *Mâyâ*, instead of being a horrible, hopeless dream as it is now, will become beautiful, and this earth, instead of being the prison-house it is now, will become our playground. Even dangers and difficulties, even all sufferings, will become deified, as it were, and show us their real nature, will show us that behind everything, as the substance of everything, He is standing, and that He is the One Real Self.

VII. THE ABSOLUTE AND MANIFESTATION.

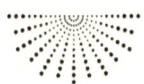

The one question that is most difficult to grasp in understanding the Advaita Philosophy, and the one question that will be asked again and again and that will always remain after thinking of it all our life, is—"How has the Infinite, the Absolute, apparently become the finite?" I will take up this question, and, in order to illustrate it better, I will use a figure.

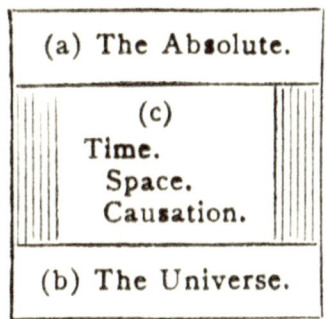

Here is the Absolute (a), and this is the Universe (b). The Absolute has become the Universe. By this is not only meant the material world, but the mental world, the spiritual world —everything, heavens and earths, and all that exists. Mind is the name of a change, and body the name of another change, and so on, and all these changes compose our universe. The Absolute (a) appears to have become the Universe (b) by coming through time, space, and causation (c).

This is the central idea of Advaita. Time, space, and causation are like the glass through which the Absolute is seen, and when It is seen on the lower side It appears as the Universe. Now we at once gather from this, that in the Absolute, there is neither time, space, nor causation. The idea of time cannot be there, seeing that there is no mind, no thought. The idea of space cannot be there, seeing that there is no external change. What you call motion and causation cannot exist where there is only one. We have to understand this and impress it on our minds, that what we call causation begins after, if we may be permitted to say so, the degeneration of the Absolute into the phenomenal, and not before; that our will, our desire, and all these things always come *after* that. I think Schopenhauer's philosophy makes a mistake in its interpretation of Vedânta, for it seeks to make the will everything. Schopenhauer makes the will stand in the place of the Absolute. But the Absolute cannot be presented as will, for will is something changeable and phenomenal, and over the line drawn above time, space and causation, there is no change, no motion. It is only below the line that external motion and internal motion, called thought, begin. There can be no will on the other side, and will, therefore, cannot be the cause of this universe. Coming nearer, we see in our own bodies that will is not the cause of every movement. I move this chair; will was the cause of that movement, and that will became manifested as muscular motion at the other end. But the same power that moves the chair is moving the heart, the lungs, and so on, but not through will. Given that the power is the same, it only becomes will when it rises to the plane of consciousness, and to call it will before it has risen to this plane is a misnomer. This makes a good deal of confusion in Schopenhauer's philosophy.

A stone falls and we ask why. This question is possible only on the supposition that nothing happens independently, that every motion must have been preceded by a cause of some kind. I request you to make this very clear in your minds, for whenever we ask why anything happens, we are taking for granted that everything that happens must have a *why*, that is to say, it must have been preceded by something else which acted as cause. This precedence and succedence are what we call the law of causation. It means that everything in the Universe is by turn a cause and an effect. It is the cause of certain things which come after it and is itself the effect of something else which has preceded it. This is called the law of causation, and is a necessary condition of all our thinking. We believe that every particle in the universe, whatever it be, is in relation to every other particle. There has been great discussion as to how this idea arose. In Europe there have been so-called intuitive philosophers who believed that it was constitutional in humanity, others have believed that it comes from experience, but the question has never been settled. We shall see later on what Vedânta has to say about it. But first we have to understand this, that the very asking of the question "why" presupposes that everything round us has been preceded by certain things, and will be succeeded by certain other things. The other belief involved in this question is that nothing in the universe is independent, everything can be acted upon by something outside itself. Inter-dependence is the law of the whole universe. In saying, "What caused the Absolute?" what error are we making! We are applying the same supposition in this case. To ask this question we have to suppose that the Absolute also is bound by something else, and that the Absolute also is dependent on something else. That is to say, in so using the word Absolute, we drag the Absolute down to the level of the universe. For above that line there is neither time, space, nor causation, because it is all one. That which exists by itself alone cannot have any cause. That which is free, cannot have any cause, else it would not be free, but bound. That which has relativity cannot be free. Thus, we see that the very question, why the infinite became the finite, is an impossible one, it is self-contradictory. Coming from subtleties to the logic of our common plane, to common sense, we can see this from another side, when we seek to know how the Absolute has become the relative. Supposing we knew the answer, would the Absolute remain the Absolute? It would have become the relative. What is meant by knowledge in our common sense idea? It is only something that has become limited by our mind, that we know, and when it is beyond our mind, it is not knowledge. Now if the Absolute becomes limited by the mind, it is no more Absolute; it has become finite. Everything limited by the mind becomes finite. Therefore, to know the Absolute is again a contradiction in terms.

That is why this question has never been answered, because if it were answered there would no more be an Absolute. A God known is no more God; He has become finite like one of us. He cannot be known, He is always the Unknowable One. But what Advaita says is that God is more than knowable. This is a great fact to learn. You must not go home with the idea that God is unknowable in the sense in which Agnostics put it. For instance, here is a chair, it is known to me. On the contrary what is beyond ether, or whether people exist there or not is possibly unknowable. But God is neither known nor unknowable in this sense. He is something still higher than known; that is what is meant by God being unknown and unknowable; the expression is not used in the sense in which it may be said that some questions are unknown and unknowable. God is more than known. This chair is known; but God is intensely more than that, because in and through Him we have to know this chair itself. He is the witness, the Eternal Witness of all knowledge. Whatever we know, we have to know in and through Him. He is the essence of our own Self. He, the "I," is the essence of this ego; we cannot know anything excepting in and through that "I." You have to know everything in and through the *Brahman*. To know the chair, therefore, you have to know it in and through God. Thus God is infinitely nearer to us than the chair, yet He is infinitely higher. Neither known, nor unknown, but something infinitely higher than either. He is your Self. "Who would live a second, who would breathe a second in this universe, if that Blessed One were not filling it, because in and through Him we breathe, in and through Him we exist?" Not that he is standing somewhere and making my blood circulate. What is meant is that He is the essence of all this, the Soul of my soul. You cannot by any possibility say you know Him; it would be too much of a degradation. You cannot jump out of yourself, so you cannot know Him. Knowledge is objectification. For instance, in memory you are objectifying many things, projecting them out of yourself. All memory, all the things which I have seen and which I know are in my mind. The pictures, the impressions of all these things are in my mind, as it were, and when I would try to think of them, to know them, the first act of knowledge would be to project them outside. This cannot be done with God, because He is the essence of our souls; we cannot throw Him out. This is said to be the holiest word in Vedânta: "He that is the essence of your soul, He is the Truth, He is the Self, Thou that art, O Svetaketu." This is what is meant by "Thou art Brahman." You cannot describe Him by any other language. All attempts of language, calling Him father, or brother, or our dearest friend, are attempts to objectify God, which cannot be. He is the Eternal Subject of everything. I am the subject of this chair; I see the chair, so God is the Eternal Subject of my soul. How can you objectify Him, the Essence of your souls, the Reality of everything? Thus, I would repeat to you once more, God is neither knowable nor unknowable, but something infinitely higher than these. He is one with us, and that which is One is neither knowable, nor unknowable, just as my own self, or your own self. You cannot know your own self, you cannot move it out, and make it an object to look at, because you are that, and cannot separate yourself from it. Neither is it unknowable, for what is more known than yourself? It is really the centre of our knowledge in exactly the same sense that God is neither unknowable nor known, but infinitely higher than that, your real Self.

Thus we see, that, first, the question: "What caused the Absolute" is a contradiction in terms, and secondly, we find that the idea of God in the Advaita is His Oneness, and therefore we cannot objectify Him, for we are always living and moving in Him; whether we know it or not does not matter. Whatever we do is always through Him. Now the question is what are time, space, and causation? Advaita means non-duality; there are no two, but One. We see that here is a proposition that the Absolute, the One is manifesting Itself as many through the veil of time, space, and causation. Therefore it seems that here are two, the Absolute, and *Mâyâ* (the sum-total of time, space, and causation). It seems apparently very convincing that there are two. To which the Advaitist replies that it cannot be called two. To have two, we must have two independent existences, just as that of the Absolute, which cannot be caused. In the first place, this time, space, and causation cannot be said to be an independent existence. Time is entirely a dependent existence; it changes with every change of our mind. Sometimes in a dream one imagines that he has lived several years; at other times several months were passed as one second. So that time has entire dependence on our state of mind. Secondly, the idea of time vanishes altogether sometimes. So with space, we cannot know what space is. Yet it is there, indefinable, and cannot live separate from anything else. So with causation.

The one peculiar attribute we find in all this time, space, and causation, is that they cannot live separate from other things. Try to think of space which has neither color, nor limits, nor any connection with the things around, just abstract space. You cannot think of it thus; you have to think of it as the space between two limits, or between objects. It has to cling on to some object to have its existence. So with time; you cannot have any idea of abstract time, but you have to take two events, one preceding and the other succeeding, and join the two events by the idea of succession. Time depends on two events, just as space has to relate itself to outside objects. And the idea of causation is inseparable from time and space. This is the peculiar thing about them, that they have no independent existence. They have not even the existence which the chair or the wall has. They are as a shadow around everything, but you cannot catch it. It has no real existence; we see that it has not. Yet a shadow is not non-existence, seeing that through this shadow all things are manifesting as this universe. Thus we see first that this combination of time, space, and causation, has neither existence nor non-existence. It is like a shadow which comes around things. Secondly, it sometimes vanishes. To give an illustration, there is a wave on the sea. The wave is the same as the ocean, certainly, and yet we know it is a wave, and as such different from the ocean. What makes this difference? The form and the name, the idea in the mind and the form. Now can we think of a wave form as anything separate from the ocean? Certainly not. It always clings on to the ocean idea. If the wave subsides, the form vanishes in a moment, and yet the form was not a delusion. So long as the wave existed the form was there, and you were bound to see the form. This is *Mâyâ*.

The whole of this universe, therefore, is as it were, a peculiar form; the Absolute is that ocean, while you and I, the suns, and stars, and all things are various waves of the ocean. And what makes the waves different? Only form, and that form is just time, space, and causation, all entirely dependent on the wave. As soon as you take away the wave, they vanish. As soon as the individual gives up this *Mâyâ*, it vanishes for him, and he becomes free. The whole struggle is to get rid of this clinging on to time, space, and causation. It is always throwing obstacles in our way, and we are trying to get free. What do they call the theory of evolution? What are the two factors? There is a tremendous potential power which is trying to express itself, and circumstances are holding it down, the environments will not allow it to express itself. So, in order to fight with these environments, the power is getting newer and newer bodies. A little amoeba, in the struggle, gets another body and conquers some obstacles, then gets other bodies, until it becomes man. Now if we carry that logic to its conclusion, there must come a time when that power that was in the amoeba and which came out as man will have conquered *all* the obstructions that nature can bring before it, and will have escaped from all its environments. This idea brought into metaphysics would be expressed thus: there are two components of every action, the one the subject, the other the object. For instance, I feel unhappy because a man scolds me. These are the two parts; and what is my struggle all my life? To make myself strong enough to conquer that environment, so that he may scold and I shall not feel. That is how we are trying to conquer. What is meant by morality? Making the subject strong, inuring ourselves to the hardships of temptation until it ceases to have power over us and it is a logical conclusion of our philosophy, that there must come a time when we shall have conquered all environments, because Nature is finite.

That is another thing to learn. How do you know that Nature is finite? You can only know this through metaphysics. Nature is that infinite under limitations. Therefore it is finite. So there must come a time when we have conquered all environments. And how are we to conquer them? We cannot possibly conquer all the objective environments. No. The little fish wants to fly from its enemies which are in the water. How does it conquer? By flying up into the air, becoming a bird. The fish did not change the water, or the air; the change was in itself. Change is always subjective. So on, all through evolution you find that the conquest of nature comes by change in the subjective. Apply this to religion, and morality, and you will find that the conquest of evil comes by the change in the subjective also. That is how the Advaita system gets its whole force, on the subjective side of man. To talk of evil and misery is nonsense, because they do not exist outside. If I am inured against all anger, I never feel angry. If I am proof against all hatred, I never feel hatred, because it cannot touch me.

This is therefore the process by which to achieve that conquest— through the subjective, by perfecting the subjective.

Therefore, you find one more thing, that the only religion, I may make bold to say, which agrees with and even goes a little further than modern researches, both on physical and moral lines, is the Advaita, and that is why it appeals to modern scientists so much. They find that the old dualistic theories are not enough for them, do not satisfy their necessities. A man must not only have faith, but intellectual faith too. Now, in this latter part of the nineteenth century, such ideas as that a religion coming from any other source than one's own forefather's religion must be false, show that there is still weakness left, and such ideas must be given up. I do not mean that it is in this country alone, but in every country, and nowhere more than in my own. This Advaita was never allowed to come to the people. At first some monks got hold of it, and took it to the forests, and so it came to be called the Forest Philosophy. By the mercy of the Lord, the Buddha came and preached it to the masses, and the whole nation arose to Buddhism. Long after that, when atheists and agnostics had destroyed the nation again, the old preachers found out that Advaita was the only thing to save India from materialism.

Twice has Advaita saved India from materialism. Just before the Buddha came, when materialism had spread to a fearful extent, and it was of a most hideous kind, not like that of the present day but of a far worse nature. I am a materialist of a certain kind, because I believe that there is only One. That is what the materialist wants to tell you, only he calls it matter and I call it God. The materialists admit that out of this one matter, all hope, and religion, and everything have come. I say that all these have come out of *Brahman*. I allude to the old crude sort of materialism—eat, drink and be merry; there is neither God, nor soul, nor heaven; religion is a concoction of wicked priests; the materialism which said to man: "As long as you live, try to live happily; eat, though you may have to borrow money for it, and never mind about repaying." That was the old materialism, and that kind of philosophy spread so much that even to-day it has got the name of "popular philosophy." Buddha brought the Vedânta out, gave it to the people and saved India. Then a thousand years after his death a similar state of things prevailed; the mobs, the masses, and the various races, had been converted to Buddhism, and naturally the teachings of the Buddha became in time degenerated because most of these people were very ignorant. Buddhism taught no God, no Ruler of the universe, so gradually the masses brought their gods, and devils, and hobgoblins, out again, and a tremendous hotch-potch was made of Buddhism in India. Then again Materialism came to the fore, taking the form of license with the higher classes, and superstition with the lower, when Sankarâcharya arose, and once more revivified the Vedânta philosophy. He made it a rationalistic philosophy. In the Upanishads the arguments are often very obscure. By Buddha the moral side of the philosophy was emphasized, and by Sankarâcharya, the intellectual side. He collected all the obscure and apparently contradictory texts of the Upanishads and showed the harmony between them. He worked out, rationalized and placed before men a wonderful, coherent whole.

Materialism prevails in Europe to-day. You may pray all the world over for the salvation of these sceptics, but they do not yield, they want reason. The salvation of Europe depends on a rationalistic religion, and Advaita—the non-duality, the Oneness, the idea of the impersonal God—is the only religion that can keep any hold on intellectual people. It comes whenever religion seems to disappear, and irreligion seems to prevail, and that is why it is gaining ground in Europe and America. One thing more has to be added to it. In the old Upanishads we find sublime poetry; these "Seers of Truth" were poets. Plato says, inspiration comes to people through poetry, and it seemed as if these ancient *Rishis* were raised above humanity to show these truths through poetry. They never preached, nor philosophized, nor wrote. Strains of music came out of their lips. In Buddha we had the great, universal heart, infinite patience making religion practical, bringing it to every one's door; in Sankarâcharya we saw tremendous intellectual power, throwing the scorching light of reason over everything. We want to-day that bright sun of intellectuality, and joined to it the heart of Buddha, that wonderful, infinite heart of love and mercy. This union will give us the highest philosophy. Science and religion will meet and shake hands. Poetry and philosophy will become friends. This will be the religion of the future, and if we can work it out, we may be sure that it will be for all times and professions. This is the one way that will be acceptable to modern science, for it has almost fallen into it. When a great scientific teacher asserts that all things are the manifestation of one force, does it not remind you of the God of whom you hear in the Upanishads: "As the one fire entering into the universe is expressing itself in various forms, and yet is infinitely more besides, even so that one Soul is expressing itself in every soul and yet is infinitely more besides." Do you not see how science is going? The Hindu nation proceeded through the study of the mind, through metaphysics and logic. The European nations start from external nature, and now they, too, are coming to the same results. We find that searching through the mind we at last come to that Oneness, that Universal One, the Internal Soul of everything, the Essence, the Reality of everything, the Ever-Free, the Ever-Blissful, the Ever-Existing. Through material science we come to the same Oneness. Science to-day is telling us that all things are but the manifestation of one energy, which is the sum-total of everything which exists, and the trend of humanity is towards freedom, and not towards bondage. Why should men be moral? Because through morality is the path towards freedom, and immorality leads to bondage.

Another peculiarity of the Advaita system is that from its very start it is non-destructive. That is another glory, that boldness to preach: "Do not disturb the faith of any, even of those who through ignorance have attached themselves to lower forms of worship." That is what it says: "Do not disturb, but help every one to get higher and higher; include all humanity." This philosophy preaches a God who is a sum-total.

If you seek a universal religion which can apply to every one, that religion must not be partial and one-sided, it must always be the sum-total and be able to include all degrees of religious development.

This idea is not clearly found in any other religious system. They are all parts which have not yet grasped the idea of absolute Unity. The existence of the part is merely for this, that it is always struggling to attain to the whole. So, from the very first Advaita had no antagonism with the various sects existing in India. There are dualists existing to-day, and their number is by far the largest in India, because dualism naturally appeals to less educated minds. It is a very handy, natural, common-sense explanation of the universe. But with these dualists, Advaita has no quarrel. The one thinks the God of the universe is outside the universe, somewhere in heaven, and the other that the God of the universe is his own soul, and that it would be a blasphemy to call Him anything more distant. Any idea of separation would be terrible. We can only be the nearest of the near. There are not words in any language to express this nearness, except this one word—Oneness. With any other idea the Advaitist is frightened, just as the dualist is frightened with the concept of the Advaita, and thinks it blasphemy. At the same time the Advaitist knows why these other ideas must be and so has no quarrel with the dualist; the latter is on the right road. From his standpoint, as soon as he looks from the part, he will have to see many. Any view of God looked at from a part of this universe can only be that projecting outside. It is the constitutional necessity of the dualistic standpoint. Let them have it. The Advaitist knows that whatever may be their defects or mistakes, they are all going to the same goal. There he differs entirely from the dualist, who is forced by his very point of view to believe that all opposing views are wrong. The dualists all the world over naturally believe in a personal God who is purely anthropomorphic; and just as a great potentate here is pleased with some and displeased with others, the same idea attaches to the personal God of the dualist. He is arbitrarily pleased with some person, or race, and showers blessings upon them. Naturally the dualist comes to the conclusion that God has certain favorites, and hopes to be one of them. You will find in almost every religion the idea that "we are the favorites of our God, and only by believing as we do can you be taken into favor with Him." Some dualists are so narrow as to insist that only the few who have been predestined to the favor of that God can be saved, the rest may try ever so hard, but they cannot come in. I challenge you to show one dualistic religion which has not more or less of this exclusiveness. And because of it, they are in the nature of things bound to fight and quarrel with each other, and this they have ever been doing. Again, these dualists win popular favor, for the vanity of the uneducated is appealed to. They like to feel that they enjoy exclusive privileges. The dualist thinks you cannot have morality until you have a God with a rod in his hand, ready to punish you. The unthinking masses are generally dualists, and they, poor fellows, have been persecuted for thousands of years in every country, therefore their idea of salvation is absence from the fear of punishment. I have been asked by a clergyman in America: "What, no devil in your religion? How can that be?" But, on the other hand, we find that the best and greatest men that have been born in the world have worked with that high impersonal idea. It is the Man who says in the New Testament, "I and my Father are One," whose power descends unto millions. For thousands of years it has worked for good. And we know that the same Man, because he was a non-dualist, was merciful to others. To the masses who cannot conceive of anything higher than a personal God, he says: "Pray to your Father in heaven." To others, who could grasp a higher idea, he said: "I am the Vine, ye are the branches;" but to his disciples to whom he revealed himself more fully he proclaimed the highest truth: "I and my Father are One."

It was the great Buddha, in India, who never cared for the dualist gods, and who has been called an atheist and a materialist, who yet was ready to give up his body for a poor goat. That man set in motion the highest moral ideas any nation can have. Wherever there is a moral code, it is a ray of light from that man. We cannot force the great hearts of the world into little narrow limits and keep them there, especially at this time in the history of humanity, when there is a degree of intellectual development such as was never dreamed of, even a hundred years ago; a wave of scientific knowledge which nobody, even fifty years ago, would have dreamed of. Do you want to kill people by forcing them into narrow limits? It is impossible until you degrade them into animals and unthinking masses. What is now wanted is a combination of the highest intellectuality with the greatest heart expansion, infinite love and infinite knowledge. The Vedantist gives no other attribute to God except these three, that He is Infinite Existence, Infinite Knowledge, Infinite Bliss; and he regards these three as One. Existence without knowledge and love cannot be. Knowledge without love cannot be, and Love without knowledge cannot be. That is what we want, that harmony of Existence, Knowledge and Bliss Infinite. Our goal is that perfection of Existence, Knowledge, and Bliss. We want harmony, not one-sided development. It is possible to have the intellect of a Sankara with the heart of a Buddha, and I hope we shall all struggle to attain to that blessed combination.

VIII. UNITY IN DIVERSITY.

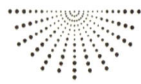

"The Self-Existent One projected the senses outwards and therefore a man looks outward, not within himself. A certain wise one, desiring immortality, with inverted senses perceived the Self within." As we have been saying, the first inquiry that we find in the *Samhita*, and in the other books, was concerning outward things, and then a new idea came, that the reality of things is not to be found in the external world; not by looking out, as it were, but by turning the eyes, as it is literally expressed, inwards. And the word used for the soul is very significant, it is "He who has gone inward," the innermost reality of our being, the heart centre, the core, from which, as it were, everything comes out; the central sun, of which the mind, the body, the sense organs, and everything else that we have, are but rays going outwards. "Men of childish intellect, ignorant persons, run after desires, which are external, and enter the trap of far-reaching death, but the wise, understanding immortality, never seek for the eternal in this life of finite things." The same idea is here made clear, that in this external world, which is full of finite things, it is impossible to see and find the Infinite. The Infinite must alone be sought in that which is infinite, and the only thing infinite about us is that which is within us, our own soul. Neither the body, nor the mind, nor the world we see around us, not even our thoughts, are infinite. They all have beginning in time and finish in time. The Seer, He to whom they all belong, the soul of man, He who is awake in the internal man, alone is infinite, and to seek for the infinite cause of this whole universe we must go there; in the infinite soul alone can we find it. "What is here is there too, and what is there is here also. He who sees the manifold is going from death to death." We have seen how at first there was the desire to go to heaven. When these ancient Âryans became dissatisfied with the world around them naturally they thought that after death they would go to some place where there would be all happiness without any miseries; these places they multiplied and called *Svargas*—the word may be translated as heavens— where there would be joy for ever; the body would become perfect, and also the mind, and there they would live with their forefathers. But as soon as philosophy came, men found that this was impossible and absurd. The very idea of an infinite in place would be a contradiction in terms. A place must begin and continue in time, therefore they had to give that up. They found out that the gods who lived in these heavens had once been human beings on earth, and through their good works, or something else, had become gods, and the godhoods, as they called them, were different states, different positions; none of the gods spoken of in the Vedas are permanent individuals.

For instance, Indra and Varuna are not the names of certain persons, but the names of conditions, as governors and so on. The Indra who had been before is not the same person as the Indra of the present day; according to them, he has passed away, and another man from earth has gone up and filled the place of Indra. So with all the gods. They are certain positions, which are filled successively by human souls, who have raised themselves to the condition of gods, and yet—even they die. In the old Rig Veda we find the word immortality used with regard to these gods, but later on it is dropped entirely, for they found that immortality, which is beyond time and space, cannot be spoken of with regard to any physical form, however subtle it may be. However fine it may be it must have a beginning in time and space, for the necessary factors that enter into the production of form are in space. Try to think of having form without space; it is impossible. Space is one of the materials, as it were, which makes up the form, and this is continually changing. Space and time are in *Mâyâ*, and this idea is related in the line —"What is here, that is there too." If there are these gods they must be bound by the same laws that apply here, and the one end of all laws, in their development, involves destruction and renewal again and again. These laws are taking the whole of matter to pieces, as it were moulding out of it different forms, and inversely crushing them out into matter again. Everything born must die, and so, if there are heavens, the same laws must hold good there.

In this world we find that all happiness is followed by some sort of misery as its shadow. Life has its shadow death. They must go together, because they are not contradictory, not two separate existences, but different manifestations of the same unit factor, life and death, sorrow and happiness, good and evil.

The dualistic conception that good and evil are two separate identities, and that they are both going on eternally, is absurd on the face of it. They are the diverse manifestations of one and the same fact, at one time appearing as bad, and at another time as good. The difference does not exist in kind, but only in degree. They differ from each other in degree of intensity. We find as a fact that the same nerve systems carry good and bad sensations alike, and when the nerves are injured neither sensation comes to us. If a certain nerve is paralyzed, we do not get the pleasurable feelings that used to come along that wire, and at the same time we do not get the painful feelings either. They are never two, but the same. Again, the same thing produces pleasure and pain at different times of life. The same phenomenon will produce pleasure in one, and give pain to another. The eating of meat produces pleasure to the man, but pain to the animal which is being eaten. There has never been anything which has pleased every one alike. Some are pleased, others displeased. So it goes on. Therefore, on the face of it, this duality of existence is denied, and what follows from this? I told you in my last lecture that we can never ultimately have everything good on this earth and nothing bad. This may have disappointed and frightened some, but I cannot help it and I am open to conviction when I am shown the contrary; but until that can be proved to me, and I can find that it is true, I cannot say so.

The general argument against my statement and apparently a very convincing one, is this, that in the course of evolution, all that is evil in what we see around us is gradually being eliminated, and the result is that if this elimination continues after millions of years a time will come when all the evil will have been eliminated, and the good alone will remain. This is apparently a very sound argument, would to God it were true, but there is a fallacy, and it is this, that it takes for granted that good and evil both are quantities that are eternally fixed. It takes for granted that there is a definite mass of evil which may be represented by 100, and likewise of good, and that this mass of evil is being diminished every day, leaving only the good remaining. But is this so? The history of the world shows that evil is a continuously increasing quantity as well as good. Take the lowest man; he lives in the forest. His sense of enjoyment is very small, and so also is his power to suffer. His misery is entirely on this sense plane. If he does not get plenty of food he is miserable, give him plenty of food and freedom to rove and to hunt, and he is perfectly happy. His happiness consists only in the senses, and his misery also. See that man increasing in knowledge; his happiness is increasing, intellect is opening to him, sense enjoyment is evolving into intellectual enjoyment. He now feels wonderful pleasure in reading a beautiful poem. A mathematical problem takes up his whole life, and he is absorbed in the intense pleasure of it. But, with that, the finer nerves are becoming more and more susceptible to intense miseries of which the savage did not think, and he suffers mental pain. The sense of separation when the husband does not love the wife, quarrels, and in a dozen things intense desires seize upon him, causing pain which was unknown to the savage. Take a very simple illustration. In Thibet there is no marriage, and there is no jealousy; yet we know that marriage is a much higher state.

The Thibetans have not known the wonderful enjoyment, the blessing of chastity, the happiness of having a chaste, virtuous wife, and a chaste, virtuous husband. These people cannot feel that. And similarly they do not feel the intense jealousy of the unchaste wife or husband, of unfaithfulness on either side, with all the heart-burnings and miseries which believers in chastity experience. On one side the latter gain happiness, but on the other they gain misery too.

Take your country, which is the richest the world ever knew, and which is more luxurious than any other country, and see how intense is the misery, how many more lunatics you have, compared with other races, only because the desires are so keen. A man must keep up a high standard. The amount of money you spend in one year would be a fortune to a man in India, and you cannot preach to him because the surroundings are such, that that man must have so much money or he is crushed.

The wheel of society is rolling on; it stops not for widows' tears or orphans' wails. You must move on, or you will be crushed under it. That is the state of things everywhere. Your sense of enjoyment is developed, your society is very much more beautiful than some others. You have so many more things to enjoy. But those who have fewer have much less misery than you have in this country. You can argue thus throughout. The higher the ideal you have in the brain, the greater is your enjoyment, and the more profound your misery. One is like the shadow of the other, so to say; that evils are being eliminated may be true, but if so, the good also must be dying out. But are not evils multiplying fast, and diminishing on the other side, if I may so put it? If good increases in arithmetical proportion, evil increases in geometrical proportion. And this is *Mâyâ*. It means that it is neither optimism nor pessimism. It is not the position of Vedânta that this world is a miserable world. That would be a lie. At the same time we say it is not true, it is a mistake to say that this world is full of happiness and blessings. So it is useless to tell children that this world is all good, all flowers, and milk and honey. That is what we have all dreamed. At the same time it is erroneous to think because one man has suffered more than another that all is evil. It is this duality, this play of good and evil, that misleads us. We must always remember the warning of Vedânta not to think that good and evil are two, not to believe that good and evil are two separate essences, for they are one and the same thing appearing in different degrees and in different guises, and producing differences of feeling in the same mind. So, the first thought of Vedânta is the finding of unity in the external, the One Existence manifesting Itself, however different It may appear in manifestation. Think of the old crude theories of the Persians—two gods creating this world. The good god doing everything that is pleasurable, and the bad one everything else. On the very face of it you find the absurdity, for if it be carried out every law of nature must have two parts, and this law of nature is sometimes manipulated by one god, and then he goes away and the other manipulates it. It is the law of Unity that gives us our food, and the same law kills many men through accidents or misadventure. Then the difficulty comes, that both are working at the same time, and these two gods keep themselves in harmony, by injuring one and doing good to another. This was a crude case, of course, the crudest way of expressing the duality of existence. But then, take the more advanced philosophy, the abstract cases, of telling people that this world is partly good and partly bad.

This again is absurd, arguing from the same standpoint. As such, we find first of all that this world is neither optimistic nor pessimistic; it is a mixture of both, and as we go on we shall find that the whole blame is taken out of the hands of nature and put upon us. And again, the Vedânta offers a great hope. It is not a denial of evil; it analyzes boldly the fact as it is, and does not seek to conceal anything. It is not hopeless; it is not agnostic. It finds out a remedy, but it wants to place that remedy on adamantine foundations, not by shutting the child's mouth and blinding its eyes with something which is transparently untrue, and which the child will find out in a few days. I remember when I was a young child, a young man's father died and left him poor, and with a large family to support. He found that his father's friends were his worst enemies in reality, and one day he had a conversation with a clergyman who offered this consolation, "Oh, it is all good, all is sent for our good." That is the old method of trying to put a piece of gold cloth on an old sore. It is a confession of weakness, of absurdity. Then this young man went away, and six months afterwards the clergyman had a son born, and the young man was invited to the party for thanksgiving. Then the clergyman began to pray, "Thank God for His mercies." And the young man stood up and said, "Stop; this is all misery." The clergyman asked why. "Because when my father died it was all good, though apparently evil; so now this is apparently good, but really evil." Is this the way to cure the misery of the world? Be good and have mercy to those who suffer. Do not try to patch it up, nothing will cure this world; go beyond it.

This world is a world of good and evil always. Wherever there is good, evil follows, but beyond and behind all the manifestation, all the contradiction, the Vedânta finds that Unity. It says give up what is evil and give up what is good. What then remains? It says good and evil are not all we have. Behind these stands something which is yours, the real you, beyond every evil, and beyond every good too, and it is that which is manifesting itself as good and bad. Know that first, and then, and then alone, you will be an optimist, and not before; for you will then control the whole thing. Control these manifestations and then you will be at liberty to manifest the real "you" just as you like. Then alone you will be able to manifest it only as good, or only as evil, just as you like; but be first master of yourself, stand up and be free; go beyond the pale of these laws, for these laws do not absolutely govern you, they are only part of your being. First find out that you are not the slave of nature, never were and never will be; that this nature, infinite as you may think it, is only finite, but one drop in the ocean, and your nature is as the ocean; you are beyond the stars, or the sun, or the moon. They are like mere bubbles compared with your infinite being. Know that and you will control both good and evil. Then alone the whole vision will change and you will stand up and say, how beautiful is good and how wonderful is evil.

That is what the Vedânta teaches you to do. It does not propose any slipshod remedy by covering things over with gold paper, and the more the wound festers putting on the more gold paper. This life is a hard fact; work out of it if you can, boldly, though it may be adamantine; no matter, the soul is greater. It lays no responsibility on little gods; but you are the makers of your fortunes. You make yourselves suffer, you make good and evil, and it is you who put your hands before your eyes and say it is dark. Hands off and see the light; you are effulgent, you are perfect already, from the very beginning. We understand it now. "He goes from death to death who sees the many here. See that One and be free."

How are we to see it? Nay, even this very mind, so deluded, so weak, so easily led, even this mind can be strong and may catch a glimpse of that knowledge, that Oneness, and then it saves us from dying again and again. "As water which falls upon a mountain breaks into pieces, and in many various streams runs down the sides of the mountain, so all the energies which you see here are that one Unit beginning." It has become manifold falling upon *Mâyâ*. Do not run after the manifold; go towards the One. "He is in all that moves; He is in all that is pure. He fills the Universe; He is in the sacrifice; He is the Guest in the house; He is in man, in water, in animals, in truth; He is the Great One; He is the One Fire coming into this world. He is manifesting Himself in various forms. Even so that one Soul of the Universe is manifesting Himself in all these various forms. As the one air coming into this universe manifests itself in various forms, even so the One Soul of all souls of all beings, is manifesting Himself in all forms." This is true for you when you have understood this Unity, and not before. Then all is optimism, because He is seen everywhere. The question is, that if all this be true, that that Pure One, the Self, the Infinite, has entered all this, how is it that He suffers, how is it that He becomes miserable, impure? He does not, says the Upanishad. "As the sun is the cause of the eye-sight of every being, yet is not made defective by the defect in any eye, even so the Self of all is not affected by the miseries of the body, or by any misery that is around you." I may have some disease, and see everything yellow, but the sun is not affected. "He is the One, the Creator of all, the Ruler of all, the internal Soul of every being, He who makes His Oneness manifest. Thus sages who realize him as the Soul of their souls, unto them belong eternal peace; unto none else, unto none else. He who in this world of evanescence finds Him who never changes, he who in this universe of death finds that one life, he who in this manifold finds that oneness, and all those who realize Him as the soul of their souls, to them belongs eternal peace; unto none else, unto none else. Where to find Him in the external world, where to find Him in the suns, and moons, and stars? There the sun cannot illumine, nor the moon, nor the stars, the flash of lightning cannot illumine the place; what to speak of this mortal fire. He shining, everything else shines. It is His light that they have borrowed, and He is shining through them." Here is another beautiful simile. Those of you who have been in India and have heard of the Banyan tree, how it comes from one root, and spreads far around, will understand. He is that Banyan tree; His root is above, and has branched out until it has become this universe, and however far it extends, every one of these trunks and branches is connected. He is the root of all.

Various heavens are spoken of in the *Brâhmana* portion of the Vedas, and the philosophical teaching of the Upanishads implies giving up the idea of going to heaven. All the work is not in this heaven, or that heaven, it is here in the soul; places do not signify anything. Here is another passage which shows these different states. "In the heaven of the forefathers, as a man sees things in a dream, so the real truth is seen." As in dreams we see things hazy and indistinct, so we see things there. There is another heaven called the *Gandharva;* there it is still less distinct; as a man sees his own reflection in the water, so is the reality seen there. The highest heaven that the Hindûs conceive is called the *Brahmaloka*, and in this the truth is seen much more clearly but not yet quite distinctly, like light and shade; but as a man sees his own face in a mirror, perfect, distinct, and clear, so is the truth shining in the soul of man.

The highest heaven, therefore, is here in our own souls, the greatest temple of worship is the human soul, greater than all heavens, says the Vedânta, for in no heaven anywhere can we understand the reality as distinctly and clearly as here in this life, in our own soul. You may change places, just as we have seen. I have thought while in India that the cave would give clearer vision. I found it was not so. Then I thought the forest would be better. Then I thought Benares. The difficulty exists everywhere, because we make our own worlds. If I am evil the whole world is evil to me. That is what the Upanishad says. And the same thing applies to all. If I die and go to heaven, I should find the same. Until you are pure it is no use going to caves, or forests, or to Benares, or to heaven; and if you have polished your mirror it does not matter where you live, you get the reality just as it is. So it is useless work, running hither and thither, spending energy in vain, which should be spent only in polishing the mirror. The same idea is expressed again.

"None see Him, none see His form with the eyes. It is in the mind, the pure mind, He is seen, and thus immortality is gained." Those that were at the summer lectures on *Râja Yoga* will be interested to know that what was taught then was a different kind of *Yoga*. Here in philosophy there is also a *Yoga*, but this is what is meant, that where there is control of all our senses, when these are held as slaves by the human soul; when they can no longer disturb his mind, then the *Yogin* has reached the goal.

"When all vain desires of the heart have been thrown out, then this very mortal becomes immortal, then here he becomes one with God. When all the knots of the heart are cut asunder, then the mortal becomes immortal, and he enjoys *Brahman*." Here on earth, nowhere else.

A few words ought to be said here. Generally you will hear that this Vedânta, this philosophy and these Eastern systems look only to something beyond, letting go the enjoyments and struggles of this life. This idea is entirely wrong. Ignorant people who do not know anything of Eastern thought, and never had brain enough among them all to understand anything of the real teaching, tell you that you are going outside to the other world. On the other hand, we read in black and white here that they do not desire to go to any other world, but depreciate these worlds as places where people weep or laugh for a little while and then die. So long as we are weak, we shall have to go through the same thing there, but whatever is true is here, and that is the human soul. And this also is insisted upon, that we cannot escape the inevitable by committing suicide; we cannot evade it. But the right path is hard to find. The Hindû mind is just as practical as the Western, only we differ in our views of life. One man says build a good house, and have good clothes and good food, and intellectual knowledge, knowledge of science and so on, this is the whole of life; and in that he is immensely practical. But the Hindû says true knowledge of the world means knowledge of the soul, metaphysics, and he wants to enjoy that life. In America there was a great Agnostic orator,

a very noble man, a very good man, and a very fine speaker. He lectured on religion and said it was no use, we need not bother our heads about other worlds, and he employed this simile: we have an orange here, and we want to squeeze all the juice out of it. I met him once and said, "I agree with you entirely. I have this orange and I want to squeeze the juice out too. Only we differ as to the fruit. You think it is an orange; I think it is a mango. You think it is only necessary to live here and eat and drink and have a little scientific knowledge, but you have no right to say, that is the whole idea of life. To me such a conception is nothing. If I had only to know how an apple falls to the ground, or how an electric current shakes my nerves, I would commit suicide the next moment. I want to know the heart of things, the very life itself. Your study is the manifestation of life, mine is the life itself. I want to squeeze the juice out of my fruit even in this life. My philosophy says you must know the whole of it and drive out your heavens and hells and all these superstitions, even if they exist in the same sense that this world exists. I would know the heart of this life, its very essence, how it is, not only how it works and what are its manifestations. I want the 'why' of everything, I leave the 'how' to children. As one of your countrymen said, 'While I am smoking a cigarette, if I were to write down everything that happens, it would be the science of the cigarette.' It is good and great to be scientific. Lord bless them in their search, but when a man says that is all, he is talking foolishly, not caring to know the *raison d'être* of life, never studying existence itself. I may argue that all your knowledge is nonsense without basis. You are studying the manifestations of life, and when I ask you what life is you say you do not know. You are welcome to your study, but leave me mine."

Yet I myself am practical, very practical, in my own way. So all these ideas about being practical are nonsense. You are practical in one way, and others in another. But a man of another type of mind does not talk. If he is told that he will find out the truth standing on one leg, he will find it that way. Another kind of man hears there is a gold mine somewhere, with savages all round. Three men go. Two perish, but one succeeds. The same man has heard there is a soul, and is content to leave it to the clergyman to preach. But the first man will not go near the savages. He says it may be dangerous, but if you tell him that on the top of Mount Everest, 30,000 feet above the sea level, there is a wonderful sage who can give him knowledge of the soul, he tries to climb there—40,000 may be killed, but one finds out the truth. These are practical, too, but the mistake lies in regarding what you term the world, as the whole of life. Yours is the vanishing point of enjoyment of the senses; there never was anything permanent in it, it can only bring more and more misery. Mine brings eternal peace, and yours brings only perpetual sorrows.

I do not say your view of what is practical is wrong. You are welcome to your interpretation. Great good and man's blessing come out of it, but do not therefore condemn my view. Mine also is practical in its own way. Let us all work according to our own plans. Would to God all of us were equally practical on both sides. I have seen some scientists who were equally practical scientists and spiritual men, and it is my great hope that in course of time the whole of humanity will be efficient in all such things. When a kettle of water is boiling, if you watch the phenomenon you find a bubble rising in one corner, and another in an opposite corner, then the bubbles begin to multiply, and four or five join together, and at last they all join, and a tremendous motion goes on. This world is very similar. Each individual is like a bubble, and the nations resemble many bubbles. Gradually these nations are joining, and I am sure the day will come when such a thing as a nation will vanish, and this separation will vanish; that Oneness to which we are all going, whether we like it or not, will become manifest; we are brothers by nature, and have become separate. A time must come when all these ideas will be joined, and every man and woman in this world will be as intensely practical in the scientific world as in the spiritual, and then that Oneness; the harmony of oneness, will pervade the whole world. The whole world will become *jīvanmuktas*—"free whilst living." And we are all fighting towards that one end through all our jealousies and hatreds, through co-operation and antagonism. A tremendous stream is flowing towards the ocean. There are little bits of paper and straw in the stream. They may struggle to go back, but, in the long run, must follow down to the ocean. So you and I and all nature are like these little bits of paper rushing in mad currents towards that ocean of Life, Perfection and God; we may struggle to go back, to get up or down, and play all sorts of pranks, but in the long run we must go and join this ocean of Life and Bliss.

IX. GOD IN EVERYTHING.

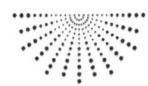

We have seen how the greater portion of our life must of necessity be filled with evils, however we may resist, and that this mass of evil is practically almost infinite for us. We have been struggling to remedy this since the beginning of time, yet everything remains very much the same. The more we discover remedies, the more we find subtle evils existing in the world. We have also seen that all religions propose a God, as the one way of escaping from these difficulties. All religions tell us that if you take the world as it is, as most practical people would advise us to do in this age, then nothing would be left to us but evil. But all religions assert that there is something beyond this world. This life in the five senses, life in the material world, is not all that we have, it is only a small portion, and merely superficial. Behind and beyond is the Infinite where there is no more evil. Some people call this Infinite God, some Allah, some Jehovah, and so on. The Vedântin calls It *Brahman*.

The first impression of the advice given by religions is that we had better terminate our existence. Yet we have to live. The question is how to cure the evils of life, and the answer apparently is, give up life. It reminds one of the old story. A mosquito settled on the head of a man, and a friend, wishing to kill the mosquito, gave it such a blow that he killed both man and mosquito. The remedy seems to suggest a similar course of action. Life is full of ills, the world is full of evil; that is a fact which no one who is old enough to know the world can deny. But what is the remedy proposed by all the religions? That this world is nothing. Beyond this world is something which is very real. And here is the real fight. The remedy seems to destroy everything. How can that be a remedy? Is there no way out? Another remedy is proposed. The Vedânta says that what all the religions advance is perfectly true, but it should be properly understood. Often it is misunderstood, because the various religions are not very explicit, not very clear. What we want is head and heart together. The heart is great indeed; it is through the heart that come the great inspirations of life. I would a hundred times rather have a little heart and no brain, than be all brains and no heart. Life is possible, progress is possible for him who has heart, but he who has no heart and only brains dies of dryness.

At the same time we know that he who is carried along by his heart alone has to undergo many ills, for now and then he is liable to fall into pits. The combination of heart and head is what we want. I do not mean that a man should have less heart or less brain, and make a compromise, but let every one have an infinite amount of heart and feeling, and at the same time an infinite amount of reason. Is there any limit to what we want in this world? Is not the world infinite? There is room for an infinite amount of feeling, and so also for an infinite amount of culture and reason. Let them all come together without any limit, let them be running together, as it were, in parallel lines each with the other.

Most religions understand this fact and state it in very clear and precise language, but the error into which they all seem to fall is the same; they are carried away by the heart, the feelings. There is evil in the world; give up the world: that is the great teaching, and the only teaching, no doubt. Give up the world. There cannot be two opinions that, to understand the truth, every one of us must give up error. There cannot be two opinions that every one of us, in order to have good must give up evil; there cannot be two opinions that every one of us to have life, must give up what is death. And yet, what remains to us, if this theory involves giving up the life of the senses, life as we know it, and what do we mean by life? If we give up all this, nothing remains. We shall understand this better, when, later on, we come to the more philosophical portions of the Vedânta. For the present, however, I beg to state that in Vedânta alone we find a rational solution of the problem. Here I can only lay before you what the Vedânta seeks to teach, and that is, the deification of the world.

The Vedânta does not, in reality, denounce the world. The ideals of renunciation nowhere attain such a climax as in the teachings of the Vedânta, but, at the same time, dry suicidal advice is not intended, it really means deification of the world— to give up the world as we think of it, as we seem to know it, as it is appearing, and to know what it really is. Deify it; it is God alone, and, as such, we read at the commencement of the oldest of the Upanishads, the very first book that was ever written on the Vedânta—"Whatever exists in this Universe, whatever is there, is to be covered with the Lord."

We have to cover everything with the Lord Himself, not by a false sort of optimism, not by blinding our eyes to the evil, but by really seeing God in everything. Thus we have to give up the world, and when the world is given up, what remains? God. What is meant? You can have your wives; it does not mean that you are to abandon them, and leave them to go away, but that you are to see God in the wife. Give up your children; what does that mean? Take your children and throw them into the street, as some human brutes do in every country? Certainly not. That is diabolism; it would not be religion. But see God in your children. So in everything. In life and in death, in woe and in joy, in misery and in happiness, the whole world is full of the Lord. Open your eyes and see Him. That is what Vedânta says. Give up the world which you have conjectured, because your conjecture was based upon very partial experience; your conjecture was based upon poor reasoning, and upon your own weakness. Give that up; the world we have been thinking of so long, the world to which we have been clinging so long, is a false world of our own creation. Give that up; open your eyes and see that as such it never existed; it was a dream, *Mâyâ*. What existed was the Lord Himself. It is He in the child, He in the wife, and He in the husband, He in the good, and He in the bad, He in the murderer, He in the sin, and He in the sinner, He in life, and He in death. A tremendous proposal indeed! Yet that is the theme which the Vedânta wants to demonstrate, to teach, to preach, and to prove. This is just the opening theme.

Thus we avoid the dangers of life and its evils. Do not want anything. What makes us miserable? The cause of all miseries from which we suffer has been made by desire, want. You want something, and the want is not fulfilled; the result is distress. If there be no want there will be no more suffering. When we shall give up all our desires, what will be the result? The walls have no desires and they never suffer. No, and they never evolve. This chair has no desires; it never suffers, and it is a chair, too, all the time. There is a glory in happiness, there is a glory in suffering. If I may dare to say so, there is a utility in evil, too. The great lesson in misery we all know. Hundreds of things we have done in our lives which we wish we had never done, but which, at the same time, have been great teachers. As for me, I am glad that I have done good things, and glad I have done something bad; glad I have done something right, and glad I have committed many errors, because every one of them has been a great lesson.

I, as I am this minute, am the resultant of all I have done, all I have thought. Every action and every thought has had its effect, and these effects are the sum-total of my progress.

The problem becomes difficult. We all understand that desires are wrong, but what is meant by giving up desires? How can life go on? It would be the same suicidal advice, which means killing the desire and the patient too. So the answer comes. Not that you should not have property, not that you should not have things which are necessary, and things which are even luxuries. Have all that you want, and everything that you do not want sometimes, only know the truth and realize the truth. This wealth does not belong to anybody. Have no idea of proprietorship, possessorship. You are nobody, nor am I, nor anyone else. It all belongs to the Lord, because the opening verse told us to put the Lord in everything. God is in that wealth that you enjoy, He is in the desire that rises in your mind, He is in these things you buy because you desire them; He is in your beautiful attire, in your handsome ornaments. That is the line of thought. All will be metamorphosed as soon as you begin to see things in that light. If you put God in your every movement, in your clothes, in your talk, in your body, in your mind, in everything, the whole scene changes, and the world, instead of appearing as woe and misery, will become a heaven. "The kingdom of heaven is within you," says Jesus; it is already there, says the Vedânta; so say others, so says every great teacher. "He that hath eyes to see, let him see," and "he that hath ears to hear, let him hear." It is already here. And that is one of the themes which the Vedânta undertakes to prove. It will prove also, that the truth for which we have been searching all this time is already present, it was all the time with us. In our ignorance, we thought we had lost it, and went about in the world crying and weeping, suffering misery, struggling to find the truth, and all the time it was dwelling in our own hearts.

There alone can we find it.

If giving up the world is true, and if it is taken in its crude, old sense, then it would come to mean this: that we must not work, that we must become idle, that we must sit like lumps of earth, and neither think nor do anything, but become fatalists, driven about by every circumstance, ordered about by the laws of nature, drifting from place to place. That would be the result. But that is not what is meant. We must work. Ordinary mankind, driven everywhere by false desires, what do they know of work?

The man propelled by his own feelings and his own senses, what does he know about work? He works who is not propelled by his own desires, or by any selfishness whatsoever. He works who has no ulterior motive in view. He works who has nothing to gain from work.

Who enjoys a picture, the seller of the picture or the seer? The seller is busy with his accounts, computing what his gain will be, how much profit he will realize on the picture. His brain is full of that. He is looking at the hammer, and watching the bids. He is intent on hearing how fast the bids are rising. That man is enjoying the picture who has gone there without any intention of buying or selling. He looks at the picture and enjoys it. So this whole universe is a picture, and when these desires have vanished, men will enjoy the world; and this buying and selling, and these foolish ideas of possession will be ended. The money-lender gone, the buyer gone, the seller gone, this world remains the picture, a beautiful painting. I never read of any more beautiful conception of God than the following: "He is the great poet, the ancient poet: the whole universe is his poem, coming in verses and rhymes and rhythms, written in infinite bliss." When we have given up desires, then alone shall we be able to read and enjoy this universe of God. Then everything will become deified. Nooks and corners, by-ways and shady places, which we thought so unholy, spots on its surface which appeared so black, will be all deified. They will all reveal their true nature, and we shall smile at ourselves, and think that all this weeping and crying has been but child's play, and we were standing there watching.

Thus, says the Vedânta, do you work. It first advises us how to work—by giving up—giving up the world, the apparent, illusive world. What is meant by that? Seeing God everywhere, as said already. Thus do you work. Desire to live a hundred years, have all the earthly desires, if you will, only deify them, convert them into heaven, and live a hundred years. Have the desire to live a long life of helpfulness, of blissfulness and activity on this earth.

Thus working, you will find the way. There is no other way. If a man plunges headlong into foolish luxuries of the world without knowing the truth, he has not reached the goal, he has missed his footing. And if a man curses the world, mortifies his flesh, goes into a forest, and kills himself bit by bit by starving himself, makes his heart a barren waste, a desert, kills out all his feeling, becomes stern, awful, dried-up, that man also has missed the way. These are the two extremes, the two mistakes at either end. Both have lost the way, both have missed the goal.

Thus, says the Vedânta, thus work, putting God in everything, and knowing Him to be in everything, thus work incessantly, holding life as something deified, as God Himself, and knowing that this is all we have to do, this is all we have to ask for, because God is here in everything; where else shall we go to find Him? In every work, in every thought, in every feeling, He is already there. Thus knowing, we must work; this is the only way, there is no other. Thus the effects of work will not bind us down. We shall not be injured by the effects of work. We have seen how these false desires are the causes of all the misery and evil we suffer, but when they are thus deified, purified through God, when they come they bring no evil, they bring no misery.

Those who have not learned this secret will have to live in a demoniacal world until they discover the secret. Many do not know what an infinite mine of blissfulness and pleasure and happiness is here, in them, around them, everywhere; they have not yet discovered it. What is a demoniacal world? The Vedânta says a world of ignorance.

Says the Vedânta, we are dying of thirst sitting on the banks of the mightiest river. We are dying of hunger sitting near piles of food. Here is the blissful universe. We do not find it. We are in it; it is around us all the time, and we are always mistaking it. Religions propose to find this out for us. This blissful universe is the real search in all hearts. It has been the search of all nations, it is the one goal of religion, and this ideal is expressed in various languages; all the petty differences between religions and religions are mere word struggles, nonsense. It is only difference of language that makes all these apparent divergences; one expresses a thought in one way, another a little differently, yet perhaps each is saying exactly what the other is expressing in different language. That is how struggles come in this life of ours.

More questions arise in connection with this. It is very easy to talk about. From my childhood I have heard of this putting God everywhere and everything will become deified, and then I can really enjoy everything, but as soon as I come into this world, and get a few blows from it, this idea vanishes. I am out in the street thinking that God is in every man, and a strong man comes and gives me a push and I fall flat on the footpath.

Then I rise up quickly, the blood has rushed into my head, and my fist clinches and reflection goes. Immediately I become mad.

Everything is forgotten, instead of encountering God I see the devil. We have been told since we were born to see God in all; every religion has taught that—see God in everything and everywhere. Do you not remember in the New Testament how Christ explicitly says so? We have all been taught this, but it is when we come to the practical side that the difficulty begins. You all remember how in "Æsop's Fables" a fine big stag is looking at his picture reflected in a lake, and saying to his child, "How powerful I am, look at my splendid head, look at my limbs, how strong and muscular they are; how swiftly I can run," and in the meantime he hears the barking of dogs in the distance, and immediately takes to his heels, and after he has run several miles he comes back panting. The child says, "You just told me how strong you were, how was it that when the dogs barked you ran away?" "That is it, my son; when the dogs bark all my confidence vanishes. I forget my strength; my courage forsakes me and I flee for my life." So are we all our lives. We are all thinking highly of poor humanity, we feel ourselves strong and valiant in the right; we make grand resolves, but when the "dogs" of trial and temptation bark, we are like the stag in the fable. We forget our power to overcome, we waver and for a time we are vanquished. Then if such is the case, what is the use of teaching all these things? There is the greatest use. The use is this, that perseverance will finally conquer. Nothing is to be done in a day.

"This Self is first to be heard, then to be thought upon, and then meditated upon." Everyone can see the sky, even the very worm crawling upon the earth, as soon as he looks up, sees the blue sky, but how very far away it is. The mind goes everywhere, but the poor body takes a long time to crawl on the surface of the earth. So it is with all our ideals. The ideal is far away, and we are here far below. At the same time we know that we must have an ideal. We must even have the highest ideal. And we know that unfortunately the vast majority of persons are groping through this dark life of ours without any ideal at all. If a man with an ideal makes a thousand mistakes, I am sure the man without an ideal makes fifty thousand. Therefore it is better to have an ideal. And this ideal we must hear as much as we can, hear till it enters into our hearts, enters into our brains, hear until it enters into our very veins, until it tingles in every drop of our blood, until it fills every pore in our body. We must meditate upon it. "Out of the fulness of the heart the mouth speaketh," and out of the fulness of the heart the hand works, too.

It is thought which is the propelling force in us. Fill the mind with the highest thoughts, hear them day after day, think of them month after month. Never mind failures; they are quite natural, they are the beauty of life, these failures. What would life be without these failures? It would not be worth having if it were not for the struggle. Where would be the poetry of life? Never mind the struggles, the mistakes. I never heard a cow tell a lie, but it is a cow— never a man. So never mind these failures, these little backslidings, hold the ideal a thousand times, and if you fail a thousand times make the attempt once more. This is the ideal of man, to see God in everything. If you cannot see Him in everything, see Him in one, in that thing which you like best, and then see Him in another. So on you can go. There is infinite life before the soul. Take your time and you will achieve your desire.

"He, that One who vibrates more quickly than mind, who attains to more speed than mind can ever attain, to whom even the gods attain not, nor thought grasps, He moving, everything moves. In Him all exists. He is moving, He also is immovable. He is near and He is far. He is inside everything. He is the outside of everything, interpenetrating everything. Whoever sees in every human being that same Âtman, and whoever sees everything in that Âtman, he never goes far from that Âtman." When all life and the whole universe are seen in this Âtman, then man has attained the secret. There is no more delusion for him. Where is any more misery for him who sees this oneness in the universe?

This is another great theme of the Vedânta, this Oneness of life, Oneness of everything. We shall see how it demonstrates that all misery comes through ignorance, for this ignorance creates the idea of manifoldness, of separation between man and man, between nation and nation, between earth and moon, between moon and sun. Out of this idea of separation between atom and atom arises all misery, but the Vedânta says this separation does not exist, that it is not real. It is merely apparent, on the surface. In the heart of things there is Unity still. If you go inside you find that Unity between man and man, between races and races, high and low, rich and poor, gods and men, and animals too. If you go deep enough all will be seen as only variations of the One, and he who has attained to this conception of Oneness has no more delusion. He has reached that Unity which we call God in theology. Where is there any more delusion for him? What can delude him? He knows the reality of everything, the secret of everything. Where is there any more misery for him? What does he desire? He has traced the reality of everything unto the Lord, that centre, that Unity of everything, and that is Eternal Existence, Eternal Knowledge, Eternal Bliss. Neither death nor disease, nor sorrow nor misery, nor discontent is there. All is Perfect Union and Perfect Bliss. For whom should he mourn then? In reality there is no death, there is no misery; in the centre, the Reality, there is no one to be mourned for, no one to be sorry for. He has penetrated everything, the Pure One, the Formless, the Bodiless, the Stainless, He the Knower, He the Great Poet, the Self-Existent, He who is giving to every one what he deserves. They are groping in darkness who are worshipping this ignorant world, the world that is produced out of ignorance. Those who are worshipping this world, thinking of it as Existence, are groping in darkness, and those who live their whole lives in this world, and never find anything better or higher, are groping in still greater darkness.

But he who knows the secret of beautiful nature, thinking of pure nature through the help of nature, he crosses death, and through the help of that which is pure nature, he enjoys Eternal Bliss. "Thou Sun, thou hast covered the truth with thy golden disk. Do thou open that for me so that I may see the truth which is inside thee. I have known the truth that is inside thee, I have known what is the real meaning of thy rays and thy glory, and have seen that which shines in thee; the truth in thee I see, and that which is within thee is within me also, and I in thee."

X. REALIZATION.

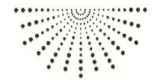

I will read to you from one of the simplest, but, I think, one of the most poetical of the Upanishads. It is called the Katha Upanishad. Some of you, perhaps, have read the translation by Sir Edwin Arnold, called "The Secret of Death." In our last lecture we saw how the inquiry which started with the origin of the world, and the creation of the universe, failed to obtain a satisfactory answer from without, and how it then turned inward. This book psychologically takes up that suggestion, questioning into the internal nature of man. It was first asked who created the external world, how it came into being, and now the question is, what is that in man which makes him live and move, and what becomes of it when the man dies. The first philosophers studied the material substance, and tried to reach the ultimate through that. At the best they found a personal Governor of the Universe, a human being immensely magnified, but yet to all intents and purposes a human being. But that cannot be the whole of truth; at best it can only be partial truth. We see this universe as human beings, and our God is our human explanation of the universe.

Suppose a cow were philosophical and had religion, it would have a Cow Universe, and a cow solution of the problem, and it would not be necessary that it should see our God. Suppose cats became philosophers, they would see a Cat Universe and have a cat solution of the problem of the universe, some Cat ruling it. So we see from this that our explanation of the universe is not the whole of the solution. Neither does our conception cover the whole of the universe. It would be a great mistake to accept that tremendously selfish position which man is apt to take. Such a solution of the universal problem as we can get from the outside, labors under this difficulty, that in the first place the universe we see is our own particular universe, our own view of the Reality. That Reality we cannot see through the senses; we cannot comprehend it. We only know the universe from the point of view of beings with five senses. Suppose we obtain another sense, the whole universe must change for us. Suppose we had a magnetic sense; it is quite possible that we might find millions and millions of varieties of forces in existence which we do not yet know, for which we have no present sense or feeling. Our senses are limited, very limited indeed, and within those limitations exists what we call our universe, and our God is the solution of our universe, but that cannot be the solution of the whole problem. It cannot be; it is nothing, so to say. But man cannot stop. He is a thinking being, and he wants to find a solution which will comprehensively explain all universes. He wants to see a world which is at once the world of men and of God, and of all beings possible and impossible, and he wants to find one solution which will explain all phenomena.

We see we must first find the Universe where all universes are one; we must find something which, by itself, of a logical necessity must be the background, the material running through all these various planes of existence, whether we apprehend it through the senses or not. If we could possibly find something which we could know as the common property of the lower worlds, as also of the higher worlds, although we do not see them, but by the sheer force of logic could understand that this must be the basis of all existence, then our problem would approach to some sort of solution; but this solution certainly cannot be obtained from the world we see and know, because that is only one view of the whole.

The only hope then lies in penetrating deeply. The early thinkers discovered that the further they were from the centre, the more marked were the variation and differentiation, and the nearer they approached the centre the nearer they were to unity. The nearer we are to the centre of a circle the nearer we are to the common ground in which all the radii meet, and the farther we are from the centre, the more differentiated is our radical line from the others. The external world is farther and farther away from the centre, and so there is no common ground where all the phenomena of existence meet. At best the external world is but one part of the whole of phenomena. There are other parts, the mental phenomena, the moral phenomena, the intellectual phenomena, the various planes of existence, and to take up only one, and find a solution of the whole out of that one, would be simply impossible. We first, therefore, want to find somewhere a centre from which, as it were, all the other planes of existence start, and standing there we will try to find a solution. That is the proposition. And where is that centre? It is inside, internal man. Going deeper and deeper inside, the ancient sages found that there, in the innermost core of the human soul, is the centre of the whole universe. All the planes gravitate towards that one point; there is the common ground, and standing there alone can we find a common solution. So the question who made this world is not philosophical, nor does its solution amount to anything.

This Katha Upanishad speaks in very figurative language. There was in ancient times, a very rich man, who made a certain sacrifice which required that he who made it should give away everything that he had. Now this man was not sincere. He wanted to get the fame and glory of having made the sacrifice, which required the giving away of everything, but at the same time he was only giving things which were of no further use to him—old cows, half dead, barren, with one eye, and lame. Now he had a boy called Nachiketas. This boy saw that his father was not doing what was right, that he was breaking his vow, and he did not know what to say. In India the father and mother are living gods; a child dare not do anything before them, or speak before them, but simply stands. And so the boy approached the father, and because he could not make a direct inquiry he asked him, "Father, to whom are you going to give me? Your sacrifice requires that everything shall be given away." The father became very much vexed. "What do you mean, boy? A father giving away his own son?" The boy asked the question a second and a third time, and then the angry father answered, "Thee I give unto Death" (*Yama*). And the story goes on to say that the boy went unto Death. There is a god called *Yama*, the first man who died. He went to heaven and became the governor of all the *Pitris;* all the good people who die, go and live with him for a long time. He is a very pure and holy person (*i.e., yama*), chaste and good and pure is this *Yama*. The boy went to *Yama's* world. Even gods are sometimes not at home, and so three days this boy had to wait there. After the third day *Yama* returned.

"O, learned one," says *Yama*, "you have been waiting here for three days without food, and you are a guest worthy of respect. Salutation to thee, O Brâhman, and welfare to me. I am very sorry I was not at home. But for that I will make amends. Ask three boons, one for each day." And the boy asked. "My first boon is that my father's anger against me may pass away, that he be kind to me and recognize me when you allow me to depart." *Yama* granted this fully. The next boon was that he wanted to know about a certain sacrifice which took people to heaven. Now we have seen that the oldest idea which we got in the *Samhita* portion of the Vedas was only about heaven, where they had bright bodies, and lived with the fathers. Gradually other ideas came, but they were not sufficient; there was need for something higher yet. Living in heaven would not be very different from life in this world. At best it would only be a very healthy rich man's life, plenty of enjoyment of the senses, plenty of things to enjoy, a sound body which knows no disease.

It would be this material world a little more refined, and just as we have seen, there is this difficulty, that this external material world can never solve the problem. So it would be there; no heaven can solve the problem. If this world cannot solve the problem no multiplication of this world can do so, because we must always remember that matter is only an infinitesimal part of the phenomena of nature. The vast part of phenomena which we actually see is not matter.

For instance, in every moment of our life how much is our own feeling, how much is thought phenomena, and how much is actual phenomena outside? How much do we feel and touch and see? How vast is the external world with its tremendous activity! And the sense phenomena are very small compared with the mental phenomena. The heaven solution commits this mistake; it insists that the whole of phenomena is only in touch, taste, sight, etc., so this idea of heaven where we are to live with very bright bodies, did not give full satisfaction to all. Yet Nachiketas asks as the second boon for some sacrifice through which people might attain to this heaven. There was an idea in the Vedas that these sacrifices pleased the gods and took human beings to heaven. Now, in studying all religions you will find the inevitable fact that whatever is old becomes holy. For instance, our forefathers in India used to write on birch bark, but in time they learned how to make paper. Yet the birch bark is still looked upon as very holy. When the utensils in which they used to cook in the most ancient times were improved upon, the old became holy, and nowhere has this idea been more kept up than in India. Old methods, which must be nine or ten thousand years old, of rubbing two sticks together to make fire, are still kept up. At the time of sacrifice no other method will do. So with the other branch of the Asiatic Âryans.

Their modern descendants still like to preserve fire that comes from lightning, showing that they used to get fire in this way, afterwards learning to obtain it by rubbing two pieces of wood, and when they learned other customs they kept up the old customs, which then became holy.

So with the Hebrews. They used to write on parchment. They now write on paper, and the other method is very holy. So with all nations, every rite which you now consider holy was simply an old custom, and these sacrifices were of this nature. In course of time, as they found better methods of life, their ideas were much improved, still, these old forms remained, and from time to time they were practised, and received a holy significance. Then a body of men made it their business to carry on these sacrifices. These were the priests, and they speculated on the sacrifices, and the sacrifices became everything to them. The gods came to enjoy the fragrance of the sacrifices, and everything in this world could be got by the power of sacrifices. If certain oblations were made, certain hymns chanted, certain peculiar forms of altars made, the gods would grant everything. So Nachiketas asks by what form of sacrifice a man will go to heaven. This second boon was also readily granted by *Yama*, who promised that this sacrifice should henceforth be named after Nachiketas.

Then the third boon comes, and with that the Upanishad proper begins. The boy says: "There is this difficulty; when a man dies some say he is, others that he is not. Instructed by you, I desire to understand this."

Yama is frightened. He was very glad to satisfy the other two boons. Now he says, "The gods in ancient times were puzzled on this point. This subtle law is not easy to understand. Choose some other boon, O Nachiketas, do not press me, release me on this point." The boy was determined and said, "What thou hast said is true, O Death, that even the gods doubted on this point, and it is no easy matter to understand. But I cannot obtain another exponent like you and there is no other boon equal to this."

Death said: "Ask for sons and grandsons who will live one hundred years, many cattle, elephants, gold and horses. Ask for empire on this earth and live as many years as you like. Or choose any other boon which you think equal to these— wealth and long life. Or be thou a king, O Nachiketas, on the wide earth I will make thee enjoyer of all desires. Ask for all those desires which are difficult to obtain in this world. These heavenly maidens with chariots and music which are not to be obtained by men. Let these, which I will give to you, serve you, O Nachiketas, but do not ask me what comes after death."

Nachiketas said: "These are merely things of a day, O Death, they bear away the energy of all the sense-organs. The longest life even is very short. These horses and chariots and dances and maidens may remain with thee. Man cannot be satisfied by wealth.

Shall we retain wealth when we behold Thee? We shall live only so long as Thou desirest. Only the boon which I have asked is to be chosen by me."

Yama is pleased with this answer and replies: "Perfection is one thing and enjoyment another, these two having different ends, bind a man. He who chooses perfection becomes pure. He who chooses enjoyment misses his true end. Both perfection and enjoyment present themselves to man; the wise man having examined both distinguishes one from the other. He chooses perfection as being superior to enjoyment, but the foolish chooses enjoyment for the benefit of his body. O Nachiketas, having thought upon the things which are desirable or apparently so, thou hast abandoned them." Death then proceeds to teach Nachiketas.

We now get a very developed idea of renunciation and Vedic morality—that until one has conquered the desire for enjoyment the truth will not shine in him. So long as the vain desires of our senses are clamoring and, as it were, dragging us every moment outward, making us slaves to everything outside, a little bit of color, a little bit of taste, a little bit of touch, dragging the human soul out, notwithstanding all our pretensions, how can the truth express itself in our hearts? "That which is to follow never rises before the mind of a thoughtless child deluded by the folly of riches. This world exists, the other does not, thinking thus they come again and again under my power," says Yama.

To understand this truth is very difficult. Many, even hearing it continually, do not understand, for the speaker must be wonderful, so must be the hearer. The teacher must be wonderful, so must be the taught. Neither is the mind to be disturbed by vain argument, for it is no more a question of argument, it is a question of fact. We have always heard that there is a path in every religion which insists on our faith. We have been taught to believe blindly. Well, this idea of blind faith is objectionable, no doubt—no doubt it is very objectionable—but analyzing it we find that behind it is a very great truth. What it really means is what we read now. The mind is not to be ruffled by vain arguments, because argument will not bring us to know God. It is a question of fact, and not of argument. All argument and reasoning must be based upon certain principles. Without these principles there cannot be any argument. Reasoning is the method of comparison between certain facts which we have already absolutely perceived. If these absolutely perceived facts are not there already, there cannot be any reasoning. Just as it is true in the external sense, why should it not be at the same time true in the internal? The external sensations all depend on actual experiences. You are not asked to believe in any assertions, but the rules become established by actual demonstration, not in the form of argument, but by actual perception.

All arguments are based upon certain perceptions. The chemist takes certain things and certain results are produced. This is a fact; you see it, sense it, and make that the basis on which to build all your chemical arguments. So with the physicists, so with all other sciences, all knowledge must stand on certain perception of facts, and upon that we have to build our reasoning. But, curiously enough, the vast majority of mankind think, especially at the present time, that no such perception is possible in religion, that religion can only be apprehended by vain arguments outside. Therefore we are told, the mind is not to be disturbed by vain arguments. Religion is a question of fact, not of talk. We have to analyze our own souls and to find what is there. We have to understand it and to realize what is understood. That is religion. No amount of talk will make religion. So the question of whether there is a God or not can never be proved by argument, for the arguments are as much on one side as the other. But if there be a God, He is in our own hearts. Have you ever seen Him? Just as the question as to whether this world exists or not has not yet been decided, so the debate between the idealists and the realists is eternal. It is a fact, yet we only know that the world exists, that it goes on. We only change the meaning of the word. So with all the questions of life, we must come back to facts. There are certain facts which are to be perceived, and there are certain religious facts, as in external science, that have to be perceived, and upon them religion will be built. Of course the extreme claim that you must believe any dogma of a religion is degrading to the human mind. That man who asks you to believe anything degrades himself, and, if you believe, degrades you too. The only right that the sages of the world have to tell us anything, is that they have analyzed their own minds and have found these facts, and if we do the same, we shall believe, and not before. That is all that there is in religion. But you must always remember this, that as a matter of fact 99.9 per cent. of those who attack religion have never analyzed their minds, have never struggled to get at the facts. So their arguments do not have any weight against religion, any more than those of a blind man who cries against the sun, "You are all fools who believe in the sun." That would have no weight with us. So the arguments of these people who have not gone to work to analyze their own minds, yet at the same time try to pull down religion, should have no weight with us.

This is one great idea to learn and to hold on to, this idea of realization. This turmoil and fight and difference in religions will only cease when we understand that religion is not in books, neither in temples, nor in the senses. It is an actual perception, and only the man who has actually perceived God and perceived soul, has religion, while all men who have not done that are alike. There is no real difference between the highest ecclesiastical giant, who can talk by the volume, and the lowest, most ignorant materialist. We are all atheists; let us confess it. Mere intellectual assent will not make us religious, and it does not. Take a Christian, or a Mohammedan, or a follower of any religion in the world. See the Sermon on the Mount. Any man who truly realized it would be a god immediately, would be perfect, and yet it is said that there are many millions of Christians in the world. Do you mean to say they are all Christians? What is meant is, that mankind may at some time try to realize that sermon. Not one in twenty millions is a real Christian.

So, in India, there are said to be three hundred millions of Vedântins. If there were one in a thousand who had actually realized religion, this world would soon be greatly changed. We are all atheists, and yet we try to fight the man who admits it. We are all in the dark; religion is to us a mere nothing, mere intellectual assent, mere talk—this man talks well, and that man ill—this to us is religion. "Wonderful methods of joining words, rhetorical powers, and explaining texts of the books in various ways, these are for the enjoyment of the learned, not religion." Religion will begin when that actual realization in our own souls begins. That will be the dawn of religion; then we shall become religious; then, and then alone, morality will begin. Now we are not much more moral than the animals in the streets. We are only held down by the whips of society. If society said to-day I will not punish you if you go and steal, we should just make a rush for every one's property. It is the policeman that makes the majority of us moral. It is social opinion that makes a great deal of our morality, and really we are little better than the animals. We understand how much this is so, in the secret of our own rooms. So let us not be hypocrites. Let us confess that we are not religious and have no right to look down on others. We are all brothers, and we shall be moral, we hope, when we have realized religion.

If you have seen a certain country, a man may cut you to pieces, but you will never in your heart of hearts say you have not seen the country. Extraordinary physical force may compel you to say you have not seen it, but in your own mind you know you have seen it. When you see Religion and God in a more intense sense than you see this external world, nothing will be able to shake your belief. Then will real faith begin. That is what is meant by the words in your Gospel: "He who has faith even as a grain of mustard seed." Then you will know the truth because you have become the truth, for mere intellectual assent is nothing.

The one idea is, does this realization exist? This is the watchword of Vedânta, realize religion, no talking will do, but it is only to be done with great difficulty. He has hidden Himself inside the atom, the Ancient One who resides in the inmost recess of every human heart. The sages realized Him through the power of introspection, and then they got beyond both joy and misery, beyond what we call virtue, beyond what we call vice, beyond our bad deeds, beyond our good deeds, beyond being and non-being, he who has seen Him has seen the Reality. But what then about the idea of heaven? It was the idea of happiness minus unhappiness. That is to say, what we want, is all the joys of this life minus its sorrows. That is a very good idea, no doubt; it comes naturally; but it is a mistake throughout, because there is no such thing as absolute good, nor any such thing as absolute sorrow.

You have all heard of that very rich man in Rome who learned one day that he had only about a million pounds left of his property, and said: "What shall I do to-morrow?" and forthwith committed suicide. A million pounds was poverty to him. What is joy, and what is sorrow? It is a vanishing quantity, continually vanishing. When I was a child I thought if I could become a cabman that would be the very acme of happiness for me, just to drive about. I do not think so now. To what joy will you cling? This is one point we must all try to understand, and it is one of the last superstitions to leave us. Everyone's pleasure is different. I have seen a man who is not happy unless he swallows a lump of opium every day. He may dream of a heaven where the land is made of opium. It would be a very bad heaven for me. Again and again in Arabian poetry we read of heaven full of gardens, where rivers run below. I have lived much of my life in a country where there is too much water; some villages and a few thousand lives are sacrificed to it every year. So my heaven would not have gardens beneath which rivers flow; I would have dry land where very little rain falls. So with life, our pleasures are always changing. If a young man dreams of heaven he dreams of a heaven where he will have a beautiful wife. Let that very man become old and he does not want a wife. It is our necessities which make our heaven, and the heaven changes with the change of our necessities. If we had a heaven where all these things were intensified, the heaven desired by those to whom this sense enjoyment is the very end of existence, we should not progress. That would be the most terrible curse we could pronounce on the soul. Is this all we can come to? A little weeping and dancing, and then to die like a dog. What a curse you pronounce on the head of humanity when you long for these things! That is what you do when you cry after the joys of this world, for you do not know what joy is. What philosophy insists on is not to give up joys, but to know what joy really is. The Norwegian heaven is a tremendous fighting place, where they all sit before Wodin, and then comes a wild boar hunt, and then they go to war and slash each other to pieces. But somehow or other, after a few hours of such fighting the wounds are all healed up, and they go into a hall, where the boar has been roasted, and have a carousal. And then the wild boar is made up again to be hunted the next day. That is quite the same thing, not a whit worse than our ideas, only our ideas are a little more refined. We want to hunt all these wild boars, and get to a place where all the enjoyments will continue, just as they imagine that the wild boar is hunted and eaten every day, and recovers the next day.

Now philosophy insists that there is a joy which is absolute, which never changes, and therefore that joy cannot be the joys and pleasures we have in this life, and yet it is Vedânta alone that proves that everything that is joyful in this life is but a particle of that real joy, because that is the only joy there is. Every moment we are really enjoying the absolute bliss, covered up, misunderstood, caricatured. Wherever there is any blessing, any blissfulness, any joy, even the joy of the thief in stealing from somebody else, it is that absolute bliss coming out through him, only it has become obscured, muddled up as it were, with all sorts of extraneous circumstances, caricatured, misunderstood, and that is what we call the thief. But, to understand that, we have first to go through the negation, and then the positive side will begin. First we have to give up all that is ignorance, all that is false, and then truth will begin for us. When we have grasped the truth these things which we have given up at first will take a new shape and form, will appear to us in a new light, they will all have become deified. They will have become sublimated, we shall understand them then in their real light. But to understand them we have first to get a glimpse of truth, and we must give them up first, and then take them back again deified. Therefore we have to give up all our miseries and sorrows, all our little joys. They are but different degrees of happiness or misery as we may call it. "That which all the Vedas declare, which is proclaimed by all penances, seeking which men lead lives of continence, I will tell you in one word— it is 'Om.'" You will find this word "Om" praised very much in the Vedas, and it is held to be very sacred.

Now *Yama* answers the question—"What becomes of a man when the body dies?" "This Wise One never dies, is never born; it arises from nothing, nothing arises from it. Unborn, Eternal, Everlasting, this Ancient One can never be destroyed with the destruction of the body. If the killer thinks he can kill, or if the killed thinks he is slain, they both do not know the truth, for the Self neither kills nor is killed." A most tremendous position. The one adjective in the first line is "wise" One. As you go on you will find that the ideal of Vedânta is, that all wisdom, and all purity are in the soul already—dimly expressed, or better expressed— that is the only difference. The difference between man and man, and all things in the whole creation is not in kind but only in degree. The background, the reality of every one is that same eternal, ever blessed, ever pure, and ever perfect One. That is the *Atman*, the soul, in the sinner or the sinless, in the happy or the unhappy, in the beautiful or the ugly, in man or animals, it is the same throughout. He is the Shining One. The difference is caused by the power of expression. In some it is expressed more, in others less, but this difference of expression has no effect upon Him, the *Atman*. If in his clothing one shows more of his body, and another less, it would not make any difference in the bodies. The difference is in the clothes that cover or do not cover the body. According to the covering, the body and the man, its powers, its purity begin to shine. Therefore we had better remember here also, that throughout the Vedânta philosophy, there is no such thing as good and bad, they are not two different things; the same thing is good or bad, and the difference is only in degree, and that we see to be an actual fact. The very thing I call pleasurable to-day, to-morrow under better circumstances, I may call pain. So the difference is only in the degree, the manifestation, not in the thing itself. There is no such thing as what we call good or bad. The fire that warms us, would also consume us; it would not be the fault of the fire. Thus, the soul being pure and perfect, the man who wants to do evil is giving the lie unto himself, he does not know the nature of himself. Even in the murderer the pure soul is there; it dies not. It was his mistake; he could not manifest it; he had covered it up. Nor in the man who thinks that he is killed is the soul killed; it is the eternal, never killed, never destroyed. "Infinitely smaller than the smallest, infinitely larger than the largest, yet this Lord of all is present in the depths of every human heart.

The sinless, bereft of all misery, see Him through the mercy of the Lord; the bodiless, yet living in the body, the spaceless, yet seeming to occupy space, infinite, omnipresent; knowing such to be the soul, the sages never are miserable."

This *Atman* is not to be realized by the power of speech, nor by a vast intellect, nor by the study of the Vedas. This is a very bold thing. As I told you before, the sages were very bold thinkers, never stopped at anything. You will remember that in India these Vedas are regarded in such a light as the Christians never regarded the Bible. Your idea of revelation is, that a man was inspired by God; but their idea was, that things exist because they are in the Vedas. In and through the Vedas the whole creation has come. All that is called knowledge is in the Vedas. Every word is sacred and eternal, eternal as the created man, without beginning and without end. As it were, the whole of the Creator's mind is in this book. That was the light in which they held the Vedas. Why is this moral? Because the Vedas say so. Why is this immoral? Because the Vedas say so, and in spite of that, see these bold men. No, the truth is not to be found by much study of the Vedas. "With whom the Lord is pleased, unto that man He expresses Himself." But then, the objection may be advanced—this is something like partisanship. But *Yama* explains: "Those who are evil doers, whose minds are not peaceful, can never know the light." It is those who are true in heart, pure in their deeds, whose senses have become controlled, unto them this Self manifests Itself.

Here is a beautiful figure. Picture the Self to be the rider and this body the chariot, the intellect to be the charioteer, the mind the reins, and the senses the horses. In that chariot, where the horses are well broken, where the reins are strong and kept well in the hands of the charioteer (the intellect), that chariot reaches the goal which is the state of Him the Omnipresent. But where the horses (the senses), are not controlled, nor the reins (the mind), well managed, that chariot comes to destruction. This *Atman* in all beings does not manifest Himself to the eyes or the senses, but those whose minds have become purified and refined, they see Him. Beyond all sound, all sight, beyond form, absolute, beyond all taste and touch; infinite, without beginning and without end, even beyond nature, the unchangeable, he who realizes Him, frees himself from the jaws of death. But it is very difficult. It is, as it were, walking on the blade of a razor; the way is long and perilous, but struggle on, do not despair. "Awake, arise, and stop not till the goal is reached."

Now you see that the one central idea throughout all the Upanishads is that of realization. A great many questions will arise from time to time, and especially to the modern man.

There will be the question of utility, there will be various other questions, but in all we shall find, that we are prompted by our past associations. It is association of ideas that has such a tremendous power in our mind. To those who from childhood have always heard about a personal God and the personality of the mind, these ideas will of course appear very stern and harsh, but if we listen to them, think of them for a long time, they will become part and parcel of our lives, and will no longer frighten us. The great question that generally arises of course is the utility of philosophy. To that there can be only one answer, that if on the utilitarian ground it is good for men to seek for pleasure, why should not those whose pleasure is in religious speculation seek that? Because sense enjoyments please many, they seek for them, but there may be others whom they do not please, who want higher enjoyment. The dog's pleasure is only in eating and drinking. The dog cannot understand the pleasure of the scientist who gives up everything, and perhaps dwells on the top of a mountain to observe the position of certain stars. The dog may smile at him and think he is a madman. Perhaps this poor scientist never had money enough to marry even; he eats a few bits of bread and drinks water and sits on the top of a mountain. Perhaps this dog laughs at him. But the scientist will say, "My dear dog, your pleasure is only in the senses; you enjoy it; you know nothing beyond it, but for me this is the most enjoyable thing, and if you have the right to seek your pleasure in your own way so have I, in my own way." The mistake is that we want to tie the whole world down to our own plane, we want to make our minds the measure of the whole universe. To you the old sense things are perhaps the greatest pleasure,

but it is not necessary that my pleasure should be the same, and when you insist upon that, I differ from you. That is the difference between the worldly utilitarian and the religious man. The worldly utilitarian says: "See how happy I am. I get a little money, but about all these other things I do not bother my head. They are too unsearchable, and so I am happy." So far, so good; good for all you utilitarians. This world is terrible. If any man gets happiness in any way excepting by injuring his fellow beings, God speed him, but when this man comes to me and says you too must do these things; you will be a fool if you do not, I say you are wrong, because the very things which are pleasurable to you, have not the slightest attraction for me. If I had to go after a few handfuls of gold, my life would not be worth living! I would die. That is the answer the religious man would make to him. The fact is that religion is only possible for those who have finished with these lower things. We must have our experiences, must have our full run. It is only when we have finished this run that the other world opens.

There is a great problem that arises in my mind. It is a very harsh thing to say, and yet a fact. These enjoyments of the senses sometimes assume another phase which is very dangerous and tempting. This idea you will always hear—it was in very old times, in every religion—that a time will come when all the miseries of life will cease, and only its joys and pleasures will remain, that this earth will thus become a heaven. That I do not believe. This earth of ours will always remain this same world. It is a most terrible thing to say, yet I do not see my way out of it. It is like rheumatism; drive it from the head, it goes to the legs, drive it from there it goes to other parts. Whatever you do is there. So is misery. In olden times people lived in forests, and they ate each other up; in modern times they do not eat each other's flesh, but they cheat one another. They ruin whole countries and cities by cheating. That is not great progress; I do not see that what you call progress in the world is other than multiplication of desires. If one thing is obvious to me it is this, that desires bring all misery, the state of the beggar, always begging for something, unable to see anything without the idea of having it; having, having, everything. The whole life is the life of the thirsty, thirsty beggar, unquenchable thirst of desire. If the power to satisfy our desires is increased in arithmetical progression, the power of desire is increased in geometrical progression. The sum-total of happiness and misery in the world is at least the same throughout. If a wave rises in the ocean it makes a hollow somewhere. If happiness comes to a man unhappiness comes to some other, or to some animal. Men are increasing and animals are vanishing; we are killing them, and taking their land; we are taking all means of sustenance from them. How can we say that happiness is increasing? The strong race eats up the weaker, but do you think that the strong race will be very happy? No; they will begin to kill each other. I do not see how it can be on practical grounds. It is a question of fact. On theoretical grounds, also, I see it cannot be.

Perfection is always infinite. We are this infinite already, and we are trying to manifest that infinity. You and I and all beings are trying to manifest this infinity. So far it is all right. But from this fact, some German philosophers have tried to make out a very peculiar theory of philosophy—that this manifestation will become higher and higher until we attain perfect manifestation, until we have become perfect beings. What is meant by perfect manifestation? Perfection means infinity, and manifestation means limit, and so it means that we shall become unlimited limiteds; which is self-contradictory. Such a doctrine may please children; it may be very nice to please children, to give them a comfortable religion, but it is poisoning them with lies, and it is bad for religion. We are told that this world is a degradation, that man is a degradation of God, that Adam fell. There is no one religion to-day which does not teach you that man is a degradation. We have been degraded down to the animal; now we are going up, to emerge again, to get away from this bondage, but we shall never be able to manifest the infinite here. We shall struggle hard, and then find it impossible. There will come a time when we shall find that it is impossible to be perfect here, while we are bound by the senses. And then the march back will be sounded.

This is renunciation. We shall have to get out of the difficulty as we got in, and then morality and charity will begin. What is the watchword of all ethical codes? "Not I, but thou," and this "I" is the outcome of the infinite behind, trying to manifest itself on the outside world. This little "I" is the result. This is the result that has been obtained, and this little "I" will have to go back and join the infinite, its own nature. It will find that it has been making a false attempt. It has put its foot into the wheel and will have to get out, and this is being discovered every day. Every time you say: "Not I, my brother, but thou," you are trying to go back, and every time you forget the ideal, you say: "I, not thou." Struggles and evils are in the world, but after that must begin renunciation, eternal renunciation. Why care for this little life? All these vain desires of living here and enjoying this life, this thinking I will live and enjoy again in some other place—living always in the senses and in sense enjoyment— these ideas bring death.

If we are developed animals the very same argument can be worked out on the other side; the animals also may be degraded men. How do you know it is not so? You have seen that the proof of evolution is simply this, that you find a series of bodies, one near to the other, from the lowest body to the highest body, but from that argument how can you insist that it is from the lower up, and not from the top down? The argument applies to both sides, and if anything is true I believe it is going up and down, the series repeating itself. How can you have an evolution without going back in the same series in which we came up? However it may be, the central idea to which I am referring is there.

Of course I am ready to be convinced the other way, that the infinite can manifest itself. As to the other idea—that we are going ever and ever in a straight line—I do not believe it; it is too nonsensical to believe. There is no motion in a straight line. If you could throw a stone forward with sufficient force, a time would come when it would complete the circle and return to its starting place. Do you not read the mathematical axiom, a straight line infinitely projected becomes a circle? It must be so, only it may vary as to details. So I always cling to the side of the old religious ideas, when I hear Christ preach, and Buddha assert, and the Vedânta declare, and the Bible proclaim, that we must all come to perfection in time, but only by giving up this imperfection. This world is nothing. It is at best only a hideous caricature, a shadow of the reality. All the fools are rushing after sense-enjoyments.

It is easy to live in the senses. It is easier to run in the old groove, eating and drinking; but what these modern philosophers want to tell you is to take these comfortable ideas and put the stamp of religion on them. Such a doctrine is dangerous. Death is in the senses. We must go beyond death. It is not a reality. Renunciation will take us to the reality. Renunciation is meant by morality. Renunciation is the very basis of our true life; every moment of goodness and real life that we enjoy, is when we do not think of ourselves. This little separate self must die; and then we shall find that we are in the Real, and the Vedânta says, that Reality is God, and He is our own real nature, and He is always in us and with us. Live in Him and stand in Him; although it seems to be so hard, it will become easier by-and-by. You will find that it is the only joyful state of existence; every other existence is of death. Life on the plane of the spirit is the only life, life on any other plane is mere death; the whole of this life can be only described as a gymnasium. We must go beyond it to enjoy real life. We must attain to Realization.

XI. THE FREEDOM OF THE SOUL.

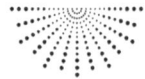

The Katha Upanishad, which we have been studying, was written much later than that to which we now turn— the Chândogya. The language is more modern, and the thought more organized. In the older Upanishads the language is very archaic, like that of the hymn portions of the Veda, and one has to wade sometimes through quite a mass of unnecessary things to get at the essential doctrines. The ritualistic literature about which I told you, which forms the second division of the Vedas, has, to a large extent, left its mark upon this old Upanishad, so that more than half of it is still ritualistic. There is, however, one great gain in studying the very old Upanishads; you trace, as it were, the historical springing up of spiritual ideas. In the more recent Upanishads the spiritual ideas have been collected and brought into one place, just as in the Bhagavad Gîtâ, for instance, which we may perhaps look upon as the last of the Upanishads, and you do not find in them any inkling of these ritualistic ideas. Every verse of the Gîtâ has been collected from some portion of the Upanishads, and made into a sort of bouquet. But therein you cannot understand the rise of the idea, you cannot trace it to its source, and to do that is, as has been pointed out by many, one of the great benefits of studying the Vedas; for the great idea of holiness that has been attached to these books has preserved them, more than any other book in the world, from mutilation. There, thoughts at their highest and at their lowest level have all been preserved, essential and non-essential. The most ennobling teachings and simple matters of detail stand side by side, for nobody has dared to touch them. The commentators came, of course, and tried to smooth them out, and to bring out wonderful new ideas from very old things; they tried to find spiritual ideas in even the most ordinary statements, but the texts remained, and, as such, they are the most wonderful historical study. We all know that in every religion in later times, as thoughts began to grow and develop there came this spiritual progress. One word is changed here and one put in there; another is thrown out, apart from the commentators. This, probably, has not been done with the Vedic literature at all, or if ever done, it is almost imperceptible. So we have this great advantage, we are able to study thoughts in their original significance, to note how they developed, how from materialistic ideas, finer and finer spiritual ideas evolved, until they attained their greatest height in the Vedânta. Some of the old manners and customs are also there, but not very much in the Upanishads. The language is a peculiar terse mnemonic.

The writers of these books simply jotted down these lines as helps to remember certain facts which they supposed were already well known. In a narrative, perhaps, as they are telling a story they take it for granted that it is well known to every one they are addressing, and thus a great difficulty arises; we scarcely know the real meaning of any one of these stories, because the traditions have nearly died out, and the little that is left has been very much exaggerated. So many new interpretations have been put on them that when you find them in the Puranas, they have already become lyrical poems. Now, just as in the West, we find one fact in the political development of western races: that they cannot bear absolute rule, that they are always trying to throw off any sort of bondage, to prevent any one man from ruling over them, and are gradually advancing to higher and higher democratic ideas, higher and higher ideas of physical liberty, so in metaphysics exactly the same phenomenon appears in the development of spiritual life. Multiplicity of gods gives place to one God of the Universe, and in the Upanishads there is a rebellion against that one God. Not only was the idea of so many governors of the universe ruling their destinies unbearable, but it was also intolerable to them that there should be one person ruling this universe. This is the first thing that strikes us. The idea grows and grows, until it attains its climax. In almost all of the Upanishads we find the climax coming at the last, and that is the dethroning of this God of the Universe. The personality of God vanishes, the impersonality comes. God is no more a person, no more a human being, however magnified and exaggerated, ruling this universe, but God has become an embodied Principle in us, in every being, immanent in the whole universe. And of course it would be illogical to go from the personal God to the impersonal, and at the same time to leave man as a person. So the personal man has to be broken down, man is also a principle. The person is without, the principle is within.

Thus from both sides simultaneously we find the breaking down of personalities and the approach towards principles, the personal God approaching the impersonal, the personal man approaching the impersonal man, and then come the succeeding stages of delineating the difference between the two advancing lines of impersonal God and impersonal Man. And the Upanishads embody these succeeding stages, by which these two lines at last become one, and the last word of each Upanishad is, "Thou art That." There is but One eternally blissful, and that One Principle is manifesting Itself as all this variety.

Then came the philosophers. The work of the Upanishads seems to have ended at that point; the next was taken up by the philosophers. The framework was given them by the Upanishads, and they had to work out the details. So, many questions would naturally arise. Taking for granted that there is but one impersonal Principle which is manifesting Itself in all these manifold forms, how is it that the One becomes many? It is another way of putting the same old question which in its crude form comes into the human heart in the shape of an inquiry into the cause of evil and so forth. Why does evil exist in the world, what is its cause? But the same question has now become refined, abstracted. No more is it asked from the platform of the senses why we are unhappy, but from the platform of philosophy. How is it that this one Principle becomes manifold? And the answer, as we have seen, the best answer that India produced, was the theory of *Mâyâ*, that it really has not become manifold, that it really did not lose a bit of its real nature. This manifold is only apparent. Man is only apparently a person, and in reality he is the Impersonal Being. God is a person only apparently, but really He is the Impersonal Being of the Universe.

Even in this answer there have been succeeding stages—philosophies have varied. All Indian philosophers did not admit this theory of *Mâyâ*. Possibly most of them did not. There are the dualists, with a very crude sort of dualism, who would not allow the question to be asked, stifled it at its very coming into existence. They said you have no right to ask such a question, you have no right to ask for an explanation; it is simply the will of God, and we have to submit quietly. There is no liberty for the human soul. It is all predestined—what we shall do, and have, and suffer, and enjoy, and it is our duty quietly to suffer, and if we do not we shall be punished all the more. How do we know that? Because the Vedas say so. And so they have their texts, their meanings, and they want to enforce them. The idea here is much like the theory of predestination preached by St. Paul.

There are others who, though not admitting the *Mâyâ* theory, stand midway, and try to explain all this by succeeding manifestations, succeeding development and degradation of the nature of man. All souls are metaphorically expanded and contracted in turn. The whole of this creation forms, as it were, the body of God. God is the Soul of all souls and of the whole of nature. Creation means the expansion of this nature of God, and after it is expanded for a certain time it again begins to contract. In the case of individual souls the contraction comes from evil doing. When a man does anything evil his soul begins to contract in its power, and so on it goes, until it does good works, and then it expands again. One idea seems to be common in all these various Indian systems, and to my mind in every system in the world, whether they know it or not, and that is what I should call the Divinity of Man. There is no one system in the world, no proper religion, which does not hold somewhere or other, either expressed in the language of mythology or in the language of allegory, or in the polished, clear language of philosophy, the one idea that the human soul, whatever it be, or whatever its relation to God, is essentially pure and perfect. Its real nature is blessedness and power, not weakness and misery. Somehow or other this misery has come.

The crude systems may call in a personified evil, a devil, or an Ahriman to explain how this misery came. Other systems may try to make a God and a devil in one, making some people miserable and some happy, without any explanation whatever. Others again, more thoughtful, bring in the theory of *Mâyâ* and so forth. But one fact stands out clearly, and it is with this that we have to deal. After all, these philosophical ideas and systems are but the gymnastics of the mind, intellectual exercises. The one great idea that to me seems to be clear, and comes out through masses of superstition in every country and every religion, is the one luminous idea that man is divine, that that divinity is our nature.

Whatever else comes is a mere super-imposition, as the Vedânta calls it. Something has been superimposed, but that Divine Nature never dies. In the most degraded, as well as the most saintly, it is ever present. It has to be called out, and it will work itself out. We have to ask and it will manifest itself. The people of old fancied that fire lived in the flint, and that friction of the steel was necessary to call that fire out. Others believed that fire lived in two dry pieces of stick and that friction alone was necessary to cause it to manifest itself. So this fire of natural freedom and purity is the nature of every soul, not a quality, because qualities can be acquired and therefore can be lost. The soul is one with freedom, and the soul is one with existence, and the soul is one with knowledge; this *Sat-Chit-Ananda*—Existence-Knowledge-Bliss Absolute—is the nature, the birthright of the soul, and all the manifestations that we see are the expressions of this nature of the soul, dimly or brightly manifesting itself. Even death itself is but the manifestation of that Real Existence. Birth and death, life and decay, degradation and degeneration, or regeneration, are all only the manifestations of that Oneness. So, knowledge, however it manifests itself, either as ignorance or as learning, is but the manifestation of that same Chit, that essence of knowledge; the difference is only in degree, and not in kind. The difference in knowledge between the lowest worm that crawls under our feet and the highest genius that the heavens may produce, is only one of degree, and not of kind. So the Vedântin thinker says boldly that the bliss of the enjoyments in this life, even the most degraded joy, is but the manifestation of that one Divine Bliss, the essence of the soul.

This one idea seems to be the most prominent, and, as I have said, to me it appears that every religion holds this same doctrine. I have yet to know the religion which has not that as its basis. It is the one universal idea working through all religions. Take the Bible for instance. You find there the allegorical statement, how Adam came first and was pure, and that purity was obliterated by his evil deeds afterwards. It is clear from this allegory that they thought that the nature of the primitive man, or however they may have put it, the real man, was already perfection. The impurities that we see, the weaknesses that we feel, are but super-impositions, and the subsequent history of that very religion shows that they also believe in the possibility, nay, the surety of regaining that old state. This is the whole history of the Bible, Old and New Testament together. So with the Mohammedans, they also believed in Adam and the purity of Adam, and since Mohammed came the way opened to regain that lost state. So with the Buddhists, they also believed in the state called *Nirvâna*, which is beyond this relative world of ours. It is exactly the same which the Vedântins called the *Brahman*, and the whole system of the Buddhists is advice to regain that lost state of *Nirvâna*. So in every system, we find this one doctrine always present, that you cannot get anything which is not yours already. You are indebted to nobody in this universe. You will claim your own birthright, or as it has been most poetically put by the great Vedântin philosopher, by making it the title of one of his books—"The attaining to our own empire." That empire is ours; we have lost it and we have to regain it. The *Mâyâ-âvdin*, however, says that this losing of the empire was an hallucination; you never lost it. This is the only difference.

Although all the systems agree so far, that we had the empire, and that we have lost it, they give us varied advice how to regain it. One says that you must perform certain ceremonies, pay certain sums of money to certain idols, eat certain sorts of food, live in a peculiar fashion to regain that empire. Another says that if you weep and prostrate yourselves and ask pardon of some Being beyond nature you will regain that empire. Another says, if you love such a Being with all your heart you will regain that empire. All this varied advice is in the Upanishads. As I go on you will find it so. But the last and the greatest counsel is, that you need not weep at all. You need not go through all these ceremonies, and need not take any notice of how to regain your empire, because you never lost it. Why should you go to seek for what you never lost. You are pure already, you are free already. If you think you are free, free you are this moment, and if you think you are bound, bound you will be. Not only that: it is a very bold statement—as I told you at the beginning of this course, I shall have to speak to you most boldly. It may frighten you now, but you will come to know by-and-by that it is true, when you think of it, and when you realize in your life the truth of it. For, supposing it is not your nature, that freedom is not your nature; by no manner of means can you become free. Supposing you were free and in some way you lost the freedom, then you cannot regain it, because that shows you were not free to commence with. Had you been free what could have bound you? The independent can never be made dependent, otherwise it was not independent, it was an hallucination.

So, of the two sides which will you take? If argument is stated it comes to this. If you say that the soul was by its own nature pure and free, it naturally follows that there was nothing in this universe which could make it bound or limited. But if there was something in nature which could bind you, it naturally follows that the soul was not free, and your statement that it was free is a delusion. So you have to come to this idea, that the soul is by its nature free. It cannot be otherwise. Freedom means independence of anything outside, and that means that nothing outside itself could work upon it as a cause. The soul is causeless, and hence come all the great ideas that we have. You cannot establish any idea of immortality unless you grant that the soul is by its nature free, or in other words, that it cannot be acted upon by anything outside. For death is an effect produced by something outside of man, showing that he can be acted upon by something else. I drink some poison and I am killed, showing that my body can be acted upon by something outside that is called poison. If this be true of the soul, the soul is bound. But if it be true that the soul is free it naturally follows that nothing outside can work upon the soul, and never will; therefore the soul will never die, it is beyond the law of causation. Freedom, immortality, blessedness, all depend on this, that the soul is beyond the law of causation, beyond this *Mâyâ*. Very good. Now if your nature was originally perfectly free and we have become bound, that shows that we were not really free. It was untrue. But, on the other side, here is this proposition, that we *are* free, and that this idea of bondage is but a delusion. Of these two, which will you take? Either make the first a delusion, or make the second a delusion. Certainly I will make the second a delusion. It is more consonant with all my feelings and aspirations. I am perfectly aware that I am free by nature, and I will not admit that this bondage is true and my freedom a delusion.

This discussion you see going on in all philosophies, taken in the crude form. Even in the most modern philosophies you find the same discussion entering. Here are the two parties. One party says that there is no soul, soul is a delusion. That delusion is being produced by the repeated transit of particles of matter, this combination which you call the body or the brain, and so on; its vibrations and motions and continuous transit of particles here and there, leaving that impression of freedom. There were Buddhistic sects who said, if you take a torch, and whirl it round you rapidly, there will be a circle of light. That does not exist, because the torch is changing place every moment. We are but bundles of little particles, which in the rapid whirling produce this delusion. On the other hand there is the statement, that this body is true, and the soul does not exist. Another explanation is, that in the rapid interchange of thought matter occurs as a delusion, but matter does not really exist.

These remain to the present day, one side claiming that spirit is a delusion and the other that matter is a delusion. Which side will you take? Of course we will take the spirit side and deny the matter side. The arguments are the same for both sides, only on the spirit side the argument is a little stronger. For nobody has even seen what matter is. We can only feel ourselves. I never saw a man who could feel matter outside of himself. Nobody was ever able to jump outside his own soul.

Therefore the argument is a little stronger on the side of the spirit. Secondly, the spirit thought explains the universe, while materialism does not. Therefore the materialistic explanation is illogical. This is a crude form of the same thought. If you boil all these philosophies down and analyze them, you will find these two things in collision. So here, too, in a more intricate form, in a more philosophical form, we find the same question about natural purity and freedom, and natural bondage. One side says that the first is a delusion, and the other that the second is the delusion. And here, too, we side with the second, that our bondage is a delusion.

So the solution of the Vedânta is that we are not bound, we are free already. Not only so, but to say or to think that we are bound is dangerous; it is a mistake; it is self-hypnotism. As soon as you say, "I am bound," "I am weak," "I am helpless," woe unto you; you rivet one more chain upon yourself. Do not say that, do not think it. I have heard of a man who lived in a forest and used to repeat day and night, "*Śivoham*"—I am the Blessed One—and one day a tiger fell upon the man and dragged him away to kill him, and people on the other side of the river saw it, and heard the voice as long as voice remained in him saying, "*Śivoham*"—even in the very jaws of the tiger. There have been many such men. There have been cases of men who, while being cut to pieces, have blessed their enemies. "I am He, I am He; and so art thou." I am pure and perfect, and so are all my enemies. You are He, and so am I. That is the position of strength. Nevertheless, there are great and wonderful things in the religions of the dualists; wonderful is the idea of the personal God apart from this nature, whom we are to worship and whom we are to love. Sometimes it is very soothing. But, says the Vedânta, that soothing is something like morphia, the soothing that comes from an opiate, not natural. It brings weakness in the long run, and what this world wants to-day more than it ever did is strengthening. It is weakness, says the Vedânta, which is the cause of all misery in this world. Weakness is the one cause of suffering. We become miserable because we are weak. We lie, steal, kill, or commit any crime, because we are weak. We suffer because we are weak. We die because we are weak. Where there is nothing to weaken us, there is no death or sorrow. We are miserable through delusion. Give up the delusion and the whole thing vanishes. It is plain and simple indeed. Through all these philosophical discussions and tremendous mental gymnastics we come back to this one religious idea, the simplest in the whole world. The Monistic Vedânta is the simplest form in which you can put a truth. To teach dualism was the tremendous mistake made in India, made everywhere else, because people did not look at the principles they arrived at, but only thought of the process, which is very intricate indeed. These tremendous philosophical and logical propositions were alarming to them. They thought these things could not be made universal, could not be made teachings of everyday practical life, and that under the guise of such a philosophy much laxity of living would arise.

But I do not believe at all that Monistic ideas preached to the world would produce immorality and weakness. On the contrary, I have reason to believe that it is the only remedy there is. If this be the truth, why let people drink ditch water when the stream of life is flowing by? If this be the truth, that they are all pure, why not at this moment teach it to the whole world? Saints and sinners, men, women and children, great or small, why not teach it with the voice of thunder, teach it to every man that is born or ever will come into the world, to the man on the throne and to the man sweeping the streets, rich or poor?

It appears now a very big and a very great undertaking, to many it appears very startling, but that is because of superstition, nothing else. By eating all sorts of low and indigestible food, and by starving ourselves, we have made ourselves incompetent to eat a good meal. We have listened to words of weakness from our childhood. It is just the same with ghosts. You always hear people say they do not believe in ghosts, but, at the same time, there are very few who do not get a little creepy sensation in the dark. It is simply superstition. So with all these things. This is the one idea that will come out of Vedânta, and the one idea that deserves to live. These books may perish tomorrow. Whether this idea first flashed into the brains of Hebrews or of people living at the North Pole nobody cares. But this is truth and truth is eternal, and truth itself teaches that it is not the special property of any being. Men and animals and gods are all common recipients of this one truth. Teach it to them. Why make life miserable? Why let people fall into all sorts of superstition? I will give ten thousand lives if twenty of them will give up their superstitions. Not only in this country, but in the land of its very birth, if you tell people this they are frightened. They say that this idea is for Sannyâsins, who give up the world and live in forests; for them it is all right. But for us poor householders, we must all have some sort of fear, we must have ceremonies, and so on.

Dualistic ideas have ruled the world long enough, and this is the result. Why not make a new experiment? It may take millions of years perhaps for all minds to receive it, but why not begin now? If we have told it to twenty persons in our lives we have done a great work. There is generally one idea in India which militates against it. It is this. It is all very well to say, "I am the Pure, the Blessed," but I cannot show it always in my life. That is true; the ideal is always hard. Every child that is born sees the sky over head very far away, but is that any reason why we should not strike towards the sky? Would it mend matters to go towards superstition? If we cannot get nectar, will it mend matters for us to drink poison? Would it be any help for us because we cannot realize truth immediately to go into darkness and weakness and superstition?

I have no objection to dualism in many of its forms. I like most of them, but I have objections to every form of teaching which inculcates weakness. That is the one question I put to every one, man, woman or child, when they are in training, physical, mental or spiritual. The question is: Are you strong? Do you feel strength?—for I know it is truth alone that gives strength. I know that truth alone gives life, and nothing but going towards reality will make us strong, and none will reach truth until he is strong. Every system, therefore, which weakens the mind, weakens the brain, makes one superstitious, makes one mope in darkness, makes one desire all sorts of morbid impossibilities and mysteries and superstitions, I do not like, because its effect is dangerous on the human being. Such teachings never bring any good.

Some may agree with me, that such things create morbidness in the human being, make him weak, so weak that in course of time it will be almost impossible for him to receive truth or live up to it. Strength, therefore, is the one thing that we want. Strengthening is the great medicine for the world's disease. Strengthening is the medicine which the poor must have when tyrannized over by the rich. Strength is the medicine that the ignorant must have when oppressed by the learned; and it is the medicine that sinners must have when tyrannized over by other sinners, and nothing gives such strength as this idea of Monism. Nothing makes us so moral as this idea of Monism. Nothing makes us work so well at our best and highest, as when all the responsibility is thrown upon us. I challenge every one of you. How will you behave if I put a little baby in your hands?

Your whole life will be changed for the moment; whatever you may be you must become selfless for the time being. You will give up all your criminal ideas; as soon as responsibility is thrown upon you, your whole character will change. So, if the whole responsibility is thrown upon our own shoulders we shall be at our highest and best. When we have nobody to grope towards, no one to lay all our blame upon; when we have neither the devil nor a personal God to lay all our evils upon, when we are alone responsible, then we shall rise to our highest and best. I am responsible for my fate, I am the bringer of good unto myself, I am the bringer of evil. I am the Pure and Blessed One. We must reject all thoughts that assert the contrary. "I never had death nor fear, I have no difference of caste or creed, I had neither father nor mother, nor birth nor death, nor friend nor foe, for I am the Existing-Knowledge-Bliss Absolute; I am the Blissful One, I am the Blissful One. I am not bound either by virtue or vice, by happiness or misery. Pilgrimages and book and the Vedas, and all these ceremonials can never bind me. I do not eat, the body is not mine, nor the superstitions that come to the body, nor the decay that comes to the body, for I am Existence-Knowledge-Bliss Absolute; I am the Blissful One, I am the Blissful One."

This, says the Vedânta, is the only prayer that the masses should have. This is the only way to reach the goal, to tell ourselves, and to tell everybody else that we are divine. And as we go on repeating, strength comes. He who limps at first will get stronger and stronger, the voice will increase in volume until it takes possession of our hearts and ideas, and will course through our veins, and permeate all our body. The delusion will vanish as the sunlight becomes more and more effulgent, load after load of ignorance will vanish, and then will come a time when the whole has disappeared and the Sun alone will be left.

This Vedantic idea of course to many seems very terrible, but that is, just as I have said, on account of superstition. There are people in this country who, if I tell them there is no such being as the devil, will think all religion has gone too. Many people have said to me, how can there be religion without a devil? They say, how can there be a religion without some one to direct us? How can we live without being ruled by somebody? We like to be so treated. We have become used to it and like it. We are not happy until we feel we have been reprimanded by somebody every day. The same superstition! But however terrible it may seem now, the time will come when we shall look back, each one of us, and smile at every one of those superstitions which covered the pure and eternal soul, and repeat with gladness, with truth, and with strength, "I am free, and was free, and always will be free."

XII. PRACTICAL VEDÂNTA. PART I.

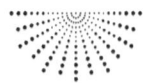

I have been asked to say something about the practical position of the Vedânta Philosophy. As I have told you, theory is very good indeed, but how are we to carry it into practice? If it be absolutely impracticable no theory is of any value whatever, except as intellectual gymnastics. The Vedânta, therefore, to become a religion, must be intensely practical. We must be able to carry it out in every part of our lives. And not only this, the fictitious differentiation between religion and the life of the world must vanish, for the Vedânta teaches Oneness—one life throughout. The ideals of religion must cover the whole field of life, they must enter into every one of our thoughts, and more and more into our practice. I will enter gradually into the practical side as we go on. But this series of lectures is intended to be a basis, and so we must first apply ourselves to theories, and understand how they are worked out, proceeding from forest caves, to busy streets, and cities; and one peculiar feature we find is that many of these thoughts have been the outcome, not of retirement into forests, but have emanated from thrones—from persons whom we expect to be the busiest in this life of ours, from ruling monarchs.

Śvetaketu was the son of *Aruni*, a sage, most probably a recluse. He was brought up in the forest, but he went into the city of the Panchâlas and there went to the court of the king, *Pravâhana Taivali*, and the king asked him: "Do you know how beings depart hence at death?" "No, Sir." "Do you know how they return hither?" "No, Sir." "Do you know the way of the fathers and the way of the gods?" "No, Sir." Then the king asked other questions. Śvetaketu could not answer them. Then the king told him that he knew nothing. The boy went back to his father and the father admitted that he could not answer these questions. It was not that he had not taught the boy, but he did not know these things himself. So Śvetaketu returned to the king with his father and they both asked to be taught this secret. The king said this secret, this philosophy, was only known among kings hitherto; the priests never knew it. He, however, proceeded to teach them what he knew about these things. Thus we find in various Upanishads the same idea, that this Vedânta philosophy is not the outcome of meditation in the forests only, but that the very best parts of it were thought out and expressed by brains which were busiest in the affairs of this life of ours. We cannot conceive any man busier than an absolute monarch, one man who is ruling absolutely over millions of people, and yet some of these rulers were deep thinkers.

Everything goes to show that this philosophy must be very practical, and later on, when we come to the Bhagavad Gîtâ— most of you, perhaps, have read it; it is the best commentary we have on the Vedânta philosophy—curiously enough the scene is laid on the battle field, where *Krishna* teaches this philosophy to Arjuna, and the doctrine which stands out luminously in every page of the Gîtâ is intense activity, but in the midst of that, eternal calmness. And this idea is called the "Secret of Work," to attain which is the goal of the Vedânta. Inactivity as we understand it, in the sense of passivity, certainly cannot be the goal. Were it so then the walls around us would be the most intelligent; they are inactive. Clods of earth, stumps of trees, would be the greatest sages in the world; they are inactive. Nor does inactivity become activity when it is combined with passion. Real activity, which is the goal of Vedânta, is that which is combined with eternal calmness, the calmness which cannot be ruffled, the balance of mind which is never disturbed, whatever happens around it. And we all know from our experience in life that that is the best attitude for work.

I have been asked many times how we can work if we do not feel the passions which we generally feel for work. I also thought in that way years ago, but as I am growing older, getting more experience, I find it is not true. The less passion there is, the better we work. The calmer we are, the better for us, and the more the amount of work we do. When we let loose our feelings we spoil so much of energy, shatter our nerves, disturb our minds, and accomplish very little work. The energy which ought to have gone out as work is spent as mere feeling, which counts for nothing. It is only when the mind is very calm and collected that the whole of its energy is spent in doing good work. And if you read the lives of the great workers which the world has produced, you will find that they were wonderfully calm men. Nothing, as it were, could throw them off their balance. That is why the man who becomes angry never does a great amount of work, and the man whom nothing can make angry accomplishes much more. The man who gives way to anger, or hatred, or any other passion, cannot work in this life of ours; he only breaks himself to pieces, and does nothing practical. It is the calm, forgiving, equable, well-balanced mind that does the greatest amount of work.

The Vedânta preaches the ideal, and the ideal, as we know, is always far ahead of the real, of the practical, as we may call it. There are two tendencies in this life of ours, one to harmonize the ideal with the life, and the other to elevate the life to the ideal. It is a great thing to understand this, for the former tendency is the temptation of our lives. I think that I can only do a certain class of work. Most of it, perhaps, is bad; most of it, perhaps, has a motive power of passion behind it, anger, or greed, or selfishness. Now if any man comes to preach to me a certain ideal, and the first step is to give up selfishness, to give up self-enjoyment, I think that is impractical. But when a man comes to bring an ideal which reconciles my selfishness, which reconciles all my vileness to itself, I am glad at once, and jump at the ideal. That is the ideal for me. As the word "orthodox" has been manipulated into various forms, so has been the word "practical." "My doxy is orthodoxy; your doxy is heterodoxy." So with practicality. What I think is practical is the only practicality in the world. If I am a shopkeeper I think shopkeeping the only practical religion in the world. If I am a thief I think the best means of stealing is the only practical thing; the others are not practical. You see how we all use this word practical for things *we* can do, as we are at present situated, and circumstanced. Therefore I will ask you to understand that Vedânta, though it is intensely practical, is always so in the sense of the ideal. It does not preach an impossible ideal however high it is, and it is high enough for an ideal. In one word, its ideal is that "Thou art That," you are divine. That is the result of all this teaching; after all its ramifications and intellectual gymnastics you arrive at the human soul as pure and omniscient; you see that such superstitions as birth and death would be entire nonsense when spoken of the soul. The soul was never born and will never die, and all these ideas that we are going to die and are afraid to die are mere superstitions. And all such ideas, as we can do or cannot do, are also superstition. We can do everything. The Vedânta preaches to men to have faith in themselves first. As certain religions of the world say a man who does not believe in a personal god outside of himself is an atheist, so the Vedânta says, a man who does not believe in himself is an atheist. Not believing in the glory of your own soul is what the Vedânta calls atheism. To many this is, no doubt, a terrible idea, and most of us think that this ideal can never be reached, but the Vedânta insists that it can be realized by everyone. There is neither man nor woman nor child, nor difference of race or sex, nor anything that stands as a bar to the realization of the ideal, because Vedânta shows that it is realized already, it is already here.

All the powers in the universe are already ours. It is we who have put our hands before our eyes, and cry that it is dark. Know that there is no darkness round us. Take the hands off and there is light from the beginning. Darkness never existed, weakness never existed. We who are fools cry that we are weak; we who are fools cry that we are impure. Thus not only Vedânta insists that the ideal is practical, but it has been so all the time, and this apparent Ideal, this Reality, is our own nature. Everything else that you see is false, untrue. As soon as you say "I am a little mortal being," you are saying something which is not true, you are giving the lie to yourselves, you are hypnotizing yourselves into something vile and weak and wretched.

It recognizes no sin, it recognizes error: and the greatest error, says the Vedânta, is to say you are weak, and a sinner, and a miserable creature, and that you have no power, and cannot do this and that. Every time you think in that way you, as it were, rivet one more link in the chain that holds you down, you add but one more layer of hypnotism to your own soul. Therefore, whosoever thinks he is weak is wrong, whosoever thinks he is impure, is wrong, and is throwing a bad thought into the world.

This we must bear in mind always: that in the Vedânta there is no attempt at reconciling the present life, the hypnotized life, this false life which we have assumed, with the ideal, but this false life must go, and the real life, which is always existing, must manifest itself, must shine out. No man becomes purer and purer: it is more or less of manifestation. The veil goes away, and the native purity of the soul begins to manifest itself. All is ours already, infinite purity, freedom, love and power.

Also, the Vedânta says, not only can this be realized in the depths of forests, or hidden in caves, but just as we have seen, the first people who discovered these truths for us were neither living in caves nor forests, nor were they ordinary persons in life, but persons whom we have every reason to believe had the busiest lives to lead, persons who had to command armies, to sit on thrones, and look to the welfare of their subjects—and in those days of absolute monarchs, not in these days when a king is to a great extent a mere figure head. Yet they could find time to think out all these thoughts, to realize them, and to teach them to humanity. How much more then should it be practical for us whose lives, compared with theirs, are lives of leisure? That we cannot realize them is a shame to us, seeing that we are comparatively free all the time, have very little to do. My wants are as nothing to the wants of one of those ancient absolute monarchs. My wants are as nothing to the wants of Arjuna on the battle-field at *Kurukshetra*, commanding a huge army, and yet finding time in the midst of the din of battle to talk of the highest philosophy, and to carry it into his life also: and we ought to be able to do as much in this life of ours, comparatively free, mostly of ease and comfort. Most of us here have more time than we think of, or know of, if we really want to use it for good. We can attain two hundred ideals in this life of ours, if we want them, with the amount of freedom we have, but we must not degrade the ideal to the actual. This is one of the most insinuating things that comes to us in the shape of persons who apologize for us here, and teach us how to make special excuses for all our foolish wants, foolish desires, and we think that this is the only ideal we can have, but it is not so. The Vedânta teaches no such thing. The actual is to be reconciled to the ideal, the present life is to be made to coincide with the eternal life.

For you must always remember that the one central ideal of Vedânta is this Oneness. There are not two in anything, no two lives, or two kinds of life for two worlds even. You will find the Vedas speaking of heavens and all these things at first, but later on, when they come to the highest ideals of their philosophy, they brush off all these things. There is but One Life, and One World, and One Existence. Everything is that Oneness, and the difference is in degree and not of kind. The difference between our lives is not of kind. The Vedânta entirely denies such ideals as that the animals are separate from men, and that they were made and created by God to be used for our food.

Some people have been kind enough to start an antivivisection society. I asked a member, "Why, my friend, do you think it is quite lawful to kill animals for food, and not to kill one or two for scientific experiments?" He replied, "That vivisection is most horrible, but animals have been given to us for food." The Oneness includes all animals. If man's life is immortal so is the animal's. The difference is only in degree and not in kind. The amœba is the same as I am; the difference is only in degree, and from the standpoint of the highest life all these little differences vanish. A man may see a great deal of difference between grass and a little tree, but if you climb a very high mountain, grass and the biggest tree will appear much the same. So, from the standpoint of the highest, all these ideals are the same, and if you believe there is a God, the animals and the highest creatures must be the same. A God who is partial to his children called men, and so cruel to his children called brute-beasts, is worse than a demon. I would rather die a hundred times than worship such a God. My whole life would be a fight with such a God. But it is not so. Those who say so do not know, they are irresponsible, heartless people, who do not know. Here is again a case of the practical used in the wrong sense. We want to eat. I myself may not be a very strict vegetarian, but I understand the ideal. When I eat meat I know it is wrong. Even if I were bound to eat it under certain circumstances I know it is cruel. I must not drag the ideal down to the actual and try to apologize for my weak conduct in this way. The ideal is not eating flesh, not injuring any being, for the animal is my brother; so is the cat and the dog. If you can think of them as that, you have arrived a little towards the brotherhood of all souls, not to speak of the brotherhood of man! That is child's play. You generally find that this is not very acceptable to many, because it teaches to give up the actual, and go up higher to the ideal; but if you bring out a theory which reconciles their present conduct they regard that as entirely practical.

There is this strongly conservative tendency in human nature: we do not like to move one step forward. I think of mankind just as I read of persons who have become frozen in snow; all such, they say, want to go to sleep, and if you try to drag them up they say, "Let me sleep. It is so beautiful to sleep in the snow," and they die there in that sleep. So is our nature. That is what we are doing all our life, getting frozen from the feet upwards, and yet wanting to sleep. Therefore you must struggle towards the ideal, and if there comes anyone to bring the ideal down to your level, if a man comes to teach you a religion that is not the highest ideal, do not listen to him. That is impracticable religion for me. But if a man comes and says religion is the highest work in life, I am ready for him. This is one thing to be guarded against, one thing to be taken care of. Beware when anyone is trying to apologize for sense vanities and sense weaknesses. If anyone wants to preach that way, sense-bound clods of earth as we have made ourselves, if we follow in that teaching, we shall never progress. I have seen a number of these things, I have had some experience of the world, and my country is the land where religious sects grow like mushrooms. Every year new sects arise. But one thing I have marked, that it is only those that never want to reconcile the man of flesh with the man of truth that make progress. Wherever there is this false idea of reconciling fleshly vanities with the highest ideals, of dragging down God to the level of man, there comes decay. Man should not be degraded to man where he is; he should be raised up to God.

At the same time, there is another side to the question. We must not look down with contempt on others. All of us are going towards the same goal. The difference between weakness and strength is one of degree; the difference between light and darkness is one of degree; the difference between virtue and vice is one of degree; the difference between heaven and hell is one of degree; the difference between life and death is one of degree; all difference in this world is one of degree, and not of kind, because Oneness is the secret of everything. It is all One, either as thought, or as life, or as soul, or as body, and the difference is only of degree. As such we have no right to look down with contempt upon those who are not exactly in the same degree that we are. Condemn none; if you can stretch out a helping hand, do so. If you cannot, fold your hands, bless your brothers and let them go their own way. Dragging down and condemning is not the way to work. Never is work accomplished in that way. We spend our energies in condemning others. Criticism and condemnation is a vain way of spending our energies, for in the long run we come to learn that all are seeing the same thing, are more or less approaching the same ideal, and that most of our differences are merely differences of language.

Take even the idea of sin, what I was telling you just now, the Vedânta idea and the other idea, that man is a sinner; they are practically the same, only the one is a mistaken direction. One takes the negative side and the Vedânta the positive. One shows to man his weakness, the other says weakness there may be, but never mind, we want to grow. Disease was found out as soon as man was born. Every one knows his disease; it requires no one to tell us what our diseases are. We may forget anything outside, we may try to become hypocrites to the external world, but in the heart of our hearts we all know our weakness. But, says the Vedânta, being reminded of weakness will not help much; give medicine, medicine is not making man think that he is diseased all the time. The remedy for weakness is not by making men think of their weakness all the time, but letting them think of their strength. Teach them of the strength that is already within them. Instead of telling men they are sinners, the Vedânta takes the opposite stand, and says, "You are pure and perfect, and all you call sin does not belong to you." Sins are very low degrees of manifestation; manifest yourself in a higher degree if you can. That is one thing to remember; all of us can. Never say no; never say, "I cannot." It must not be, for you are infinite. Time and space even are nothing compared to your nature. You can do anything and everything, you are almighty.

These of course are the principles of ethics. We shall have to come down still lower and work into the details. We shall have to see how this Vedânta can be carried into this everyday life of ours, the city life, the country life, life in every nation, the home life of every nation. For, if a religion cannot help man wherever he may be, wherever he stands, it is not much use; it will remain only a theory for a chosen few. Religion, to help mankind, must be ready and able to help him wherever he is; in servitude or in the full freedom of life, in the depths of degradation or in the heights of purity, everywhere equally it should be able to help mankind, and then alone the principles of Vedânta, or the ideal of Religion, or however you may call it, will be fulfilled.

The one ideal of faith in ourselves is the greatest help that can come to mankind. Had faith in ourselves been more extensively taught and practiced I am sure a very large portion of the evils and miseries that we have would have vanished. Throughout the history of mankind, if any motive power in the lives of all great men and women from their very birth has been more potent than another it is that of faith in themselves; born in the consciousness that they were to be great, they became great. Let a man go down as low as he likes, but there must come a time when out of sheer desperation an upward curve will be taken and he will learn to have faith in himself. But for us it is better that we know it from the very first. Why should we be compelled to have all this bitter experience in order to have faith in ourselves? We can see that all the difference between man and man is owing to the existence or non-existence of faith in himself. Faith in ourselves will do everything. I have experienced it in my own life, and am doing so continually, and as I grow older that faith becomes stronger and stronger. He is an atheist who does not believe in himself. The old religions said he was the atheist who did not believe in God. The new religion says he is the atheist who does not believe in himself. But it is not selfish faith, because the Vedânta, again, is the doctrine of oneness. It means faith in all, because you are pure. Love for yourselves means love for all, for you are one; faith in animals, faith in everything. This is the great faith which will make the world better. I am sure of that. He is the highest man who dares to say "I know all about myself." Do you know how many powers, how many forces, how many energies are still lurking behind that frame of yours? What scientist has yet known all that is in man? Millions of years have passed since man was here, and yet but one infinitesimal part of his power has been manifested. Therefore, how dare you say you are weak? How do you know what is behind that degradation on the surface? How do you know everything that is within you? Behind you is the ocean of infinite power and blessedness.

"This *Atman* is first to be listened to, to be heard." Hear day and night that you are that Soul. Repeat it to yourselves day and night till it enters into your very veins, till it tingles in every drop of blood, till it is in your flesh and bone. Let the whole body be full of that one ideal, "I am the birthless, the deathless, the blissful, the omniscient, the omnipotent, ever-glorious Soul."

Think on it day and night; think on it till it becomes part and parcel of your life. Meditate upon it, and out of that will come work. Out of the fulness of the heart the mouth speaketh, and out of the fulness of the heart the hand worketh also. Practice will come. Fill yourselves with the ideal; whatever you do, think well on it. All your actions will be transformed, deified, magnified, raised, by the very power of the thought. If matter is powerful, thought is omnipotent. Bring that thought, fill yourselves with the thought of your almightiness, your majesty, and your glory. Would to God all the other superstitious things had not been put into your head I Would to God we had not been born surrounded by all these superstitious influences and paralyzing ideas of our weakness and vileness I Would to God that mankind had an easier path through which to attain to the noblest and highest truths! But man has to pass through all this; do not make the path more difficult for those who are coming after you.

These are sometimes terrible doctrines to teach. I know people who get frightened, but for those who want to be practical this is the first practice. Tell not yourselves or others that you are weak. Do good if you can, but do not injure the world. You know in your inmost heart that many of your limited ideas, this humbling yourself, and weeping to imaginary beings, are superstitions. Tell me one case where these prayers have been answered. All the answers that came were from our own hearts. You all know there are no ghosts, but no sooner are you in the dark than there is a little creepy sensation. It is so because in our childhood we have all these fearful ideas put into our heads. But here is the practice. Do not do the same to others, through fear of society, through fear of public opinion, through fear of the hatred of our friends, for fear of loss of superstition. Be masters of it all. What is there more to be taught in religion? Oneness in this Universe, and to have faith in yourselves.

That is all there is to teach. All the works of mankind for thousands of years have been for this one goal, and mankind is working it out yet. It is yours now. We know it. It has been taught from all sides. Not only philosophy and psychology, but materialistic sciences have every day declared it. Where is the scientific man to-day who fears to acknowledge the truth of this oneness of the universe? Who is there who dares talk of many worlds, and so on? All these were superstitions. There is only one life and one world, and this one life and one world is appearing to us as manifold, just as when you dream, one dream passes away and another comes. You do not live in your dreams. The dreams come one after the other, scene after scene unfolds before you. So it is in this world of ours, of ninety per cent. misery and ten per cent.

happiness. Perhaps after a while it will appear as ninety per cent. happiness, and we shall call it heaven; but a time will come to the sage when the whole thing will vanish, and this very world will appear as God Himself, and our own soul as God. It is not therefore that there are many worlds, it is not that there are many lives. All this manifoldness is the manifestation of that One. That One is manifesting Himself as many, either in matter, or in spirit, or in mind, or in thought; or in any other thing. It is that One, manifesting Himself as many. Therefore the first practice for us is to teach the truth to ourselves and to others.

Let the world resound with this ideal and let superstitions vanish. Tell it to men who are weak; persist in telling it to them. You are the pure one; arise and awake, oh mighty one, this sleep does not represent you. Arise and go; it does not befit you. Think not that you are weak and miserable. Almighty, arise and awake, and manifest your own nature. It is not fitting that you think yourself a sinner. It is not fitting that you think yourself weak. Say that to the world, say it to yourselves, and see what a practical result will come, see how with an electric flash everything will be manifested, how everything will be changed. Tell that to mankind and show them their power. Then we shall learn how to practise it in our daily lives.

What we call *viveka* (discrimination), we shall come to later on, we shall learn how in every moment of our lives, in every one of our actions, to discriminate between what is right and wrong, true or false, and we shall have, therefore, to know the test of truth, which is purity, oneness. Everything that makes for oneness is truth. Love is truth, and hatred is false, because hatred makes for multiplicity. It is hatred that separates man from man; it is wrong and false therefore. It is a disintegrating power; it separates and destroys.

Love binds, love makes for that oneness. You are become one, the mother with the child, families become one with the city. The whole world becomes one with the animals. For love is existence, God Himself, and all this is the manifestation of that one love, more or less expressed. The difference is only in degree, but it is the manifestation of that one love throughout. Therefore in all our actions we have to judge whether it is making for diversity or for oneness. If for diversity we have to give it up, but if it makes for oneness we are sure it is a good action. So with our thoughts we have to understand whether they make for disintegration, the many, or for oneness, for binding soul unto soul, and bringing one influence to bear. If they do this we will take them up, and if not we will throw them off as criminal.

The whole idea of ethics is that it does not depend on anything unknowable, it does not teach anything unknown, but in the language of the Upanishad, "The God whom we worship as an unknown God, the same I preach unto thee." It is through that Self that you know anything else. I know the chair, but to know the chair I have first to know myself and then the chair. It is in and through the Self that the chair is known. It is in and through the Self that you are known to me, that the whole world is known to me, and therefore to say this Self is unknown is sheer nonsense. Take off the Self and the whole universe vanishes. In and through Self all knowledge comes. Therefore it is the most known of all. It is yourself, that which you call "I."

You may wonder how this "I" of me can be the "I" of you. You may wonder how this limited "I" can be that unlimited Infinite, and yet it is so. The limited is a mere fiction. It has been covered up, and a little of it is manifesting as the "I," but as yet it is only a part of the Infinite. The limitation never comes upon the unlimited; the limited is a fiction. The Self is known, therefore, to every one of us, man, woman or child, even to the animals. Without knowing Him we can neither live nor move, nor have our being. Without knowing this Lord of all we cannot breathe a second, or live a second, for He must be there to make us move, and think, and live. The most known of all, the God of the Vedânta, is not the outcome of imagination.

If this is not preaching a practical God, how would you teach a practical God? A God omnipresent, in every being, more real than these senses of ours. Where is there a more practical God than Him I see before me? For you are He, the Omnipresent God Almighty, the Soul of your souls, and if I say you are not I tell an untruth. I know it, whether at all times I realize it or not. He is the oneness, the unity of all, the reality of all life and all existence.

These ideas of the ethics of Vedânta have to be worked out in great detail, and therefore you must have a little patience. As I have told you, we want to take the subject in detail and work through it thoroughly, to see how the ideas grow from very low ideals, how the one great ideal of oneness has started out from all the surrounding ideas, and become shaped into that universal love, and we ought to study all these, in order to avoid dangers. But the world cannot wait for time to work up from the lowest steps. What is the use of our standing on higher steps if we cannot give the same truth to others coming afterwards.

Therefore it is better to study it in all its workings; and first, it is absolutely necessary to clear the intellectual portion, although we know that intellectuality is almost nothing, it is the heart that is of most importance. It is through the heart that the Lord is seen not through the intellect. The intellect is only the street cleaner, cleansing the path for us, a secondary worker, the watchman, the policeman; but the policeman is not a positive necessity for the workings of society. He is only to stop disturbances, to check wrong-doing, and that is all the work required of the intellect. When you read intellectual books, you think when you have mastered them: "Bless the Lord that I am out of them once more," because the intellect is blind and has no motion of itself, it has neither hands nor feet. It is feeling that is the worker, that moves with speed infinitely superior to that of electricity or any thing else. Do you feel, is the question. If you do, through that you will see the Lord. It is this feeling that you have to-day that will be intensified, deified, raised to the highest platform, till it feels everything, the oneness in everything, till it feels God in itself and in others. The intellect can never do that. "Different methods of speaking words, different methods of explaining the texts of books, these are for the enjoyment of the learned, not for the salvation of the soul."

Those of you who have read Thomas à Kempis will have found how in every page he insists on this: and almost every holy man in the world has insisted on it. Intellect is necessary, without it we fall into crude error, make all sorts of crude mistakes. Intellect checks this, but beyond that, do not try to build anything upon it. It is an inactive, secondary help; the real help is feeling, love. Do you feel for others? If you do you are growing in oneness. If you do not feel for others you may be the most intellectual giant ever born, but you will be nothing; you are but dry intellect, and you will remain so. And if you feel, even if you cannot read any book, and do not know any language, you are in the right way. The Lord is yours.

Do you not know in the history of the world the power the prophets had, and where was it? In the intellect? Did any of them write a fine book on philosophy, on the most intricate ratiocinations of logic? Not one. They spoke only a handful of words. Feel like Christ and you will be a Christ; feel like Buddha and you will be a Buddha. It is feeling that is the life, the strength, the vitality without which no amount of intellectual activity can reach God. Intellect is like limbs without power of locomotion. It is only when feeling enters and gives them motion that they move and strike others. That has been the way all over the world, and you must remember it. This is one of the most practical things in Vedantic morality, for it is the teaching of the Vedânta that you are all prophets, and all must be prophets. The book is not the proof of your conduct, but you are the proof of the book. How do you know that a book preaches truth? Because you do it and feel it. That is what Vedânta says. What is the proofs of the Christs and Buddhas of the world? That you or I feel like them. That is how I and you understand that they were true. Our prophet soul is the proof of their prophet soul. Your godhead is the proof of God Himself. If you are not a prophet there never has been anything true of God. If you are not God there never was any God, and never will be. This, says the Vedânta, is the ideal to follow. Every one of us has to become a prophet, and you are that already. Only, *know* it. Never think there is anything impossible for the soul. It is the greatest heresy to say that. If there be sin this is the only sin, to say that you are weak, or that others are weak.

XIII. PRACTICAL VEDÂNTA. PART II.

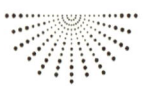

I will read to you a very ancient story from the Chândogya Upanishad, how knowledge came to a boy. The form of the story is very crude, but we shall find that it contains a principle. A young boy said to his mother, "I am going to study the Vedas. Tell me the name of my father, and my caste." The mother was not a married woman, and in India the child of a woman who has not been married is considered an outcast; he is not fit for anything, he is unable to be recognized, much less is he competent to study the Vedas. So the poor mother said: "My child, I do not know the name of your family. I was in service; I had to serve in many places; I do not know who your father is, but my name is Jabâlâ." The child went to the college of sages, and there he was asked the same question. He asked to be taken as a student, and they in turn asked him: "Say child, what is the name of your father, and what is your caste?" The boy repeated what he had heard from his mother. "Sir, I asked my mother the question, and this was her answer." Most of the sages were disappointed at the answer, and did not know what to say, but one of them stood up and asked the boy to come to him, and said: "My boy you have not swerved from the truth; you have not swerved from the path of righteousness, and this is what is called a Brahmin, so you are a Brahmin, and I will teach you." So he kept the boy with him and educated him; and because he had told the truth, gave him a new name— *Satyakâma*—the "truth desiring."

Now come some of the peculiar methods of ancient education. This teacher gave Satyakâma four hundred lean, weak cows to take care of, and sent him to the forest. There he went and lived for some time. The teacher had told him to come back when there were one thousand in the herd. So after a few years, Satyakâma heard a big bull in the herd telling him "We are a thousand now; take us back to your teacher. I will teach you a little of *Brahman*." "Say on, sir," said Satyakâma.

Then the bull said, "The east is a part of the Lord, so is the west, so is the south, so is the north. The four cardinal points are four parts of Brahman. You will be taught by the fire." Fire was the great symbol in those days, and every student had to procure fire and make offerings. So Satyakâma came back, and after performing his oblation, and worshipping at the fire, he was sitting near it, when from the fire came a voice, "O Satyakâma."

"Speak Lord," said Satyakâma. Perhaps you may remember a very similar story in the Old Testament, how Samuel heard a mysterious voice. "O Satyakâma, I am come to teach you a little of *Brahman*. This earth is a portion of that *Brahman*. The sky and the heaven are a portion of Him. The ocean is a part of that *Brahman*." Then the fire said that a certain bird would teach him something. Satyakâma continued on his journey, and when he had performed his evening sacrifice, there came a swan who said, "I will teach you something about *Brahman*. This fire which you worship, O Satyakâma, is a part of that *Brahman*. The sun is a part, the moon is a part, the lightning is a part of that *Brahman*. A bird called *Madgu* will tell you another part." The next evening that bird came, and a similar voice was heard by Satyakâma, "I will tell you something about *Brahman*. Breath is a part of *Brahman*, sight is a part, hearing is a part, the mind is a part." Then the boy returned to his teacher, and the teacher saw him from a distance, and this is what he said,

"Boy, thy face shines like a knower of *Brahman*." Then the boy asked the teacher to teach him more, and he said: "You have known some part of the truth already."

Now, apart from these allegories, what the bull taught, what fire taught, and what these others taught, we see the tendency of the thought and the direction in which it is going. The great idea of which we here see the germs, is, that all these voices are inside ourselves. As we read on we shall find how it is at last made clear that the voice is here in the heart, and the student understands that all this time he was hearing the truth, but his explanation was not correct. He was interpreting the voice as from the external world, while all the time the voice was inside him. The second idea that comes, is that of making the knowledge of the *Brahman* practical. It is always seeking the practical possibilities of religion, and we find in reading these stories how it is becoming more and more practical every day.

The idea is shown through everything with which the students were familiar. The fire with which they were worshipping was that *Brahman*. This earth is a part of *Brahman*, and so on.

The next story belongs to a disciple of this Satyakâma, who went to be taught by him and dwelt near him for some time. Now Satyakâma went away somewhere, and the student became very down-hearted, so that when the teacher's wife came and asked the boy why he was not eating, the boy said: "I am too unhappy to eat," and then a voice from the fire he was worshipping, saying: "This life is *Brahman*. *Brahman* is the ether, and *Brahman* is space. Know *Brahman*." "I know, sir, that life is *Brahman*, but that He is space and that He is ether I do not know." What is meant by ether is infinite space. Then the fire taught him the duties of the householder. "This earth, this food, this fire and this sun, whom you worship, are forms of *Brahman*.

He who inhabits these is within you all. He who knows this and meditates on Him, all his sins vanish and he has long life and becomes happy. He who lives in the cardinal points, I am He. He who lives in the breath, and in the ether, in the heavens, and in the lightning, I am He." Here too we see the same idea of practical religion. That which they were worshipping as the fire, the sun, the moon, and so forth, the voice with which they are familiar, takes up the subject, and explains it, and gives it a higher meaning, and that is the real practical side of Vedânta. It does not destroy the world, but it explains it; it does not destroy the person, but explains it; it does not destroy the individuality, but explains it, by showing the real individuality. It does not show that this world is vain, and does not exist, but it says understand what this world is, so that it may not hurt you. The voice did not say to Satyakâma that the fire which he was worshipping was all wrong, or the sun, or the moon, or the lightning, or anything else, but it showed him that the same spirit which is inside the sun, the moon, the lightning, the fire, and the earth, is in him, so that everything became transformed, as it were, to the eyes of Satyakâma. The fire which was merely a material fire before in which to make oblations, assumes a new aspect, and becomes the Lord really. The earth has become transformed, life has become transformed, the sun, the moon, the stars, the lightning, everything becomes transformed, deified. Their real nature is known. For we must know that the theme of the Vedânta is to see the Lord in everything, to see things in their real nature, not as they appear to be.

Then another lesson is taught which is very peculiar. "He who shines through the eyes is *Brahman*. He is the beautiful one, He is the shining one. He shines in all these worlds." A certain peculiar light, the commentator says, which comes to the pure man is the light in the eyes meant here, and it is said that when a man is pure, such a light will shine in his eyes, and that light belongs really to the soul within which is everywhere. It is the same light which is shining in the planets, in the stars, and suns.

The other thing that I will read to you is about some peculiar doctrines of these ancient Upanishads, about birth and death and so on. Perhaps it will interest you. Svetaketu went to the king of the *Panchâlas*, and there the king asked him, "Do you know where people go when they die? Do you know whether they come back or not? Do you know why this earth does not become full, and why it does not become empty?" The boy replied that he did not know. Then he went to his father and asked him the same questions. The father said, "I do not know," and they both returned to the king. The king said this knowledge was never among the priests, it was only among the kings, and that is why the king rules the world. But this man served the king for some time, and at last the king said he would teach him. "O Gautama, the fire that you worship outside is a very low state of things. This earth itself is that great symbol of fire. The air is its fuel. The night is its smoke. Its flame is the cardinal points. The lower part is inhabited by darkness. In this fire the gods pour the oblation, the rain out of which comes food. You need not make oblation to that little fire; the whole world is that fire, and this oblation, this worship, is continually going on. The gods, and the angels, everybody is worshipping. Man, O *Gautama*, is the greatest symbol of fire, the body of man. We get the idea becoming practical once more, the *Brahman* coming down. And the one idea that runs through all these symbolical stories is that invented symbolism may be good, and helpful, but better symbols exist already than any you can invent. If you want to invent an image to worship God, a better image still exists, the living man. If you want to build a temple to worship God, that may be good, but a better one, a much higher one, exists, the human body.

We must remember that the Vedas have two parts, the ceremonial and the knowledge portions. By that time ceremonials had become so intricate and multiplied that it was almost hopeless to disentangle them and in the Upanishads the ceremonials are almost done away with, but gently, by explaining them. We see that in old times they had these oblations and sacrifices, but here the philosophers come, and they, instead of snatching their symbols from the hands of the ignorant, instead of taking the negative position which we, unfortunately, find general in modern reforms, gave them something to take their place. Here is the symbol of fire, very good. But here is another symbol, the earth. What a grand, great symbol! Here is this little temple, but the whole universe is a temple; a man can worship anywhere. There are the peculiar figures that men, draw on the earth, and build altars, but here is the greatest of altars, the living conscious human body, and worship here is far greater than the worship of any dead symbols.

We now come to a peculiar doctrine. I do not understand much of it myself. If you can make something out of it I will read it to you. When a man who has meditated, and purified himself, and got knowledge, dies, then he first goes to light, from light to day, from day to the light half of the moon, from that to the six months when the sun goes to the north, from the months to the year, from the year to the sun, from the sun to the moon, from the moon to the lightning, and when he comes to the sphere of lightning he meets a person who is not a man, and that person helps him to meet *Brahman*, to meet God. This is the path of the gods. When sages and knowing persons die they go that way and they do not return. What is meant by this month and year and all these things, no one understands clearly. Each one makes his own meaning, and a good many say it is all nonsense. What is meant by going to the world of the moon, and of the sun, and this person who comes to help the Soul after it has reached the spheres of light, no one knows. There has been a peculiar idea among the Hindûs that the moon is a state of life, and we will see how life has come from the moon, it has rained from the moon upon this earth. Those that have not attained to knowledge, but have done good work in this life, when they die, first go through smoke, then to night, then to the dark fifteen days, then the six months when the sun goes to the south, from that they go to the region of the forefathers, then to ether, then to the region of the moon, and there they become the food of the gods, and are born as gods. There they live as long as their good works will permit. And when the effect of the good work has been finished they come back. They first become ether, and then air, and then smoke, then mist, then cloud, and then get hold of raindrops, and fall upon the earth, get into food, are eaten up by human beings, and then become their children. Those whose works have been very good take birth in very good families, and those whose works have been bad take very bad births. The animals are always dying, and are continually coming in this earth. That is why this earth is not full, and not empty.

Several ideas we can get also from this, and later on, perhaps, we shall be able to understand it better, and we can speculate a little upon what they mean. The last part, how those who have been in heaven are returning, is clearer perhaps than the first part, but the whole idea seems to be this, that there is no permanent heaven without realizing God. Now some people who have not realized God, but have done good work in this world, with the view of enjoying the results thereof, when they die go through this and that place, until they reach heaven, and there they are born in the same way as we are here, as children of the gods, and they live there as long as their good works will permit. Out of this comes one basic idea of the Vedânta, that everything which has name and form is transient. This earth is transient, because it has name and form, and so the heavens must be transient, because there also the name and form remain. A heaven which was eternal would be contradictory in terms, just as the earth cannot be eternal; because everything that has name and form must begin in time, exist in time, and finish in time. These are settled doctrines with the Vedânta, and the heavens are given up.

We have seen in the *Samhita* how the other idea was that heaven was eternal, much the same as the idea which is prevalent in Europe among Mohammedans and Christians. The Mohammedans concretize it a little more. They say it is a place where there are gardens, beneath which rivers run. In the desert of Arabia water is something which is very desirable, so the Mohammedan always conceives his heaven as full of water. I was born in a country where there are six months of rain every year. I would think of heaven, I suppose, as a dry place, and so would the English people. These heavens in the *Samhita* portion are eternal; the departed have beautiful bodies and live with their forefathers, and are happy ever afterwards. There they meet with their fathers, and children, and relatives, and lead very much the same life as here, only much happier. All the difficulties and obstructions to happiness in this life will vanish, and all its good parts and enjoyments will be left. But however comfortable mankind may consider this, there is something which is truth and something which is comfort. There are cases where truth is not comfortable until we reach the climax. Human nature is very conservative. It goes on doing something, and once having done that something it finds it hard to get out of it. The mind will not allow new thoughts to come, because they give pain.

So here, in the Upanishads, we see a tremendous departure made. It is declared that these heavens, where men used to go and live with the ancestors cannot be permanent, seeing that everything which has name and form must die. If there are heavens with forms, these heavens must vanish in course of time; it may be millions of years, but there must come a time when they will have to go. Another idea by this time has appeared, that these souls must come back: to this earth, that these heavens are places where they enjoy the results of their good works, and after these effects are finished they come back into this earth life again. One idea is clear from this, that mankind had a perception of the philosophy of causation even at that early time. Later on we shall see how our philosophers bring that out in the language of philosophy and logic, but here it is almost in the language of children. One thing you may remark in reading these books, that it is all internal perception. If you ask me if this can be practical, my answer is it has been practical first, and philosophical next. You can see that these things have been perceived and realized first, and then written. This world spoke to the early thinkers, birds spoke to them, animals spoke to them, the sun, the moon spoke to them, and bit by bit they realized things and got into the heart of nature, not by cogitation, not by the force of logic, not by picking the brains of others and making a big book, as is the fashion in modern times, not as I do, by taking up one of their writings and making a lecture; but by patient investigation and discovery. Its essential method was practice, and so it will be always. Religion will be always a most practical science. There never was or will be any theological religion. It is practice first, and knowledge afterwards. The idea that these souls come back is already there. Those persons who do good work with the idea of a result, get it, but the result is not permanent. There we get the idea of causation very beautifully put forward, that the effect is only commensurate with the cause. What the cause is, so the effect will be. The cause being finite, the effect must be finite. If the cause is eternal the effect can be eternal, but all these causes, doing good work, and all other things, are only finite causes, and as such cannot produce infinite result.

We come to the other side of the question, that as there cannot be an eternal heaven, there cannot be an eternal hell, on the same grounds. Suppose I am a very wicked man. Suppose I do evil every minute of this life of mine. Still this whole life here, compared to my eternal life, is nothing. If there be an eternal punishment it will mean that there is an infinite effect produced by a finite cause. The infinite effect of my work will be produced by the finite cause of this life, and for this infinite result I shall have a finite cause which cannot be. If I do good all my life I cannot have an infinite heaven; it would be making the same mistake. But there is the third course, for those who have known the truth, for those who have realized. That is the only way to get out, as it were, beyond this veil of *mâyâ*, to realize what truth is, and the Upanishads indicate what line these are taking, what is meant by realizing the truth.

It means recognizing neither good nor bad, but knowing all as coming from the Self; self is in everything. It means denying the universe; closing your eyes; seeing the Lord in heaven and in hell also; seeing the Lord in life and in death also. This is the line which thought is taking in the passage I have just read to you, how this earth itself is a symbol of the Lord, how the sky is said to be the Lord, how the place we fill is said to be the Lord. Everything is *Brahman*. And this is to be seen, realized, not simply talked about, or thought about. We can see as a logical consequence that when the soul has realized that everything in this universe, every place is full of the Lord, of *Brahman*; it will not mean anything to that soul whether it goes to heaven, or hell, or anywhere. It does not mean anything to it whether it be born again on this earth, or in heaven. These have ceased to have any meaning, because for the soul that has realized its real nature, every place is the same, every place is the temple of the Lord, every place has become holy, and the presence of the Lord is all that it sees in heaven, or hell, or anywhere. Neither good nor bad, neither life nor death; only one Infinite *Brahman* exists for that soul.

When a man has arrived at that perception according to the

Vedânta, he has become free, and, says the Vedânta, that is the only man who is fit to live in this world. Others are not. The man who sees evil, how can he live in this world? His life is a misery; it is a mass of misery here. The man who sees dangers here, his life is a misery; the man who sees death, his life is a misery. That man alone can live in this world, he alone can say: "I enjoy this life, and I am happy in this life," who has seen the truth, and the truth in everything. By the bye, I may tell you that the idea of hell does not occur in the Vedas anywhere. It comes into India with the *Purânas*, much later. The worst punishment described in the Vedas is coming back here, having another chance on this earth. From the very first we see the idea is taking the impersonal turn. The ideas of punishment and reward are very material, and they are only consonant with the idea of a human God, a being who loves one and not another, just as we do. Punishment and reward are only admissible with the existence of such a God. They had such a God in the *Samhita*, and there we find the idea of fear entering, but as soon as we come to the Upanishads the idea of fear vanishes, and the impersonal idea takes its place, and it is naturally the hardest thing to understand, this impersonal idea, in every country.

Man is always clinging on to the person.

On the other hand the Impersonal God is a living God, a Principle. The difference between personal and impersonal is this, that the personal is only a little man, and the impersonal idea is that he is the animal, the man, the angel, and yet something more which we cannot see, because impersonality involves all personality, is the sum-total of all personality in the universe, and infinitely more besides. "As the one fire coming into the world is manifesting itself in so many forms, and yet is infinitely more besides." Such is the Impersonal.

We want to worship a living God. I have seen nothing but God all my life, nor have you. To see this chair you first see God, and then the chair, in and through Him. He is there day and night, saying: "I am." The moment you say "I am" you are knowing existence. Where shall you go to find God if you cannot see Him in your own hearts, in living beings, in the man working in the street? "Thou art the man, Thou art the woman, Thou art the girl, and Thou art the boy. Thou art the old man tottering on a stick. Thou art the young man walking in the pride of his strength." He is all that exists, a wonderful living God, who is the only Fact in the Universe. This seems to many to be a very terrible contradiction to the traditional God, who lives behind a veil somewhere and whom nobody ever sees. The priests only give us an assurance that if we follow them, listen to their admonitions and walk in the way they mark out for us —then when we die, they will give us a passport, and we may happen to see the face of God! What are all these heaven ideas but simply modifications of this nonsensical priestcraft?

Of course the impersonal idea is very destructive; it takes away all trade from the priests, all churches and temples will vanish. If they taught this impersonal idea to the people their occupation would be gone. Yet we have to teach it unselfishly, without priestcraft. You are God and so am I; who obeys whom? Who worships whom? You are the highest temple of God; I would rather worship you than any temple or any image or bible. Why are these people so contradictory in their thought?

They are like fish slipping through our fingers. They say we are hardheaded practical men. Very good. But what is more practical than worshipping here, worshipping you? I see you, feel you, and I know you are God. The Mohammedan says there is no God but Allah. The Vedânta says there is no God but man. It may frighten many of you, but you will understand it by-and-by. The living God is within you, and yet you are building churches and temples and believing all sorts of imaginary nonsense. The only God to worship is the human soul, or the human body. Of course all animals are temples, but man is the highest, the Taj Mahal of temples. If I cannot worship that, no other temple will be of any advantage. The moment I have realized God sitting in the temple of every human body, the moment I stand in reverence before every human being, and really see God, the moment that feeling comes to me, that moment I am free from bondage, everything vanishes, and I am free.

This is practical, the most practical of all worship. It does not have anything to do with theorizing and speculation; yet, if you tell it to most men, it frightens them. They say it is not right. They go on theorizing about ideas their grandfathers told them, and their forefathers six thousand years ago, that a God somewhere in heaven told somebody that he was God. Since that time we have only theories. This is practicality according to them, and our ideas are impractical. Each one must have his way, says the Vedânta, but this is the ideal. The worship of a god in heaven, and all these things, are not bad, but they are only steps towards the truth, and not the truth itself. They are good and beautiful, and some wonderful ideas are there, but the Vedânta says at every point: "My friend, Him whom you are worshipping as unknown I worship as thee. Whom you are worshipping as unknown and trying to seek throughout the universe, He has been there all the time. You are living through Him. He is the eternal witness of the universe." "Him whom all the Vedas worship, nay, more, He who is always present in the eternal 'I,' He existing, the whole universe exists. He is the light of the universe. If the 'I' were not in you, you would not see the sun, everything would be a dark mass for you, non-existence. He shining, you see the world."

One question is generally asked and it is this, that this may lead to a tremendous amount of difficulty. Every one of us will think I am God, whatever I do or think is good; God can do no evil. In the first place, even taking this danger of misinterpretation for granted, can it be proved that on the other side the same danger does not exist? They have been worshipping a God in heaven separate from them, and of whom they are so much afraid. They have come in shaking with fear, and all their life they go on shaking. Has the world been made much better?

The same question you ask on the other side. Those who have understood and worshipped a personal God, and those who have understood and worshipped an impersonal God, on which side have been the great workers of the world? Gigantic workers, gigantic moral powers? Certainly the impersonal. How can you expect moral persons to be developed from fear? It can never be. "Where one sees another, where one hurts another, that is *Mâyâ*. When one does not see another, when one does not hurt another, when everything has become the *Atman*, who sees whom, who perceives whom?" It is all

He, and all I, at the same time. The soul has become pure. Then, and then alone we understand what is love, and can love come through fear? Its basis is in freedom; then comes love. We really begin to love the world, then we understand what is meant by brotherhood and mankind, and not before.

So it is not right to say this will lead to a tremendous amount of evil doing all over the world, as if the other doctrine never lends itself to the works of evil; as if it does not deluge this world in blood, as if it does not tear to pieces and lead to sectarianism. My God is the greatest God. Let us decide it by a free fight. That is the outcome of dualism all through the world. Come out into the broad open light of day, come out from the little narrow paths. How can the great infinite human soul rest content to live and die in small ruts? There is the universe of light, everything in the universe is ours. Try to stretch out your arms and embrace the whole universe in love. If you have ever felt that you wanted to do that, you have felt God.

You remember that passage in the sermon of Buddha, how he sent a thought of love towards the South, and the North, and the East, and the West, above and below, until the whole universe was filled with this love, grand and great and infinite. When you have that feeling that means true personality. The whole universe is one Person; let go these little things. Give up the small for this infinite enjoyment, give up small enjoyments for this infinite bliss. What use is it to have these small bits of bliss? And it is all yours, for you must remember that the impersonal includes the personal. So God is the Personal and the Impersonal at the same time. So man, the infinite, impersonal Man, is manifesting himself as this person. We the infinite have limited ourselves, as it were, into little bits. The Vedânta says this is the state of things. It will not vanish, it will remain, but now it is ourselves. We are limiting ourselves by our *Karma*, and that like a chain round our necks has dragged us into this limitation. Break that chain and be free. Trample law under your feet. There is no law in human nature, there is no destiny, no fate. How can there be law in infinity? Freedom is its watchword. Freedom is its nature, its birthright. Be free, and then have any amount of little personalities you like. Then we will play as the actor, as a king comes upon the stage and takes up the role of a beggar, and the actual beggar is walking through the streets. The scene is the same in both cases, the words are perhaps the same, but yet what a difference. The one enjoys his beggary and the other is suffering misery from it. And what makes this difference? The one is free and the other is bound. The king knows this beggary is not true, but that he has assumed it, taken it up just for play, and the beggar thinks that it is his familiar state and he has to bear it whether he will or not.

This is law, so he is miserable. You and I as long as we have no knowledge of our real nature, are these beggars, jostled about by every force in nature, made slaves by everything in nature, crying all the world over for help, and help never comes to us, trying to get help from every quarter, from imaginary fictitious beings, and yet never getting any help. Then thinking, this time it will come, and weeping and wailing and hoping, one life is passed and the same play goes on.

Be free; hope for nothing from anyone else. I am sure if you all look back upon your lives you will find that you were always vainly trying to get help from others and it never came. All the help that has been given you was from within yourselves. You only had the fruits of what you yourselves worked for, and yet strangely hoping all the time for help. Like the rich man's parlor, always full, but if you watch it you do not find the same batch of people there. Always hoping that they will get something out of these rich men, but they never do. So are our lives, hoping, hoping, hoping, never coming to an end. Give up this hope, says the Vedânta. Why should you hope? You have everything.

You are the king, the Self. What are you going to hope for? If the king goes mad, and goes about to find the king in his own country, he will never find him because he is the king himself. He may go through every village and city in his own country, seeking in every house, he may weep and wail, but will never find any king because he is the king himself. It is better that we know we are the king and give up this fool's search after the king. Thus says the Vedânta, and knowing that we are the king we become happy and contented. Give up all these fools' searches, and then play on in the universe.

The whole vision is changed. Instead of an eternal prison this world has become a playground. Instead of a land of competition it is merely a land of Springtime, where the butterflies are flitting about in mirth. This very world is then heaven, where in the first place it was hell. To the eyes of the bound it is a tremendous place of torment, and to the eyes of the free it is the only world that exists. Heavens and all these places are here. This one life is the universal life. All rebirths are here. All the gods are here, the prototypes of man. The gods did not create man after their type, but man created gods. And here are the prototypes, here is the *Indra*, the *Karma*, and all the gods of the universe sitting before him. You have been projecting your little doubles, and you are the originals, the real, the only gods to be worshipped. This is the view of the Vedânta, and this its practicability. Because we have become free, we shall not go mad and throw up society and fly off to die in the forest or the cave, we shall remain where we are, only we shall have understood the whole thing. The same phenomena will come, but with new meaning. We do not know the world yet; it is only through freedom that we see what it is, understand its nature. We shall see then that this so-called law, or fate, or destiny, occupied only an infinitesimal part of our nature. It was just one side, and on the other side there was freedom all the time, and we have been like the hunted hare putting our faces on the ground, and trying to save ourselves from evil.

We have through delusion been trying to forget our nature, and yet we could not forget, it was always calling upon us, and all our search after god or gods, or external freedom, was a search after our real nature. We mistook the voice. We thought it was from the fire, or from a god, or the sun, or moon, or stars, but at last we have found that it was from ourselves. Here is this eternal voice speaking of eternal freedom. Its music is eternally going on. Part of this music of the soul has become the earth, the law, this universe, but it was always ours and always will be. In one word the ideal of Vedânta is to know man as he really is, and this is the message, that if you cannot worship your brother man, the manifested God, neither can you worship a God who is unmanifested.

Do you not remember in the Christian Bible, if you cannot love your own brother whom you have seen, how can you love God whom you have not seen? If you cannot see God in the human face divine, how can you see Him in the clouds, or in anything dull, or dead, or in mere fictitious stories of your brain? I will call you religious, from the day you begin to see God in men and women, for then you will understand what is meant by turning the left cheek to the man who strikes you on the right. When you see man as God, everything, even the tiger, will be welcome. Everything that comes is but the Lord in various forms, the Eternal, the Blessed One, our father, and mother, and friend, our own soul playing with us.

There is still a higher ideal than calling God Father; to call Him Mother. There are other ideals; He has been called "Friend"; still higher "the Beloved." The highest point of all is to see no difference between lover and beloved. You remember the old Persian story, how a lover came and knocked at the door and was asked, "Who is that." He answered, "It is I," and there was no answer. A second time he came, and answered "I am here," but the door did not open. The third time the lover came, and the voice again asked, "Who is that." He replied, "I am thyself, my love," and the door opened. So, between God and ourselves. He is in everything, He is everything. Every man and woman is the palpable blissful living and only God. Who says God is unknown, who says He is to be searched after? We have found God eternally. We have been living in Him eternally. Everywhere He is eternally known, eternally worshipped.

A great mistake is often made, that other forms of worship than our own are all errors. That is one of the great points not to be forgotten, that those who worship God through ceremonials and forms, however crude we may think them, are not in error. It is the travel from truth to truth, from lower truth to higher truth. Darkness is less light; evil is less good; impurity is less purity. This must always be borne in mind that we have to see others with eyes of love, with sympathy, knowing that they are but going through the same path that we have trod. If you are free, you must know that all are coming up to be free sooner or later, and if you are free how do you see the impermanent? If you are really pure how do you see the impure, for what is within is without. We cannot see impurity without having it first inside. This is one of the practical sides of Vedânta, and I hope that we shall all try to carry it into our lives. The whole of life is for this to be carried into practice; but one great point we gain, that we shall work with satisfaction and contentment, instead of discontent and dissatisfaction, for we know Truth is within us, we have it, it is our birthright, and we have only to manifest it, make it tangible.

XIV. PRACTICAL VEDÂNTA. PART III.

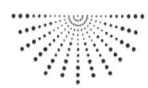

In the Chândogya Upanishad we read that a sage called *Nârada* came to another called *Sanatkumâra*, and asked various questions, and among them inquired if religion is the cause of things as they are. And Sanatkumâra takes him, as it were, step by step, tells him that there is something higher than this earth, and something higher than that, and so on, till he comes to *âkâsa*, ether. Ether is higher than light, because in the ether are the sun and the moon, lightning, the stars; it is in the ether we hear, in ether we live, and in ether we die. Then the question arises, is there anything higher than that, and he tells him of *prâna*. This *prâna*, according to the Vedânta, is the principle of life. It is like ether, an omnipresent principle, and all motion, either in the body or anywhere else, is the work of this *prâna*. *Prâna* is greater than *âkâsa*. Through *prâna* everything lives, *prâna* is in the mother, in the father, in the sister, in the teacher, *prâna* is the knower.

I will read another passage, where *Svetaketu* asks his father about the truth, and the father teaches him different things, and then at last answers "That which is the fine cause in all these things, of it are all these things made. That is the all, that is truth, thou art That, O *Svetaketu*." And then he again gives various examples. "As a bee, O *Svetaketu*, gathers honey from different flowers, and as the different honeys do not know that they are from various trees, and from various flowers, so all of us, having come out of that existence, have forgotten that we have done so. Therefore, O Svetaketu, That thou art." He gives another example of the rivers running down to the ocean, and they do not know that they have risen as various rivers, so even we come out of that Existence, and do not know that we are That. "O Svetaketu, thou art That." So on he goes.

Now there are two principles of all knowledge. The one principle is that we can know by referring the particular to the general, and the general to the universal; and the second principle is, that anything of which the explanation is sought, is to be explained so far as possible from its own nature. Taking up the first principle we see that all our knowledge really consists of that classification going higher and higher. When something happens singly we are, as it were, dissatisfied. When it can be shown that that very thing happens again and again we are satisfied, and call it law. When we find that one stone falls, or one apple falls, we are dissatisfied; when we find that all stones and all apples fall we call it the law of gravitation and are satisfied. The fact is that from the particular we deduce the general. When we want to study religion this is the scientific process.

To study religion, therefore, to make it scientific, we have to admit the same light. The same principle also holds good, and as a fact we find that that has been the course all through. In reading these books that I have been translating to you, the earliest idea that I can trace is from the particular to the general. We see how these "bright ones" become merged together and become one principle, and how in the ideas of the cosmos they are going higher and higher, how from the fine elements they are going to finer and finer, and more embracing elements, how from particulars they come to one omnipresent ether, and how from even that they went to an all embracing force, or *prâna*, and in all this the principle that runs through all, is, that one is not separate from the others. It is the very ether that exists in the higher form, or, so to say, the higher form of *prâna* concretes and becomes ether and that ether becomes still grosser, and so on.

The generalization of the personal God is another case in point. We have seen how the same generalization was reached, and how it was called the sum total of all consciousness. But a difficulty arises from that; it is not an all-sufficient generalization. We take up only one side of the facts of nature, the fact of consciousness, and out of that we generalize, and our generalization takes the form of the personal God, when the whole of nature is left aside. So, in the first place it is rather a defective generalization. There is another insufficiency, and that is the outcome of the second principle. Everything should be explained out of its own nature. There may have been people who thought that every stone that fell to the ground was dragged down by some ghost, but the explanation is the law of gravitation, and although we know it is not a perfect explanation, yet it is much better than the other, because one explanation is by some extraneous cause, and the other is by its own nature. So on, throughout the whole range of our knowledge, the explanation which is the outcome of the nature of the thing itself is a scientific explanation, and any explanation which is entirely outside of the thing in question is unscientific.

So the explanation of a personal God as the creator of the universe has to stand that test. If that God is outside of nature, having nothing to do with nature, and this nature is the outcome of the command of that God, produced from nothing, it becomes naturally, a very unscientific theory, and that has been the difficulty and the weak point of every theistic theory throughout the ages. These two defects we find therefore in what is generally called the theory of monotheism, the theory of a personal God, with all the qualities of a human being multiplied very much, and who, by his will, created this universe out of nothing, and yet is separate from it. This leads us into two difficulties.

As we have seen, it is not a sufficient generalization, and secondly it is not an explanation of nature from nature. It holds that the effect is not the cause, that the cause is entirely separate from the effect. Yet all the tendency of human knowledge shows that the effect is but the cause in another form. To this idea the discoveries in modern science are pointing every day, and the latest theory that has been granted on all sides is what we call the theory of evolution, the principle of which is that the effect is but the cause in another form, readjustment of the old cause, and the old cause takes the form of the effect. Creation out of nothing would be laughed at by modern scientific men.

Can religion stand these tests? If there be any religious theories which can stand these two tests they will be acceptable to the modern mind, to the thinking mind. Any other theory which we ask them to believe from the authority of priests, or churches, or books, the modern man is unable to accept, and the result is a hideous mass of unbelief. Even in those in whom there is an external display of belief, in their hearts there is a tremendous amount of unbelief. The rest give up religion, shrink away from it, as it were, do not want to touch it, regard it as priestcraft.

Religion has been reduced to a sort of national form. It is one of our very best social remnants; let it remain. But the real necessity which the grandfather of the modern man felt for it is gone. He no longer finds it satisfactory to his reason. The idea of such a personal God, and such a creation, the idea which is generally known as monotheism in every religion, cannot hold any longer. In India it could not hold its own because of the Buddhists, and that was the very point where the Buddhists gained their victory in ancient times. They showed that if nature is allowed its almost infinite power, and if nature can work out all its wants, it is simply unnecessary to insist that there is something beside nature. Even the soul is unnecessary. There was an old discussion, and you will sometimes find that old superstition living at the present day, the idea of substance and qualities.

Most of you have read how, during the middle ages, and, I am sorry to say, even much later, this was one of the questions of discussion, whether qualities inhered in substance, or substance in qualities; whether length and breadth and thickness form part of certain substances which we call dead matter, or if the substance remains whether the qualities are there or not. Now comes our

Buddhist, and he says you have no grounds to maintain the existence of such a substance, these qualities are all that exist. You do not see beyond them; and that is just the position of most of our modern agnostics. For, taking this fight of the substance and qualities upon a still higher plane is the fight between *noumenon* and *phenomenon*. There is this phenomenal world, the universe of continuous change, and there is something which does not change, and this duality of existence, noumenon and phenomenon, some hold is true, and others with better reason claim that you have no right to admit the two, for what we see, feel, and think is only the phenomenon. You have no right to assert there is anything beyond phenomena; and there is no answer at all. The only answer we get is from the monistic theory of the Vedânta, that it is true that only one exists, and that one is either phenomenon *or* noumenon. It is not true that there are two, something changing, and in and through that, something which does not change, but it is the one and the same thing which appears as changing, and which is in reality unchangeable.

To bring it to a concrete and philosophical conclusion, we have come to think of the body, and mind, and soul as many, but really there is only one; that one is appearing in all these various forms. Taking the well-known illustration of the monists, the rope appears as the snake. Some people mistake the rope for the snake, in the dark or through some other cause, but when knowledge comes, the snake vanishes and it is found to be a rope. By this illustration we see, that, when the snake exists in the mind, the rope has vanished, and when the rope exists, the snake has gone. When we see phenomena and phenomena only around us, the noumenon has vanished; but when we see the noumenon, the unchangeable, it naturally follows that the phenomena have vanished. We understand then better the position of both the realist and the idealist. The realist looks at phenomena only, and the idealist tries to look at the noumenon. For the idealist, the really genuine idealist, who has truly arrived at the power of perception, where he can get away from changes, for him the changeful universe has vanished, and he has the right to say it is all delusion, there was no change. The realist at the same time looks at the changeful. For him the unchangeable has vanished, and he has a right to say this is all real.

What is the outcome of this philosophy? It is that the personal idea of God is not sufficient. We have to get to something higher, to the impersonal idea. Not that the personal idea would be destroyed by that, not that we supply proof that the personal God does not exist, but it is the only logical step that we can take. Just as we say that man is a personal-impersonal being. We are the impersonal, at the same time that we are the personal. So our old idea of God must go, for it is only a repetition of the same idea on a higher plane, the anthropomorphic idea of God. To the impersonal we must go at last, therefore, for the explanation of the personal, for the impersonal is a much higher generalization than the personal. The Infinite can only be impersonal, the personal is limited. Thereby we preserve the personal and do not destroy it. Many times this doubt comes that if we arrive at the idea of the impersonal God the personal will be destroyed, if we arrive at the idea of the impersonal man the personal will be lost. But the idea is not the destruction of the individual, but its real preservation. We cannot prove the individual by any other means than by referring to the universal, by proving that this individual is really the universal. If we think of the individual as separate from everything else in the universe, it cannot stand a minute, such a thing never existed. Secondly, by the application of the second principle, that the explanation of everything must come out of the nature of the thing, we confront a still bolder idea, and one more difficult to understand. But it comes to nothing short of this, that the Impersonal Being, our highest generalization, is in ourselves, and we are That. "O Svetaketu, thou art That; thou art that Impersonal Being; that God for whom thou hast been searching all over the universe is all the time thyself"—not in the personal sense but in the impersonal sense. The man we know now, the manifested, is personalized, but the reality of this is the impersonal. To understand the personal we have to refer to the impersonal, the particular must be referred to the general, and that impersonal is the Truth, the Self of man, but this personalized manifestation is not referred to as that truth.

There will be various questions in connection with this, and I will try to answer them as we go on. Many difficulties will arise, but first let us clearly understand the position of monism.

That this universe which we see is all that exists; we need not seek elsewhere. Gross or fine it is all here: the effect and the cause are both here, the explanation is here. What is known as the particular is simply repetition in a minute form of the universal. We get our idea of the universe from the study of our own souls, and what is true there also holds good in the outside universe. The ideas of heaven and all these various places, even if they be true, are in the universe; they altogether make this unity. The first idea, therefore, is that of a whole, a unit, composed of various minute particles, and each one of us, as it were, is a part of this unit. As manifested beings we appear to be separate, but our reality is in that unit, and the less we think of ourselves as separate from that unit the better for us. The more we think of ourselves as separate from this whole the more miserable we become. From this principle we get the principle of monistic ethics, and I dare to say that we cannot get any ethics from anywhere else. We know that the oldest idea of ethics was the will of some particular being or beings, but few are ready to accept that now, because it would be only a partial generalization. The Hindûs say we must not do this, or that because the Vedas say so, but the Christian is not going to obey the authority of the Vedas. The Christian says you must do this and not do that because it is in the Bible. That will not be binding on those who do not believe in the Bible. But we must have a theory which is large enough to take in all these various grounds. Just as there are millions of people who are ready to believe in a personal Creator, there have also been thousands of the brightest minds in this world who felt that such ideas were not sufficient for them, and wanted something higher, and wherever religion was not broad enough to include all these minds the result was that the brightest minds in the society were always on the outside of religion, and never was this so marked as at the present time, especially in Europe.

To include these, therefore, religion must become broad enough. Everything it claims must be judged from the standpoint of reason. Why religions should claim that they are not bound to abide by the standpoint of reason no one knows. If one does not take the standard of reason there cannot be any true judgment, even in the case of religions. One religion may ordain something very hideous. For instance, the Mohammedan religion allows all who are not Mohammedans to be killed. It is clearly stated in the Koran, kill the infidels if they do not become Mohammedans. They must be put to fire and sword. Now if you tell a Mohammedan that this is wrong, he will naturally ask: "How do you know that? How do you know it is not good? Because your ideas of good and bad are from your books? My book says it is good." If you say your book is older, there will come the Buddhist, who says: "My book is much older still." Then there will come the Hindû, who says: "My books are the oldest of all." Therefore referring to books will not do. Where is the standard by which you can compare? You will say, look at the Sermon on the Mount, and the Mohammedan will reply, look at the Ethics of the Koran. The Mohammedan will say, who is the arbiter as to which is better of the two? Neither the New Testament nor the Koran can be the arbiter in a quarrel between them. There must be some independent authority, and that cannot be any book, but something which is universal; and what is more universal than reason? It has been said that reason is not strong enough; it does not always help us to get the Truth; many times it makes mistakes, and therefore the conclusion was, that we must believe in the authority of a church. That was said by a Roman Catholic, but I could not see the logic of it. On the other hand, if I have to state a proposition, I should say if reason be so weak, a body of priests would be weaker, and I am not going to accept their verdict, but I will yield to reason, because with all its weakness there is some chance of getting truth, while by the other means I should not get any truth.

We have to follow reason, therefore, and we have to sympathize with those who do not come to any sort of belief following reason. For it is better that mankind should become atheists by following reason, than believe in two hundred millions of gods by following anybody. What we want is progress, development, realization. No theories ever made men higher. No amount of books can help us to become purer.

The only power that lies in ourselves is in realization, and that comes from thinking. Let men think. A clod of earth never thinks; you may take it for granted that a clod of earth believes in everything, but it is only a lump of earth. The glory of man is that he is a thinking being. It is the nature of man that he differs therein from animals, and therefore man must think. I believe in reason and follow reason, having seen enough of the evils of authority, for I was born in a country where they have gone to the extreme of authority.

The Hindûs believe that creation has come out of their book.

How do you know there is a cow? Because the word cow is in the Vedas. How do you know there is a man outside? Because the word man is there. If it had not been there would have been no man outside. That is what they say. Authority with a vengeance! And it is not studied as I have studied it now, but some of the most powerful minds have taken it up and spun out some most wonderful logical theories round it. They have argued it out and there it stands, a whole system of philosophy, and thousands of the brightest intellects have been dedicated through thousands of years to the working out of this theory. Such has been the power of authority, and great are the dangers thereof! It stunts the growth of humanity, and we must not forget that we want growth. Even in all relative truth, more than the truth itself we want the exercise. That is our life.

The monistic theory has this merit, that it is the nearest to a demonstrable truth in theology that we can get. The idea of the Impersonal, and that nature is the evolution of that Impersonal, is the nearest that we can get to any truth that is demonstrable, and every other idea, every conception of God which is partial and little and personal is not rational. And it has this glory, that this rational conception of God proves that these partial conceptions which we see are yet necessary for many. For that is the only argument in their favor. You sometimes see people who say this personal explanation is irrational, but it is comfortable; they want a comfortable religion and we understand that it is necessary for them. The clear light of truth very few in this life can bear, much less work upon. It is necessary, therefore, that this comfortable religion should be there; it helps many souls, in time, to a better. The little mind whose circumference is very limited and requires little things to build it up, never dares to soar in thought. Their conceptions are very good and helpful, even of little gods and symbols and ideals, but you have to understand the impersonal, for it is in and through that alone that these others can be made helpful and good.

For instance, the man who understands and believes in the impersonal—John Stuart Mill, for example—says the personal God is impossible, cannot be proved. I admit with him, that it cannot be demonstrated, but it is the highest reading of the Absolute that can be reached by the human intellect, and what else is the universe but various readings of the Absolute. It is like a book before us, and each one has brought his intellect to read the book, and each one has to read it for himself. There is something which is similar in the intellect of all men, therefore certain things are common to the intellect of mankind. That you and I see a chair proves that there is something common to both our minds. Suppose a being comes with another sense; he will not see the chair at all, but all beings similarly constituted will see the same things. Thus this universe itself is the Absolute, the unchangeable, the noumenon, and the phenomena constitute the reading thereof. For you will first find that all phenomena are finite. Every phenomenon that we can see, feel, or think of, is finite, limited by our knowledge; and a personal God as we conceive of Him is in fact a phenomenon. The very idea of causation exists only in the phenomenal world, and God, as the cause of this universe, must naturally be thought of as limited, and yet He is the same impersonal God.

This very universe, as we have seen, is the same Impersonal Being read by our intellect. Whatever is reality in the universe is that Impersonal Being, and the forms and conceptions are given to It by our intellects. Whatever is real in this table is that Being, and the table form and all other forms are given by the intellects of men.

Now, motion, for instance, which is a necessary adjunct of the phenomenal, cannot be spoken of the universal. Every little bit, every atom inside the universe, is in a constant state of change and motion, but the universe as a whole is unchangeable, because motion or change is a relative thing, we can only think of something in motion in comparison to something not in motion. There must be two in order to understand motion. The whole mass of the universe, taken as a unit, cannot move. In regard to what will it move? It cannot be said to change. With regard to what will it change? So the whole is the Absolute, but within it every particle is in a constant state of flux and change. It is unchangeable and changeable at the same time, impersonal and personal in one. This is our conception of the universe, of motion and of God, and that is what is meant by "*Thou art That.*" For we must know our own nature.

The finite, manifested man forgets his origin, like the water that comes from the ocean forgetting its origin and thinking itself to be entirely separate. So we, as personalized beings, little, differentiated beings, forget our reality, and what is meant by the teaching of monism is not that we must give up these differentiations, but that we must learn to understand what they are. We, that infinite Being, that very Soul, are like the water, and this water starts and has its being from, and is really the ocean, not a part, but the whole of the ocean, for the infinite mass of energy which exists is yours and mine, because you and I, and every being, represent so many channels, so many paths, through which this Infinite Reality is manifesting Itself, and the whole mass of changes which we call evolution is the soul manifesting all this infinite energy, and we cannot stop anywhere on this side of the Infinite. Our power, and blessedness, and wisdom, cannot stop anywhere this side of the Infinite. Infinite power and existence and blessedness are ours, not that we will acquire them, but they are our own; we have to manifest them.

This is one great idea that comes from monism, and one that is very hard to understand. I find in myself how from childhood everyone around teaches weakness, how I have been told since I was born that I was a weak thing. It is very hard for me now to understand my own strength, but by analysis and reasoning I see I must simply gain knowledge of my own strength, must realize it. All the knowledge that we have in this world, where did it come from? It is in us. What knowledge is outside? Show me one bit. Knowledge was not in matter; it was in man all the time. Nobody ever created knowledge; man discovers it, brings it from within. It is lying there. The whole of that big banyan tree, which covers miles of ground perhaps, was in the little seed, like one-eighth of a mustard seed—that mass of energy was there confined. The gigantic intellect we know can lie coiled up in the protoplasmic cell, and why not infinite energy? We know that it is so. It may seem like a paradox, but it is true. All of us have come out of one protoplasmic cell, and all the little powers we have were coiled up there. You cannot say it was acquired by food; for build up food mountains high and see what power comes out. The energy was there; potentially, but still there, and so is infinite power in the soul of man, if man never knows it. It is only a question of being conscious of it. Slowly this infinite giant is, as it were, arousing himself, waking up, and becoming conscious of his power, and the more he is becoming conscious the more bonds are breaking, chains are snapping all around, and there must come a day when infinite consciousness is regained; with power and wisdom this giant will stand erect. Let us all help to bring that about.

XV. PRACTICAL VEDÂNTA. PART IV.

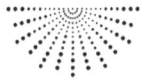

We have been dealing more with the universal so far. This morning I will try to bring before you the Vedantic ideas of the relation of the particular to the universal. As we have seen in the dualistic form of Vedic doctrines, the earlier forms, there was a clearly defined particular and limited soul for every being. There have been a great many theories about this particular soul in each individual, but the main discussion was between the ancient Buddhists and the ancient Vedantists, the one believing in the individual soul complete in itself? the other denying *in toto* the existence of such an individual soul. As I told you the other day, it is pretty much the same discussion you had in Europe as to substance and quality, one set holding that behind the qualities there is something as substance, in which the qualities inhere, and the other denying the existence of such a substance as being unnecessary; the qualities may live by themselves. The most ancient theory of the soul, of course, is based upon the argument from self-identity—"I am I"—that the "I" of yesterday is the "I" of to-day, and the "I" of to-day will be the "I" of to-morrow, that in spite of all the changes that are happening to the body, I yet believe that I am the same "I." This seems to have been the central argument with those who believed in a limited, and yet perfectly complete, individual soul.

On the other hand, the ancient Buddhists denied the necessity of such an assumption. They brought forward the argument that all that we know, and all that we possibly can know, are simply these changes. The positing of an unchangeable and unchanging substance is simply superfluous, and then, if there were any such unchangeable thing, we could never understand it, nor should we ever be able to cognize it in any sense of the word. The same discussion you will find at the present time going on in Europe between the religionists and the idealists on the one side, and the modern positivists and agnostics on the other; one set believing there is something which does not change—of whom the latest representative has been your Herbert Spencer—that we catch a glimpse of something which is, as it were, unchangeable. And the other is represented by the modern Comtists and modern Agnostics. Those of you who were interested a few years ago in the discussions between Mr. Harrison and Mr. Herbert Spencer, may have found out that it is the same old difficulty, the one party standing for a substance behind the changeful, and the other party denying the necessity for such an assumption. One party says, we cannot conceive of changes without conceiving of something which does not change, the other party brings out the argument that this is superfluous; we can only conceive of something which is changing. As to the unchanging, we can neither know, feel, nor sense it.

The great question in India did not find its solution in the very ancient times, because we have seen that the assumption of a substance which is behind the qualities, and which is not the qualities, can never be substantiated; nay, even the argument from self-identity, from memory, that I am the "I" of yesterday because I remember it, and therefore I have been a continuous something—cannot be substantiated. The other quibble that is generally put forward is a mere delusion of words. For instance, a man may take a long series of such sentences as "I do," "I go," "I dream," "I sleep," "I move," and here you will find it claimed that the doing, going and dreaming, etc., have been changing, but what remained constant was that "I." As such they conclude that the "I" is something which is constant, and an individual in itself, but all these changes belong to the body. This, though apparently very convincing and clear, is based upon word punning. The "I" and the doing, going and dreaming, may be separate in black and white, and on a piece of paper, but no one can separate them in his mind.

When I eat I think of myself as eating—I am identified with eating. When I run I and the running are not two separate things. Thus the argument from personal identity does not seem to be very strong. The other argument, from memory, is also weak. If the identity of my being is represented by my memory, many things which I have forgotten are lost from that identity. And we know that people under certain conditions will forget their whole past. In many cases of lunacy a man will think of himself as made of glass, or as being an animal. If the existence of that man depends on memory he has become glass, which not being the case we cannot make the identity of the self depend on such a flimsy argument as memory. What remains? That on the side of the soul, limited, yet complete and continuing, its identity cannot be established as separate from the qualities. We cannot establish a narrowed down, limited existence behind which there is a bunch of qualities.

On the other hand, the argument of the ancient Buddhists seems to be stronger—that we do not know, and cannot know, anything that is beyond the bunch of qualities. According to them the soul consists of a bundle of qualities called sensations and feelings. A mass of such is what is called the soul, and this mass is continually changing. The Advaitist theory of the soul reconciles both these positions.

The position of the Advaitist is that it is true that we cannot think of the substance as separate from the qualities; at the same time we cannot think of change and not change; it would be impossible; but the very thing which is substance is the same which is the quality. Substance and quality are not two. It is the unchangeable that is appearing as the changeable.

The unchangeable substance of the universe is not something separate from this changeful universe. The noumenon is not something different from the phenomena, but it is the very noumenon which has become the phenomena. There is a soul which is unchanging, and what we call feelings and perceptions, nay, even the body, is the very same soul seen from another point of view. We have got into the habit of thinking that we have bodies and souls and so forth, but really speaking we can only have one, not two even.

When I think of myself as a body I am a body alone; it is useless to say I am something else. And when I think of myself as the soul the body vanishes, perception of the body does not remain. None can get the perception of the Self without his perception of the body having vanished, none can get perception of the substance without his perception of the qualities vanishing.

The ancient illustration of the Advaita, the rope taken for a snake, may be brought in here to illustrate a little further that when a man mistakes the rope for a snake the rope has vanished, and when he takes it for a rope the snake has vanished, and the rope remains. These ideas that we have of dual existence and treble existence come from analysis, and after analysis they are written in books, and we read those books or hear about them, until we come under the delusion that we really have a dual perception of the soul and the body, but such a perception never really exists. The perception is either for body or for soul. It requires no other arguments. You can verify it in your own minds.

Try to think of yourself as a soul, as a disembodied something. You will find it is almost impossible, and those few who find it possible will find that at the time when they realize themselves as soul they have no idea of body. You have heard, or have seen, perhaps, some persons who had been at certain times in peculiar states of mind, brought about either by hypnotism or some hysterical disease, or drugs. From their experience you may gather that when they were perceiving the internal something, the external had vanished for them; it did not remain. This shows that whatever exists is one. That one is appearing in these various forms, and all these various forms give rise to the relation of cause and effect. The relation of cause and effect is one of evolution—the one becomes the other, and so on. The cause, as it were, sometimes vanishes, and in its place leaves the effect. If the soul is the cause of the body, the soul, as it were, vanishes for the time being, and the body remains, and when the body vanishes the soul remains.

This theory would meet the arguments of the Buddhists, the arguments that were levelled against the assumption of the dualism of body and soul, by denying the duality, and showing that the substance and the qualities are one and the same thing, appearing in various forms.

We have seen also that this idea of the unchangeable can only be established as regards the whole, but never as regards the part. The very idea of part comes from the idea of change, of motion. Everything that is limited we can understand and know because it is changeable, and the whole must be unchangeable because it cannot change—there is no other thing besides it. Change is always in regard to something which does not change, or which changes relatively less.

According to Advaita, therefore, the idea of the soul as universal, unchangeable and immortal, can be as far as possible demonstrated. The difficulty would be as regards the particular. What shall we do with the old dualistic theories which have got such a hold on us, which we have all to pass through, these beliefs in limited, little, individual souls?

We have seen that we are immortal with regard to the whole, but the difficulty is, we desire so much to be immortal with regard to the parts of us. We have seen that we are infinite, and that that is our real individuality. But we want so much to make these little souls individual! What becomes of them when we find in our everyday experience that these little souls are continuously growing and cannot really be individual? They are the same yet not the same. The "I" of yesterday is the "I" of to-day, and yet not. It is changed somewhat, and if we take the most modern of conceptions, that of evolution for instance, we find that the "I" is a continuously changing, expanding identity.

If it be true that man is the evolution of a mollusc, the mollusc individual is the same as the man, only it has to become expanded a great deal. From mollusc to man has been a continuous expansion towards the state of infinity. Therefore the limited soul can be styled an individual which is continuously expanding towards *the* Individual. Perfect individuality will only be reached when it has reached the Infinite, but on this side of the Infinite it is a continuously changing, growing personality.

The Advaitist system of the Vedânta has one peculiar tendency, the tendency to harmonize the preceding systems. In many cases it was very helpful; in others it hurt the philosophy.

They had the same idea that is called the theory of evolution in modern times, that all is growth, step by step, and this instrument in their hands made it easy for them to harmonize all preceding systems. Thus not one of these preceding ideas was rejected. The fault of the Buddhistic ideas was that they had neither the faculty nor the perception of this continual expansive growth, and for this reason, they never even made an attempt to harmonize their system with the pre-existing steps towards the ideal. They rejected all of them as useless and harmful.

You will find this tendency is a most harmful one in religion.

A man gets a new and better idea, and then he looks back on those he has given up, and forthwith decides that they were mischievous and unnecessary. He never thinks that however crude they may appear from his present point of view, they were very useful to him, that it was necessary for him to reach his present state through these ideas, and that every one of us has to grow in a similar fashion, living first in crude ideas, taking benefit from them, and so arriving at a higher standard. To the oldest theories, therefore, the Advaita is friendly. Dualism, and all theories that had preceded it, are accepted by the Advaita, not in a patronizing way, but with the conviction that they are truths, manifestations of the same truth; and that they have all to rise to the same conclusions that the Advaita has reached.

With words of blessing, and not of cursing, are to be preserved all these various steps through which humanity had to pass. Therefore all these dualistic systems have been kept intact in the Vedânta, and never rejected or thrown out, and the dualistic conception of an individual soul, limited, yet complete in itself, finds a place in the Vedânta. According to this conception the man dies and goes to other worlds, and so forth, and these ideas are also kept in their entirety, because with this recognition of growth behind the Advaitist system anyone of these theories can be kept in its proper place, by understanding that they represent only a partial view of the truth.

If you regard the universe from a certain point of view from which you can only look at one part, this is the way in which the universe presents itself to the mind. From the dualistic standpoint this universe can only be looked upon as a creation of matter or force, can only be looked upon as the play of a certain will, and that will again can only be looked upon as separate from the universe; thus a man from such a standpoint has to see himself as composed of a dual nature, of the body and soul, and this soul, though limited, appears individually complete in itself. Such a man's ideas of immortality and of the future life would be applied to this soul. These phases of thought have been kept in the Vedânta, and it is necessary, therefore, for me to present to you a few of the popular ideas of dualism. According to this theory we have a body, of course. Behind the body there is what they call a fine body. This fine body is also made up of materials, only very fine. It is the receptacle of all our *karma*, of all our actions; the impressions of all actions live there in that fine body, ready to spring up. Every thought that we think, every deed that we do, after a certain time becomes fine, goes into seed form, so to speak; that lives in the fine body in a potential form, and after a time it emerges again and bears its results. These results condition the life of man; thus he has moulded his own life. It is not that man is bound by any laws excepting those he makes for himself. Our works, our thoughts, our deeds, are but threads in the net which we throw round ourselves for good or for evil. Once we set in motion a certain power, we have to bear the full consequences of it. This is the law of *Karma*. Behind the subtle body lives the *jîva*, or individual soul of man. There are various discussions about the size, or the form, or the non-form, of this individual soul. According to some it is very small, like an atom; according to others it is not so small as that; according to others it is very big, and so on. This *jîva* is a part of the universal substance, and it also is eternal; without beginning it is existing as a part of the whole; it will exist without end, and it is passing through all these forms in order to manifest its real nature as purity. Every action that retards this manifestation is called an evil action; so with thoughts. And every action and every thought that helps the *jîva* to expand, to manifest its real nature, is a good action. One theory is common in India with the crudest dualists and the most advanced non-dualists—that all the possibilities and powers of the soul are always in it, and will not come from any external source. They are in the soul in potential form, and the whole work of life, or lives, is simply directed to manifesting those potentialities.

They have also the doctrine of reincarnation, that after this body has been dissolved, the *jîva* will have another body, and after that has been dissolved it will have another body, and so on, either here or in some other worlds; but this world is given the preference; it is considered as the best of worlds for all our purposes. Other worlds are conceived of as worlds where there is very little misery, but for that very reason they argue that there is less chance there of thinking of higher things. This world being nicely balanced, a good deal of misery, and some happiness, too, the *jîva* sometime or other gets awakened, as it were, and thinks of freeing itself. But just as very rich persons in this world have the least chance of thinking of higher things, so if the *jîva* goes to heaven it will have no chance, but only the same position intensified, having a very fine body which thinks of no disease, being without the necessity of eating, or drinking, and having all its desires fulfilled. The *jîva* goes there, with enjoyment after enjoyment, and forgets all its real nature. Still there are some higher worlds, where, in spite of all these enjoyments, further evolution is possible. Some dualists conceive of the goal to be reached as the highest heaven, where souls will go and live with God forever. They will have beautiful bodies there, and will know no more disease or death, or any sort of evil. They will have all their desires fulfilled, and live with God forever, and from time to time some of them will come back to this earth and take another body to teach human beings the way, and the great teachers of the world have been such. They have been already free, and were living with God in that sphere, but their mercy for suffering humanity here was very great, so they came and incarnated again, and preached unto mankind the way to heaven.

Of course we know that the Advaita holds that this cannot be the goal or the ideal; bodilessness must be the ideal. The ideal cannot be finite. Anything short of the Infinite cannot be the ideal, and there cannot be an infinite body. That would be impossible, as body comes from limitation. There cannot be infinite thought, because thought comes from limitation. We have to go beyond the body, and beyond thought too, says the Advaita. And we have also seen the other peculiar Advaitist position, that this freedom is not to be attained, it already *is*. We only forget it and deny it. This perfection is not to be attained, it already exists. This immortality and unchangeableness are not to be attained; they already exist. We have them all the time. If you dare declare of yourself that you are free, free you are this moment. If you say you are bound, bound you will remain. However, the dualists and others have these ideas. You can take up whichever you like.

This highest ideal of the Vedânta is very difficult to understand, and people are always quarrelling about it, and the greatest difficulty is that when they get hold of one set of these ideas they want to deny and fight the other sets. Take up what you are fit for, and let others take up what they are fit for. If you are desirous of clinging to this little individuality, to this limited manhood, you will have to remain in it, you will have these lower ideals, and be content and pleased with them. If your experience of manhood has been very good and nice, retain it as long as you like, for you know you are the makers of your own fortunes; none can compel you. You will be men as long as you like; none can deter you. If you want to be angels, you will be angels; that is the law. But there may be others who do not like to be angels even. What right have you to tell them that they must be? You may be frightened to lose a hundred pounds; there may be others who would not wink a bit if they lost all the money in the world. There have been such, and are still such. Why do you dare to judge them according to your standard? You cling on to your limitations, and these little worldly ideas may be your highest ideal. You are welcome. It will be to you as you wish. But there are others who have seen the truth, finished all this, and cannot rest in these limitations, who want to rush outside, and whom nothing in this world satisfies. The world with all its enjoyments is a mere mud puddle for them. Why do you want to bind them down to your ideas? You must get rid of this once for all. Give place to every one.

I once read a certain story of how some ships were caught in a cyclone in the South Sea Islands, and there was a picture in the *Illustrated London News*. All were wrecked except one, an English vessel which weathered the storm, and the picture showed those men who were getting drowned standing up on the decks and cheering the people who were sailing through the storm.[1] Be brave like that and do not try to drag others down to where you are. There is another foolish notion going on—if we are to lose our little individuality, there will be no morality, no hope for humanity. As if everybody had been dying for humanity all the time! God bless you, if in every country there were two hundred men and women really wanting to do good to humanity, the millennium would come in five days. We know how we are dying for humanity. These are tall talks and nothing else. But the history of the world shows that those who never thought of this little individuality were the greatest benefactors of the human race, and the more men and women think of themselves the less were they able to do for others. One is selfishness, the other unselfishness, clinging on to their little enjoyments, and to desire the continuation and repetition of this state of things is utter selfishness. It arises not from any desire for truth, its genesis is not kindness for other beings, but in the utter selfishness of the human heart, in this idea of "I will have everything," without caring for anyone else. This is as it appears to me. I would like to see in the world more moral men like some of those grand old prophets and sages of ancient times who would have given up a hundred lives if they could by so doing benefit one little animal! Talk of morality and doing good to others! Silly talk of the present time!

I would like to see moral men like Gautama Buddha, who did not believe in a personal God, or a personal soul, never questioned, never asked, stood there a perfect agnostic, and yet a man ready to lay down his life for anyone, and who worked all his life for the good of all, and thought only of that. Well has it been said by his biographer, describing his birth, he was born for the good of many, for a blessing to many. He never even went to the forest to meditate for his own salvation. He felt that the world was burning; some one must find a way out. Why is there so much misery was the one thought that dominated his whole life. Do you think we are so moral as that?

The more immoral is the man, the more immoral is the race, the more selfish it is. That race which is bound down to itself has been the most cruel and the most wicked in the whole world. There has not been a religion that has clung on to this dualism more than that founded by the Prophet of Arabia or which has shed so much blood and been so cruel to other beings. In the Koran there is a doctrine that a man who does not believe these teachings should be killed; it is a mercy to kill him! And the surest way to get to heaven, where there are beautiful houris, and all sorts of sense enjoyments, is by killing these unbelievers. Think of how much bloodshed there has been in consequence of such beliefs!

In the Religion of Christ there was little of crudeness, very little of difference between the pure religion of Christ and of the Vedânta. You find there the idea of oneness preached, and Christ also takes up the dualistic ideas in order to please the people, give them something to take hold of in order to come up to the highest ideal. The same prophet who preached "Our Father which art in heaven," also preached, "I and my Father are one," and the same prophet knew that through the Father in heaven lies the way to the "I and my Father are one." There was only blessing and love in the religion of Christ, but as soon as crudeness came, it was degraded into something not much better than the religion of the Prophet of Arabia. It came out of crudeness, this fight for the little self, clinging on to this "I" not only in the passage through this life, but also in the desire to continue it even after death. This they declare is unselfishness; this is the foundation of morality. Lord help us all, if this be the foundation of morality! Selfishness is made the foundation of morality, and men and women who ought to know better stand aghast, think all morality will be destroyed, if these little selves go. The watchword of all well-being, of moral good, is not I, but thou. Who cares whether there is such a thing as heaven or hell, who cares if there be a soul or not, who cares if there be an unchangeable or not? Here is the world, and it is full of misery. Come out into it as Buddha came and struggle to lessen it or die in the attempt. Forget yourselves; this is the first lesson to be learned, whether you are a theist or an atheist, whether you are an agnostic or a Vedantist, a Christian or a Mohammedan: The one lesson obvious to all is destruction of the little self and building up of the Real Self.

Two forces have been working side by side in parallel lines.

The one says "I," the other says "not I." Their manifestation is not only in man but in animals, not only in animals but in the lowest of worms. The tigress that plunges her fangs into the red hot blood of a human being, would give up her life to protect her young. The most depraved of men, who thinks nothing of taking the lives of his brother men, will perhaps do anything to save his starving wife or his little children. Thus throughout creation these two forces are working side by side, where you find the one you find the other. The one is selfishness, the other is unselfishness. The one is assumption, the other is renunciation. The one takes, the other gives up everything. From the lowest to the highest, the whole universe is the playground of these two forces. This does not require any demonstration; it is obvious to all.

What right has one section of the community to base the whole work and evolution of the universe upon one of these two, upon competition and struggle? What right has it to base the whole working of the universe upon passion, and fight, and quarrel, and struggle? That these exist we do not deny; but what right has anyone to deny the working of the other force?

Can men deny that this love, this "not I," this renunciation, is the only positive power in the universe? The other is misguided employment of the same power of love; the power of love brought competition also. The real genesis of the competition was in love. The real genesis of even evil was in unselfishness. The creator of evil is good, and the end is also good. It is only misdirection of the power of good. A man who murders another man is moved to do it perhaps, by the love of his own child. His love had become limited, and had come down to that one little baby, and been taken off from the millions of other people in the universe. Yet, limited or unlimited, it is the same love.

Thus the motive power of the whole universe, in whatever way it manifests itself, is that one wonderful thing, unselfishness, renunciation, love, the real, the only living force in existence. Therefore the Vedantist insists upon that oneness and not duality. We insist upon this explanation because we cannot admit two causes of the universe. If we simply hold that by limitation the same unit, beautiful wonderful love appears to be evil or vile, we find the whole universe explained by the one force of love. If not, two causes of the universe have to be taken for granted, one good and one evil; two forces—one love and the other hatred. Which is more logical? Certainly the one.

I have been going into things which do not belong to the dualists possibly. I cannot stand long with the dualists, I am afraid. My idea is to show that the highest ideal of morality and unselfishness goes hand in hand with the highest metaphysical conception; that you need not lower your conception to get ethics and morality; on the other hand, to reach a real basis of morality and ethics you must have the highest philosophical and scientific conceptions. Human knowledge is not antagonistic to human well-being. On the other hand, it is knowledge alone that will save us in every department of life—in knowledge is worship. The more we know the better. As the Vedantist says, the cause of all that is apparently evil is the limitation of the Unlimited. The love which gets limited into little channels and seems to be evil, eventually comes out at the other end and manifests God. And the Vedânta says that the cause of all this apparent evil is in ourselves; do not blame any supernatural being, neither be hopeless and despondent, nor think we are in a place from which we can never escape until some one comes and lends us a helping hand. That cannot be, says the Vedânta; we are like silkworms. We make the thread out of our own substance, and spin the cocoon, and in course of time are bound inside. But not forever. In that cocoon we have to develop spiritual realization and, like the butterfly, come out free. This network of *karma* we have thrown around ourselves; in our ignorance we feel as if we were bound, and sometimes weep and wail for help. But help does not come from without; it comes from within ourselves. Cry to all the gods in the universe. I cried for years, and in the end I found that I was helped; but help came from within. And I had to undo what I had done by mistake. That is the only way. I had to cut the net which I had thrown round myself, and the power to do this is within. Of this I am certain, that not one aspiration, well-guided or ill-guided, in my life has been in vain, but I am the resultant of all my past good and evil both. I have committed many mistakes in my life, but mark you, I am sure of this, without every one of those mistakes I would not be what I am to-day, and I am quite satisfied to have made them. I do not mean that you are to go home and commit mistakes; do not misunderstand me that way. But do not mope because of some mistakes you have committed, but know that in the end they will all come out straight. It cannot be otherwise, because goodness is our nature, purity is our nature, and that nature can never be destroyed. Our essential nature always remains the same.

What we are to understand is this, that what we call mistakes, or evil, we commit because we are weak, and we are weak because we are ignorant. I prefer to call them mistakes. The word sin, although originally a very good word, has got a certain flavor around it that frightens me. Who makes us ignorant? We ourselves. We throw our hands before our eyes and weep that it is dark. Take the hands off and the light exists always for us, the self-effulgent nature of the human soul. Do you not see what your modern scientific men say? What is the cause of all this evolution? Desire. The animal wants to do something else, but does not find the environment satisfactory, and therefore manufactures a new body. Who manufactures? He himself, his will. You have developed from the lowest amœba. Exercise that will and it will take you higher still. The will is almighty. If it is almighty you will say, why cannot I do many things? But you are thinking only of your little self. Look back on yourselves from the state of the amœba to the human being; who made all that? Your own will. Can you deny then that it is almighty? That which has made you come up so high can make you go higher still. What we want is character, strengthening this will, and not weakening it.

If I teach you, therefore, that your nature is evil, and tell you to go home in sackcloth and ashes and weep your lives out because you made certain false steps it will not help you, but will weaken you all the more, and I shall be showing you the road to more evil than good. If this room were full of darkness for thousands of years and you come in and begin to weep and wail "Oh, the darkness," will the darkness vanish? Bring the light in, strike a match and light comes in a moment. So what good will it do you to think all your lives "Oh, I have done evil, I have made many mistakes?" It requires no ghost to tell us that! Bring in the light and the evil goes in a moment. Strengthen the real nature, build up yourselves, the effulgent, the resplendent, the ever pure, call that up in every one that you see. I wish that every one of us had come to such a state that even when we see the vilest of human beings we could see the real Self within, and instead of condemning, say "Rise, thou effulgent one, rise thou who art always pure, rise thou birthless and deathless, rise almighty, and manifest your true nature. These little manifestations do not befit thee." This is the highest prayer that the Advaita teaches. This is the one prayer, to remember our nature, the God Who is always within us, thinking of Him always as the Infinite, the Almighty, the ever good, the ever beneficent, the selfless, bereft of all this little self, little limitations, and because that nature is selfless, it is strong and fearless; only to selfishness comes fear. He who has nothing to desire for himself whom does he fear, what can frighten him? What fear has death for him? What fear has evil for him? So we must think, if we are Advaitists, that we are dead and gone from this moment. The old Mr., Mrs. or Miss So-and-So is gone, mere superstition, and what remains is the ever pure, the ever strong, the almighty, the all-knowing—that remains for us, and then all fear has vanished from us. Who can injure us, the omnipresent? Thus all weakness has vanished from us, and our only work is to rouse this knowledge in our fellow beings. We see that they too are the same pure self, only they do not know it; we must teach them, we must help them to rouse up the infinite nature in each. This is what I feel is absolutely necessary over the whole world. These doctrines are old, older than many mountains possibly. All truth is eternal. Truth is nobody's property; no race, no individual can lay any claim to truth. Truth is the nature of all souls. Who lays any special claim to it? But it has to be made practical, to be made simple, for the highest truths are the simplest of all. It must be made thoroughly simple, so that it may penetrate every pore of human society, that it may become the property of the highest intellects and the commonest minds; of the child, the woman, and the man at the same time. All these ratiocinations of logic, all these bundles of metaphysics, all these theologies and ceremonies, may have been good in their own time, but let us try to make things simpler and bring about the golden days when every man is a worshipper, and the Reality in every man is the object of worship.

---

1. H. M. S. Calliope and the American men-of-war at Samoa.—Ed.

XVI. VEDÂNTA IN ALL ITS PHASES.

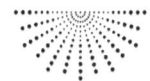

(Lecture delivered at Calcutta.)

Far back where no recorded history, nor even the dim light of tradition can penetrate, has been steadily shining a light, sometimes dimmed by external circumstances, at others effulgent, but undying and steady—a light shining not only over India, but permeating the whole thought-world with its power, silent, gentle, yet omnipotent; unperceived like the dew that falls in the evening unseen and unnoticed, yet bringing into bloom the fairest of roses—this light has been the thought of the Upanishads, the philosophy of the Vedânta. Nobody knows when it first came to flourish on the soil of India. Guessworks have been vain. The guesses, especially of the Western writers, have been so conflicting that no certain date can be ascribed to them. But we Hindus, from the spiritual standpoint, do not admit that they had any origin. This Vedânta, the philosophy of the Upanishads, I would make bold to state, has been the first as well as the final thought that on the spiritual plane has ever been vouchsafed to man. From this light have been going westward and eastward, from time to time, waves from the ocean of Vedânta. In the days of yore it traveled westward and gave its impetus to the minds of the Greeks, either in Athens, or in Alexandria, or in Antioch. The Sânkhya system clearly must have made its mark on the minds of the ancient Greeks: and the Sânkhya, and all other systems in India, had that one authority, the Upanishads, the Vedânta. In India, too, the one authority, the basis of all religious and philosophical systems, has yet been the Upanishads, the Vedânta. Whether you are a monist, or a qualified monist; an Advaitin or Dvaitin, or whatever you may call yourself, there stand behind you as your authority, your *Shâstras*, your Scriptures, the Upanishads. Whatever system in India does not obey the Upanishads cannot be called orthodox, and even the systems of the Jains and the Buddhists have been rejected from the soil of India only because they did not bear allegiance to the Upanishads. Thus, the Vedânta, whether we know it or not, has penetrated all the sects in India, and what we call Hinduism, this mighty banyan with its immense, almost infinite ramifications, has been throughout interpenetrated by the influence of the Vedânta. Whether we are conscious of it or not, we think the Vedânta, we live in the Vedânta, we breathe the Vedânta, and we die in the Vedânta, and every Hindu does that. To preach Vedânta in the land of India, and before an Indian audience, seems therefore to be an anomaly. But it is the one thing that has got to be preached, and it is the necessity of the age that it shall be preached. As I have just told you, all the Indian sects must bear allegiance to the Upanishads, but among these sects, there are many apparent contradictions. Many times the great sages of yore could not themselves understand the underlying harmony of the Upanishads. Many times even sages quarreled, and so much so that at times it became a proverb: "They are not sages who do not differ." But the time requires that a better interpretation should be given to this underlying harmony of the Upanishadic texts, whether they are dualistic, non-dualistic, or quasi-dualistic. It has to be shown before the world at large, and this work is necessary as much in India as outside of India, and I, through the grace of God, had the great good fortune to sit at the feet of one whose whole life was such an interpretation—whose life, a thousandfold more than whose teaching, was a living commentary on the texts of the Upanishads, was in fact, the *spirit* of the Upanishads living in a human form. Perhaps, I have got a little of that harmony, I do not know whether I shall be able to express it or not, but this is my attempt, my mission in life, to show that the Vedantic schools are not contradictory, that they all necessitate each other, and one, as it were, is the stepping-stone to the other, until the goal, the Advaita, is reached (the *Tat Tvam asi*). There was a time in India when the *Karma Kânda* had its sway. There have been many grand ideals, no doubt, in that portion of the Vedas. Some of our present daily worship is still according to the precepts of the *Karma Kânda*. But with all that, the *Karma Kânda* of the Vedas has almost disappeared from India. Very little of our life at the present day is bound or regulated by the orders of the *Karma Kânda* of the Vedas. In our ordinary lives, we are mostly *Paurânics* or *Tantrics*, and even where some Vedic texts are used by the Brahmins of India, the adjustment of the texts is not according to the Vedas mostly, but according to the *Tântras* or the *Purânas*. As such, to call ourselves Vaidics in the sense of following the *Karma Kânda* of the Vedas, I do not think, would be proper. But the other fact stands that we are all of us Vedântins. The people who call themselves Hindus, had better be called Vedântins, and as I have shown you just now, under that one name *Vaidântika* come all our various sects, either dualist or non-dualist.

The sects that are at the present time in India, may in general be divided into the two great classes of dualists and monists. The little differences, which some of these sects insist upon, and upon the authority of which they want to take new names, as pure Advaitins or qualified Advaitins, and so forth, do not matter much. As a classification, either they are dualists or monists, and of the sects existing at the present time, some are very new, and others seem to be reproductions of very ancient sects. The one class I would represent by the life and philosophy of Râmânuja, and the other by Sankarâchârya. Râmânuja is the leading dualistic philosopher of later India, whom all the other dualistic sects have followed directly or indirectly, both in the substance of their teaching, as well as in the organization of their sects, even down to some of the most minute points. You will be astonished if you compare Râmânuja and his works with the other dualistic *Vaishnava* sects in India, to find how much they resemble each other in organization, teaching and method. There has been the great southern preacher, Madhva Muni, and following him our great Chaitanya of Bengal taking up the philosophy of the *Madhvas*, and preaching it in Bengal. There have been some other sects in Southern India also, as the qualified dualistic Shivites. The Shivites in most parts of India are Advaitins, except in some portions of Southern India and in Ceylon. But they also only substitute Shiva for Vishnu, and are Râmânujists in every sense of the term except in the doctrine of the soul. The followers of Râmânuja hold that the soul is *anu*, like a particle, very small, and the followers of Sankarâchârya hold that it is *vibhu*, omnipresent. There have been several non-dualistic sects. It seems that there have been sects in ancient times which Sankara's movement entirely swallowed up and assimilated. In modern times the Advaitins have all ranged themselves under Sankarâchârya; and he and his disciples have been the great preachers of Advaita, both in Southern and in Northern India. The influence of Sankarâchârya did not penetrate much into our country of Bengal, or into Cashmere and the Punjab; but in Southern India the *Smârtas* are all followers of Sankarâchârya, and with Benares as the centre, his influence is simply immense even in many parts of Northern India.

Now, both Sankara and Râmânuja laid aside all claim to originality. Râmânuja expressly tells us that he is only following the great commentary of Bodhâyana. He takes it up and makes of it an abstract, and that is what we have to-day. Râmânuja is very plain on the point, and he tells us that he is taking the ideas, and sometimes even passages out of this ancient commentator and condensing them into the present Râmânuja Bhâshya. It seems that Sankarâchârya was also doing the same. There are a few places in his Bhâshya, which mention older commentaries; and when we know that his Guru and his Guru's Guru had been Vedantins of the same school as himself, sometimes even more thoroughgoing, bolder even than Sankara himself on certain points; it seems pretty plain that he also was not preaching anything very original, and that even in his Bhâshya he himself had been doing the same work that Râmânuja did with Bodhâyana, but from what Bhâshya cannot be discovered at the present time. All these *Darsanas* (schools of philosophy) that you have seen, or ever heard of, are based upon Upanishadic authority. Whenever they quote a *Sruti* (scriptural text), they mean the Upanishads. They are always quoting the Upanishads. Following the Upanishads there came other philosophies in India, but every one of them failed in getting that hold upon India which the philosophy of Vyâsa obtained. The philosophy of Vyâsa is a development out of an older one, the Sânkhya; and every philosophy and every system in India—and possibly throughout the world—owes much to Kapila, the great founder of the Sânkhya system, perhaps the greatest name in the history of India in psychological and philosophical lines. The influence of Kapila is everywhere throughout the world. Wherever there is a recognized system of thought, there you can trace his influence; it may be thousands of years back, but yet he stands there, the shining, glorious, wonderful Kapila. His psychology and a good deal of his philosophy have been accepted by all the different sects of India with but very slight differences. In our own country, our *Naiyayika* philosophers could not make much impression on the philosophical world of India. They were too busy with little species and genera and that most cumbersome terminology, which is a life's work to study. They were very busy also with logic, and left philosophy to the Vedantins, but every one of the Indian philosophic sects in modern times has adopted the logical terminology of the Naiyayikas of Bengal. The philosophy of Vyâsa as embodied in the Vyâsa Sutras is firm-seated, and has attained the permanence of that which it intended to present to men, the orthodox and Vedantic side of philosophy. Reason was entirely subordinated to the *Srutis* and as Sankarâchârya declares, Vyâsa did not care to reason at all. His idea in writing the *Sutras* was just to bring together with one thread and make a garland of the flowers of Vedantic texts. His *Sutras* are admitted so far as they are subordinate to the authority of the Upanishads and no further. And as I have said, all the sects of India now hold these Vyâsa *Sutras* to be the great authority, and every new sect in India starts with a fresh commentary on the Vyâsa *Sutras* according to its light. The difference between some of these commentators is often very great, giving rise to not a little text-torturing. The Vyâsa *Sutras* however have got the place of authority in India to-day, and no one can expect to found a new sect until he can write a fresh commentary on them.

Next in authority is the celebrated Bhagavad Gîtâ. The great glory of Sankarâchârya is his preaching of the Gîtâ. It is one of the greatest works that this great man did among the many noble works of his noble life—the preaching of the Gîtâ and the writing of a most beautiful commentary on it. And he has been followed by every founder of an orthodox sect in India, and they have each written a commentary on this Gîtâ.

The Upanishads are many in number, by some said to be one hundred and eight; others declare them to be still more numerous. Those which on the face of them bear the evidence of genuineness have been taken up by the great Teachers and commented upon, especially those upon which Sankara, and later Râmânuja wrote commentaries. There are one or two more ideas with regard to the Upanishads which I want to bring to your notice; for these are an ocean of knowledge, and to talk about the Upanishads even by an incompetent person like myself, takes years, and not one lecture only. I want therefore, to bring to your notice one or two of the more important points in the study of the Upanishads. In the first place, they are the most marvellous poems in the world. If you read the *Samhita* portion of the Vedas, you now and then find passages of most marvellous beauty. For instance, the famous *Sloka* which describes chaos—"When darkness was hidden in darkness." One reads and feels the wonderful sublimity of the poetry. Do you mark this, that outside of India, and inside of India also, there have been attempts at painting the sublime. But outside it has always been the sublime as seen in the external world, the infinite of matter, or of space. When Milton or Dante, or any other great European poet, either ancient or modern, seeks to paint a picture of the infinite, he tries to soar outside, to make you feel the infinite through the external. That attempt has been made in India also. You find in the *Samhitas*, the infinite of enumeration, the infinite of extension, most marvellously painted and placed before the readers, as has been done nowhere else. Mark that one sentence: "When darkness was hidden in darkness," and now mark the description of darkness by three poets. Take your own Kâlidasa—"Darkness which can be penetrated with the point of a needle"; Milton—"No light but rather darkness visible"; but here—"Darkness was covering darkness," "Darkness was hidden in darkness." We who live in the Tropics can understand it, the sudden outburst of the monsoon, when in a moment, the horizon becomes darkened, and the sky becomes covered with more and more rolling black clouds, and these again in denser blackness until it is literally "Darkness hidden in darkness." In India as everywhere else, attempts at finding the solution of the great problems of life have first been made through the external world. Just as the Greek mind, or the modern European mind tries to find the solution of life and of all the sacred problems of being by searching into the external world, so did our own forefathers; and just as the Europeans failed, they failed also. But the Westerners never made a move more, they remained there; they failed in the search for the solution of the great problems of life and death in the external world, and there they remained stranded; but our forefathers were bolder and declared the utter helplessness of the senses to find out the solution. Nowhere else was the fact better put than in the same Upanishad—"From whence the word comes back reflected by the mind." There are various sentences which declared the utter helplessness of the senses; but they did not stop there, they fell back upon the internal nature of man, they sought to get the answer from their own souls, they became introspective; they gave up exploring external nature as a failure, as nothing could be done there. No hope, no answer could be found; they discovered that dull dead matter would not give them truth, and they fell back upon the shining soul of man, and there the answer was found.

"Know this *Atman*," they declared; "give up all vain words and hear no other." In the *Atman* they found the solution—the greatest of all âtmans, the God, the Lord of this Universe, His relation to the âtman of man, our duty to Him, and through that our relation to each other. And herein you find the most sublime poetry in this world. No more is the attempt made to paint this *Atman* in the language of matter. Nay, they have even given up all positive language. No more do they attempt to find in the senses the idea of the Infinite, no more is there an external, dull, dead, material, spatial, sensuous Infinite; but instead of that, comes something which is as fine as that saying about darkness, and what poetry in the world can be more sublime than this?

"There the sun cannot illumine, nor the moon, nor the stars, a flash of lightning cannot illumine the place; what to speak of this mortal fire?"

Such poetry you find nowhere else. Take that most marvellous Upanishad, the *Katha*. What wonderful finish, what most remarkable art are displayed in that poem! How wonderfully it opens, with that high-minded boy, whose father devoted him to *Yama* (Death), and how that most wondrous of all teachers, Death himself, unfolds to him the great lessons of life and death. And what was the quest of that fearless youth? To know the secret of death.

The second point that I want you to remember is the perfectly impersonal character of the Upanishads. Although we find many names, and many speakers, and many teachers in the Upanishads, not one of them stands as an authority for the Upanishads, not one verse is based upon the life of anyone of them. They are simply figures like shadows moving in the background, unfelt, unseen, unrealized, but the real force is in the marvellous, the brilliant, the effulgent texts of the Upanishads, which are perfectly impersonal. If *Yagnavalkya* never lived, or died, it would not matter, the texts are there. And yet the teachings are against no personality; they are broad and expansive enough to embrace all the personalities that the world has yet produced, and all that are to be produced. Nothing is said against the worship of persons, or Avataras, or sages. On the other hand, all worship is upheld by the Upanishads. It is a most marvellous idea, like the God it preaches, the impersonal idea of the Upanishads. At the same time, for the sage, the thinker, the philosopher, for the rationalist, it is as impersonal as any modern scientist can wish. And these are our Scriptures. You must remember that what the Bible is to the Christians, what the Qu'ran is to the Mohammedans, what the Tripitaka is to the Buddhists, what the Zend Avesta is to the Parsis, these Upanishads are to us. These, and nothing but these are our Scriptures. The *Purânas*, the *Tantras*, and all the other books, even the *Vyâsa Sutras*, are of secondary, or tertiary authority, but primary are the Vedas. *Manu* and the *Purânas*, and all the other books are to be taken so far as they agree with the authority of the Upanishads, and when they disagree they are to be rejected without mercy. This we ought to remember always. The Upanishads are the words of the *Rishis*, our forefathers, and you have to believe them if you want to be a Hindu. You may even believe the most peculiar ideas about the God-head, but if you deny the authority of the Vedas, you are a *Nâstika*, an atheist. The Scriptures of other religions are all *Purânas* and not Scriptures, because they describe the history of the deluge, and the history of the kings and reigning families, and record the lives of great men, and so on. This is the work of the *Purânas*, and so far as they agree with the Vedas, very good, but when they do not agree, they are not to be accepted. So with the Qu'ran, there are many moral teachings in it and so far as they agree with the Vedas, they have the authority of the *Purânas*, but no more. The idea is that the Vedas were never written, that they never came into existence. I was told once by a Christian missionary that their Scriptures have historical character and therefore are true. To which I replied: "Mine have no historical character, and therefore they are true; yours being historical were evidently made by some man the other day. Yours are man-made but mine are not; their non-historical character is in their favor." These are the relations of the Vedas to the other Scriptures of the world.

We now return to the teachings of the Upanishads. Various texts are there. Some are entirely dualistic. There are certain doctrines which are agreed to by all the different sects in India. First there is the doctrine of *Samsâra*, or reincarnation of the soul. Secondly, they all agree in their psychology; there is the body, behind that what is called the *Sukshma Sarira* (the mind), and behind that is the *Jiva* (the soul). The great difference between Western and Indian psychology is that in the former the mind is the soul; in the latter it is not. The *antahkarana*, the internal instrument, as the mind is called, is only an instrument, in the hands of the *Jiva*, through which the *Jiva* works on the body, or on the external world. Here Hindus all agree, and they all also agree that this *Jiva* (or *Atman*, or *Jivâtman* as it is called by different sects) is eternal, without beginning or end; and that it goes from birth to birth until it gets final release.

They all agree in this, and they also all agree in one vital point which marks most characteristically, most prominently, most completely, the difference between the Indian and the Western mind, and it is this—that everything is in the soul. There is no inspiration properly speaking" but rather expiration. All power, all purity, and all greatness—everything is in the soul.

The *Yogi* would tell you that the *Siddhis* (powers) that he is striving to attain to, are not to be attained, in the proper sense of the word, but are already in the soul; the work is to make them manifest. Patanjali, for instance, would tell you that even in the lowest worm that crawls under your feet, are already existing all the eightfold powers of the *Yogi*. The difference has been made by the body; the powers are there but they will have to be brought out through the medium of a suitable body. Patanjali gives the celebrated example of the cultivator bringing water into his field from a huge tank somewhere. The tank is already filled and the water would flood his land in a moment, only there is a wall between the tank and his field. As soon as the barrier is broken, in rushes the water by its own power and force. Power and purity and perfection are in the soul already, but they are hidden by this *Avarana*—this veil—that has been cast over them. Once the veil is removed, the soul manifests its powers which are its real nature. This, you ought to remember, is the fundamental difference between Eastern and Western thought. When you find people teaching such awful doctrines as that we are all born sinners always remember that if we are by our very nature sinful, we never can become good. How can nature change? If it changes, it contradicts itself; it is not nature. We ought never to forget this. Here the Dvaitins, the Advaitins, and all others in India agree.

The next point upon which all the sects in India are agreed is belief in God. Of course, their ideas of God will be different. The dualists believe only in a personal God. I want you to understand this word personal a little more. It does not mean that God has a body, sits on a throne somewhere, and rules this world; but personal means *Saguna*, "with qualities." There are many descriptions of the personal God. This personal God as the Ruler, the Creator, the Preserver, and the Destroyer, of this universe, is believed in by all sects. The Advaitins believe something more. They believe in a still higher phase of this personal God, which is personal-impersonal. No adjective can illustrate where there is no qualification, and the Advaitin would not give God any qualities except the three—*Sat-Chit-Ananda*, Existence— Knowledge—Bliss Absolute. That is what Sankara did, but in the Upanishads themselves you find that they penetrate even further, and say nothing can be said except "*Neti, Neti,*" "Not this, Not this." According to Râmânuja the great modern representative of the dualistic system these three entities are eternal —God, Soul, and Nature. The souls are eternal, and they will remain eternally existing, and will retain their individuality forever. Your soul will be different from my soul through all eternity, says Râmânuja, and so will Nature which is an existing fact, as much so as the existence of soul, or the existence of God—Nature will remain always. And God is interpenetrating the essence of the soul. He is the *Antarayâmin* (the Soul of our souls). In this sense Râmânuja sometimes thinks that God is one with the soul, the essence of the soul, and that at the time of *Pralaya* (the end of a cycle, or dissolution of phenomena), when the whole of Nature becomes what he calls *Sankocha* (contracted), these souls become contracted, or minute, and remain so for a time. At the beginning of the next cycle, they all come out according to their past *Karma*. Every action that dims the inborn, natural purity and perfection of the soul, is a bad action; and every action that causes these to shine forth and expand the soul is a good action, says Râmânuja. And thus the soul is going on, expanding or contracting by its actions, until through the grace of God, comes salvation. And that grace comes to all souls, says Râmânuja, that are pure, and struggle to gain it.

There is a celebrated verse in the *Srutis:* "When the food is pure then the *Sattva* becomes pure, when the *Sattva* becomes pure then the *smriti* (the memory of the Lord, or the memory of our own perfection—if you are an Advaitin) becomes truer, steadier, and absolute."

Here arises a great discussion. First of all what is this *Sattva?* We know that according to the Sânkhya—and it has been admitted by all our sects of philosophy—the body is composed of three sorts of *gunas* (materials—not qualities). It is the general idea that *Sattva*, *Rajas* and *Tamas* are qualities. Not at all, they are not qualities but materials of this universe, and with *âhâra suddhi* (pure food), the *Sattva* material becomes pure. The one aim of the Vedânta is to get this *Sattva*. As I have told you, the soul is already pure and perfect but, according to the Vedânta, it is covered up by *Rajas* and *Tamas* particles.

The *Sattva* particles are the most luminous, and the effulgence of the soul penetrates through them as easily as light through glass. So if the *Rajas* and *Tamas* particles are eliminated, leaving the *Sattva* particles uncovered, the powers and purity of the soul will appear, and make the soul more manifest. Therefore it is necessary to have this *Sattva*. The text says: "When the *âhâra* becomes pure, etc." Râmânuja takes this word *âhâra* to mean food, and he has made it one of the turning points of his philosophy. Not only so, but the idea has affected the whole of India, and all the different sects. Therefore, it is necessary for us to understand what it means, for according to Râmânuja, *âhâra suddhi* is one of the principal factors in our life. "What makes food impure?" asks Râmânuja. According to him, three sorts of defects make food impure—first, *jâti*, that is, the very nature of the class to which the food belongs, as onion, garlic and so on. The next is *âsraya*, or the person from whom the food comes. A wicked person is *âsraya* and food coming from him will make you impure. I myself have seen many great sages in India following strictly that advice all their lives. The third defect is *nimitta dosha*, impurity in the food itself, as hairs dirt, etc. If only that food be taken from which these three defects have been removed, that will make *Sattva suddhi*, will purify the *Sattva*. Religion then would seem to be a very easy task! But now comes Sankarâchârya, who says this word *âhâra* does not mean pure food, but pure thought collected in the mind; when the mind becomes pure, the *sattva* becomes pure and not before that. You may eat what you like. If food alone would purify the *sattva*, then feed a monkey with milk and rice all its life, would it become a great *Yogi*? As has been said if it is by bathing much one goes to heaven, then the fishes would get there first. If by eating vegetables a man gets to heaven, the cows and the deer will get there before him. But what is the solution? Both are necessary. Of course, the interpretation that Sankarâchârya gives to the text is the fundamental and more important one. But pure food no doubt, helps pure thought, it has an intimate connection; both ideas ought to be acted upon. The defect is that many have forgotten the advice of Sankarâchârya and have taken only the "pure food" meaning of *âhara*.

According to the dualistic sects of India, the individual souls remain as individuals throughout, and God is the Creator of the universe out of pre-existing material. He is the efficient cause. According to the Advaitins, on the other hand, God is both the material and the efficient cause of the universe. He is not only the Creator of the universe, but He creates it out of Himself. The one sect of Advaitins that you see in modern India is composed of the followers of Sankara. According to Sankara, God is both the material and the efficient cause through *Mâyâ*, but not in reality. God has not become this universe, but the universe appears because God is its Background. This is one of the highest points to understand of Advaitic Vedânta, this idea of *Mâyâ*. I am afraid I have not time now to discuss this one most difficult point in our philosophy. Those of you who are acquainted with Western philosophy will find something very similar in Kant. But I must warn you, those of you, who have studied Professor Max Muller's writings on Kant, that there is one idea most misleading. It was Sankara who first found out the idea of the identity of time, space, and causation, with *Mâyâ*, and I had the good fortune to find one or two passages in Sankara's commentaries and send them to my friend the Professor. So even that idea was to be found in India. Now this is a peculiar theory— this *Mâyâ* theory of the Advaita Vedantins. The *Brahman* is all that exists, but differentiation has been caused by this *Mâyâ*. Unity, the one *Brahman*, is the ultimate, the goal, and herein is an endless dissension again between Indian and Western thought. India has thrown this challenge to the world for thousands of years, and the challenge has been taken up by different nations and the result is that they have all succumbed and you live. This is the challenge, that this world is a delusion, that it is all *Mâyâ*, that whether you eat off of the ground with your fingers, or dine from golden plates, whether you live in palaces or hovels; are the mightiest monarchs or the poorest beggars, death is the one result; it is all the same, all *Mâyâ*. That is the old Indian theme, and again and again nations are springing up trying to unsay it, to disprove it, becoming great, enjoyment their watchword, power in their hands, and they use that power to the utmost, enjoy to the utmost, and the next moment they die. We stand forever because we see that everything is *Mâyâ*. The children of *Mâyâ* live forever, but children of enjoyment die.

Here is again another great difference. Just as you find in German philosophy the attempts of Hegel and Schopenhauer you will find the very same ideas coming in ancient India. Fortunately for us Hegelianism was nipped in the bud, and not allowed to sprout out and cast its baneful shoot over this mother-land of ours. Hegel's one idea is that the One, the Absolute, is only chaos, and that the individualized form is the greater. The world is greater than the non-world, *Samsâra* is greater than Salvation. That is the one idea, and the more you plunge into this *Samsâra*, the more your soul is covered with the workings of life, the better you are. They say: "Do you not see how we build houses, cleanse the streets, enjoy the senses?" Aye, but behind that, behind every bit of that enjoyment, may lurk rancor, misery, and horror. On the other hand, our philosophers have from the very first declared that every manifestation, what is called evolution, is a vain attempt of the Unmanifested to manifest Itself. After making the attempt for a time, man finds out it is vain, and gives it up. This is *Vairâgyam*, or renunciation, and is the very beginning of religion. How can religion or morality begin without renunciation? The Alpha and Omega is renunciation. "Give up," say the Vedas, "give up."

That is the one way, give up.

"Neither through wealth, nor through progeny, but by renunciation alone immortality is to be reached." That is the dictate of the Indian Scriptures. Of course, there have been great givers up of the world even sitting on thrones, but even Janaka himself had to renounce; who was a greater renouncer than he? But in modern times we all want to be called Janakas. They are all Janakas, all over India, but unfortunately I find them only Janakas[1] of children, unclad, ill-fed, miserable children. That is all they are of Janaka, not with shining, God-like thoughts as the old Janaka was. These are our modern Janakas! If you can give up, you will have religion. If you cannot, you may read all the books that are in the world, from East to West, swallow all the libraries, and become the greatest of pandits, but with all that there will be no spirituality. "Through renunciation alone immortality is to be reached." It is the power, the great power, that cares not even for the universe. Renunciation, that is the flag, the banner of India, floating out to the world, the one undying thought which India sends again and again as a warning to dying races, as a warning to all tyranny, as a warning to wickedness in the world. Aye, Hindus, let not your hold of that banner go! Hold it aloft! Even if you are weak, and cannot renounce the world, try not to be hypocrites, torturing texts, and making specious arguments. Do not do that, but admit you are weak. For the idea is great, that of renunciation. What matters if millions fail in the attempt, if one, if two, if ten return victorious? Blessed be the millions that died; their blood has bought the victory. This renunciation is the one ideal of nearly all the different Vedic sects. We want orthodoxy, even the hideously orthodox, even those who smother themselves with ashes, even those who stand with their hands uplifted. Aye, we want them, unnatural though they be, as a warning to the race, as examples of the idea of giving up. They are to be preferred to the effeminate cravings for Western luxuries that are creeping into India; and mistaken as they are, even these crude ideas of renunciation are infinitely better than materialism, with its gross and degenerating tendencies. We want to have renunciation. It has conquered India in days of yore, it has still to conquer India. Still it stands greatest and highest of Indian ideals—Renunciation. The land of Buddha, the land of Râmânuja, of Ramakrishna Paramahamsa, the land of renunciation, the land where from the days of yore they preached against *Karma Kânda*, and where even to-day there are hundreds who have given up everything, passed everything away and became *Jivan Muktas*—shall that land give up its ideals? Certainly not. There may be people whose brains have become turned with luxurious Western ideals. There may be thousands, and hundreds of thousands, who have drunk deep of this curse of the world—enjoyment—into whose brains have come the allurements of the senses, yet for all that there will be other thousands in this Motherland of ours to whom religion will be a reality, and who will be ready to give up if need be, without counting the cost.

Another ideal very common in all our sects, I want to place before you. It also is a vast subject. This idea is unique in India, that is that religion is to be realized. "This *Atman* is not to be reached by too much talking, nor is it to be reached by the power of intellect." Nay, ours are the only Scriptures in the world that declare that not even by the study of the Scriptures themselves is the *Atman* to be realized. This power of realization comes from the teacher unto the disciple. When this insight comes to the disciple everything is cleared up and realization comes.

One more idea, what is a *Guru?* Let us go back to the *Srutis:*

"He who knows the secret of the Vedas," not book-worms, not grammarians, not pandits in general, but he who knows the meaning of the Scriptures, he alone is the *Guru.* "An ass laden with a mass of sandalwood knows only the weight of the wood, but not its precious qualities." So are these pandits (scholars); we do not want these to teach religion. What can they teach, if they have no realization? When I was a boy here in this city of Calcutta, I used to go from place to place in search of religion, and everywhere after hearing very great speakers I asked: "Have you seen God?" The men were all taken aback at the idea of seeing God, and the only man who told me, "I have," was Sri Râmâkrishna Paramahamsa, and not only so, but he said: "I will put you in the way of seeing Him too." Not a man who can twist and torture texts, is fit to be a teacher. "Different ways of throwing out words, different ways of explaining texts of the Scriptures, these are for the enjoyment of the learned, not for freedom." He who knows the secret of the *Srutis,* the sinless, and he who does not want to make money by teaching—he is the *Shanta* (saint), the *Sâdhu* (Holy one), who comes as the Spring, which brings the leaves and fruits to various plants but does not ask anything from the plant, for its very nature is to do good. It does good and that is all. Such is the *Guru*. "Who has himself crossed this ocean of life, and without any idea of gain to himself helps others to cross the ocean also;" this is the *Guru*, and mark that none else can be a *Guru*. As for others:

"Themselves steeped in darkness, but in the pride of their hearts thinking they know everything, do not stop even there, but want to help others, and, blind leading the blind, both fall into the ditch." Thus say your Vedas. You are Vedantins, you are very orthodox, are you not? Aye, what I want to do is to make you more orthodox. The more really orthodox you are the more sensible, and the more you think of modern orthodoxy the more foolish you are. Go back to your old orthodoxy, for in those days every sound that came from these books, every pulsation, was out of a strong, steady, and sincere heart; every note was true. After that came degradation in art, in science, in religion, in everything, national degradation. Go back, go back, to the old days, when there was strength and vitality. Be strong once more, drink deep out of this fountain of yore, for that is the only condition of life in India.

It has been a hard nut to crack all over the world that the idea of individuality which we have to-day is an illusion. Tell a man that he is not an individual in the ordinary sense of the word and forthwith he becomes afraid that his individuality (whatever that may be) will be lost. But the Advaitin says there never has been a finite individuality; you as a finite being have been changing every moment of your life. You have been a child, and thought in one way, you are a man, and think another way, you will be an old man, and will think yet another way. Everybody is thus changing. If so, where is your individuality? Certainly not in the body, nor in the mind, nor in thought. And beyond that is the *Atman*, and says the Advaitin: "This *Atman* is the *Brahman* Itself. There cannot be two Infinites. There is only One Individual and It is Infinite. In plain words, we are rational beings, and we want to reason. And what is reason? More or less of classification, until you cannot go any farther. And the finite can only find its ultimate rest when it is classified into the Infinite. Go on taking up a finite and finding its reasons, and you will find rest nowhere until you reach the ultimate or Infinite; and that Infinite says the Advaitin, is what alone exists. Everything else is *Mâyâ*, everything else has no real existence. Whatever of existence is in any material thing is this *Brahman;* we are this *Brahman*, and name, shape, and everything else is *Mâyâ*. Take off the name and form and you and I are all one. But we have to guard against the misuse of the word "I." Generally people say:

"If I am the *Brahman* why cannot I do this or that?" But they are using the word "I" in two different senses. You think you are a body, or a man, and as soon as you do this you are bound; no more are you *Brahman*, the Self, Who wants nothing, Whose light is within. All His pleasure and bliss are within, perfectly satisfied with Himself He wants nothing, expects nothing, is perfectly fearless, perfectly free. That is *Brahman*. That is the meaning of the real "I." In that we are all one.

Now this seems to be the great point of difference between the dualist and the Advaitin. You find even great commentators, like Sankarâchârya, making meanings of texts, which, to my mind, sometimes do not seem to be justified. Sometimes you find Râmânuja dealing with texts in a way that is not very clear. The idea has been even among our pandits that only one of these views can be true; the rest must be false. Yet they find in their *Srutis* the most wonderful idea that India has to give to the world, "*Ekam sat viprâ bahudhâ vadanti*," "That which exists is One, sages call it by various names." That has been the theme, and the working out of the whole of this life-problem of the nation is the working out of that theme: "That which exists is One, sages call it by various names." Yet, except a very few spiritual men in India, we all forget this. We forget this great idea, and you will find there are those among the pandits who are of opinion that only the Advaitin is right, or that only the *Visishtadvaitin* is right, or that only the *Dvaitin* can have the Truth. But a few years ago there came to India one whose life was the explanation of all these differences, whose life was the working out of the harmony that is the background of all the different sects of India. I mean Sri Râmâkrishna Paramahamsa. It is his life that explains that all of these are necessary; that dualism is the natural idea of the senses. As long as we are bound by the senses we are bound to see a God who is personal, and nothing but personal; we are bound to see the world as it appears. Just as says Râmânuja: "As long as you think you are a body, or think you are a mind, or think you are a *Jiva*, every act of perception will give you the three, God and Nature and something as seeing both." But yet even the idea of the body grows dimmer where the mind itself becomes finer and finer, until it has almost all disappeared; and when all the different things that bind us down to this body-life, all the things that make us fear, that make us weak, have disappeared, then comes the realization of Oneness. The *Bhagavad Gîtâ* says: "Even in this life they have conquered heaven, whose minds are firmly fixed on this sameness of everything; for God is pure, and the same to all; therefore, such are said to be living in God." And again:

"Thus seeing the same Lord everywhere he, the sage, does not hurt the Self by the self and thus goes to the highest goal."

---

1. Janaka means also "progenitor."

XVII. VEDÂNTA.

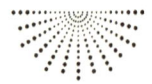

(Lecture delivered at Lahore, India.)

Two worlds there are in which we live, one the external, the other the internal. Human progress has been, from time immemorial, along parallel lines in both these worlds. The search began in the external, and man at first sought to get answers for all the deep problems from external nature. He wanted to satisfy his thirst for the beautiful and the sublime from all that surrounded him; he wanted to express himself and all that was within him in the language of the concrete; and grand indeed were the answers—most marvellous ideas of God and worship, most rapturous expressions of the beautiful, most sublime conceptions came from the external world. But the other, opening out for humanity later, laid out before him a universe yet sublimer, yet more beautiful, and infinitely more expansive. In the *Karma Kanda* (doctrines and ceremonies) portion of the Vedas we find most wonderful ideas about an over-ruling Creator, Preserver and Destroyer of this universe presented before us in language which is at times soul-stirring. Most of you, perhaps, remember that wonderful passage in the *Rig Veda Samhita*, where you get a description of chaos, possibly the sublimest that has ever been attempted by man. In spite of all this, we find it is only a painting of the sublime external, that it is still gross, that something of matter yet clings to it. It is only the expression of the Infinite in the language of matter, in the language of the finite, it is the infinite of the muscles and not of the mind. It is the infinite of space and not of thought. Therefore in the second portion of the Vedas, or *Jnâna Kanda* (philosophy), we find the method of procedure altogether different. The first attempt was to search out from external nature the truths of the universe; to get the solution of all the deep problems of life from the material world. There arose the cry—"When a man dies, what becomes of him? Some say that he exists, others that he is gone, say, O king of Death, what is truth?" The Indian mind has discovered what was to be got from the external world, but it did not feel satisfied with that; it wanted to search more deeply, to dig in its own interior, to seek from its own soul, and the answer came.

Upanishads, or Vedânta, or *Aranyakas*, is the name of this portion of the Vedas. Here we perceive at once that religion has got rid of all external formalities, that spiritual things are told not in the language of matter, but that spirituality is preached in the language of the spirit, the superfine in the language of the superfine. No more is any grossness apparent in it, no more is there any compromise with things that concern us. Bold, brave beyond our conception at the present day, stand the giant minds of the sages of the Upanishads, declaring the noblest truths that have been preached unto humanity, without compromise, without fear. This, my countrymen, I want to lay before you.

Even the *Jnâna Kanda* of the Vedas is a vast ocean; many lives are necessary to understand even a little of it. Truly has it been said by *Râmânuja* that the Vedânta is the head, the shoulders, the crested form of the Vedas, and surely enough the Upanishads that teach it have become the Scriptures of modern India. The Hindus have the greatest respect for the *Karma Kanda* of the Vedas, but for all practical purposes we know that for ages *Shruti* (sacred revelation) has meant the Upanishads and the Upanishads alone. We know that all our great philosophers, either Vyâsa or Patanjali, or Gautama, or even the great father of all philosophy, the celebrated Kapila himself, when ever they wanted an authority for what they wrote, every one of them drew it from the Upanishads and from no other source, for therein are the truths that remain forever.

There are truths that are true only in a certain line, in a certain direction, under certain circumstances and for certain times, those that are founded on the institutions of the time. There are other truths that are based on the nature of man himself that must endure as long as man himself endures. These are the truths that alone can be universal, and in spite of all the changes that we are sure must have come in India, as to our social surroundings, our methods of dress, our manner of eating, our modes of worship, these universal truths of the *Shrutis*, the marvellous Vedântic ideas, stand out in their own sublimity, immovable, unvanquishable, deathless and immortal. Yet the germs of all the ideas that are developed in the Upanishads have been taught already in the *Karma Kanda*. The idea of the cosmos which all sects of Vedântins take for granted, the psychology which has formed the common basis of all Indian schools of thought had there been worked out and presented before the world. A few words therefore about the *Karma Kanda* are necessary before we start into the spiritual portion of the Vedânta, and I want first to make clear my use of the word Vedânta. Unfortunately there is a mistake common in modern India, that the word Vedânta has reference only to the *Advaita* system, but you must always remember that in modern India there are the three *Prasthanas* (authorities) for man to study. First of all there are the Revelations (the *Shrutis*), by which I mean the Upanishads. Secondly, among our philosophies, the *Sûtras* of Vyâsa have always held great prominence on account of their being the summation of all the preceding systems of philosophy; not that these systems are contradictory to one another, but the one is based on the other. There is a gradual unfolding of the theme which culminates in the *Sûtras* of Vyâsa; and between the Upanishads and the *Sûtras*, which are the systematizing of the marvellous truths of the Vedânta, comes the divine commentary of the Vedânta *Sri Bhagavad Gîtâ*. The Upanishads, the *Gîtâ*, and the *Vyâsa Sûtras* therefore have been taken up by every sect in India which has wished to claim authority as orthodox, whether Dvaitist, or *Vaishnavist*, or

Advaitist it matters little, the authorities of each and every one are these three. We find that a *Sankarâchârya*, or a *Râmânuja*, or a *Madhvâchârya*, or a *Chaitanya*—any one who wanted to propound a new theory—had to take up these three systems and write only a new commentary on them. Therefore it would be wrong to confine the word Vedânta only to one system which has arisen out of the Upanishads. All these systems are covered by the word Vedânta. The Râmânujist has as much right to be called a Vedantist as the Advaitist; in fact I will go a little further and say that what we really mean by the word Hindu is the word Vedantist; the word Vedantist will express that too. One idea more I wish you to note, that these three systems have been current in India almost from time immemorial; for you must not believe that *Sankara* was the inventor of the Advaitist system; it existed ages before *Sankara* was born; he was one of its last representatives. So with the Râmânujist system, it existed ages before *Râmânuja* appeared, as we already know by the commentaries that were written. This is true of all the dualistic systems that have existed side by side with the others, and with my little knowledge I have come to the conclusion that they do not contradict each other. Just as in the case of our six *Darsanas* (systems of philosophy), we find that they are a grand unfolding of the highest principles, the theme beginning far back, with the uncertain utterances of early investigators, and ending in the triumphant blast of the Advaita, so also in these three main systems we trace the gradual working up of the human mind towards higher and higher ideals, until everything is merged in that wonderful unity which is reached in the Advaita. Therefore these three are not contradictory. But I am bound to tell you that this mistake has been committed by not a few. We find an Advaitist preacher keeping entire those texts which teach Advaitism especially, and getting hold of the dualistic or qualified-dualistic texts and trying to wrest them into his own meaning; We find dualistic teachers leaving alone those passages that are expressly dualistic and getting hold of Advaitic texts and trying to force them into a dualistic meaning. They have been great men, our *Gurus*, yet there is such a saying as "even the faults of a *Guru* must be told." I am of the opinion that in this only were these great teachers mistaken. We need not go into text torturing, we need not go into any sort of religious dishonesty, we need not go into any kind of grammatical twaddle, we need not go about trying to put our own ideas into texts which were never meant for those ideas, but the work is plain and it becomes easier once you understand the marvellous doctrine of *Adhikara Vedas*. It is true that the Upanishads have one theme before them. "What is that, knowing which we know everything else?" In modern language the theme of the Upanishads, like the theme of every other knowledge, is to find the ultimate unity of things, for you must remember that knowledge is nothing but discovering unity in the midst of diversity. Each science is based upon this; all human knowledge is based upon the finding of unity in the midst of diversity; and if it be the task of those small fragments of human knowledge which we call our sciences, to find unity in the midst of a few different phenomena, the effort becomes stupendous when the theme before us is to find unity in the midst of this marvellously diversified universe, differing in name and form, differing in matter and spirit, differing in everything, each thought differing from every other thought, each form differing from every other form. Yet, to harmonize these many planes, unending *lokas*—in the midst of this infinite variety to find unity, this is the theme of the Upanishads; this is the task those great sages set themselves. To show a man the Pole Star, one takes the nearest star which is bigger than the Pole Star and more brilliant, and leads him to fix his mind on that, until at last he comes to the Pole Star. This is the task before us, and to prove my idea I have simply to show you the Upanishads, and you will see it. Nearly every chapter begins with dualistic teachings. Later on God is taught as some one who is the Creator of the Universe, its Preserver, unto whom everything goes at last. He is one to be worshipped, the Ruler, the Guide of nature, external and internal. One step further, and we find the same teacher showing that this God is not outside nature, but immanent in nature. And at last both ideas are discarded and whatever is real is He; there is no difference. That immanent One is at last declared to be the same that is in the human soul. *"Tat tvam asi Svetaketo."* "Svetaketu, That thou art." Here is no compromise; here is no fear of others' opinions. Truth, bold truth, has been taught in bold language, and we need not fear to preach the truth in the same bold language to-day, and by the grace of God I hope at least to be the one who dares to be that bold preacher.

To go back to our preliminaries. There are first two things to be understood, one the psychological aspect common to all the Vedantic schools, and the other the cosmological aspect. I will first take up the latter. To-day we find wonderful discoveries of modern science coming upon us like bolts from the blue, opening our eyes to marvels we never dreamed of. Man had long since discovered what he calls force. It is only the other day that man came to know that even in the midst of this variety of forces there is a unity. Man has just discovered that what he calls heat, magnetism, electricity, and so forth, are all convertible into that one unit force, whatever you may call it. This has been done even in the *Samhita*; as ancient and hoary as the *Samhita*, is that very idea of force I was referring to. All the forces, whether called gravitation, or attraction, or repulsion; whether expressing themselves as heat, or electricity, or magnetism, are but the variations of that unit energy. They may even express themselves as thought, reflected from *antahkarana*, the mentality of man, and the unit from which they spring is what is called the *Prâna*. Again what is *prâna*? *Prâna* is *spandanam*, or vibration. When all this universe shall have resolved back into its primal state, what will become of this infinite force? Do they think that it becomes extinct? Of course not. If it became extinct, what would be the cause of the next wave, because the motion is going in wave forms, rising, falling, rising again, falling again? Here is the word *srishti*, which expresses the universe. Mark that the word is not "creation." I am helpless in talking English, I have to translate the Sanskrit words as best I can. It is *srishti*, "projection." Everything becomes finer and finer, and is resolved back to the primal state from which it sprang, and there it remains for a time, quiescent, ready to spring forth again.

That springing forth is *srishti*, projection. And what becomes of all these forces, the *prânas*? They are resolved back into the primal *prâna*, and this *prâna* becomes almost motionless—not entirely motionless, but almost motionless—and that is what is described in the Vedic hymn, "It vibrated without vibrations." There are many difficult texts in the Upanishads to understand, especially in the use of technical phrases. For instance, the word *vâyu*, to move; many times it means air and many times motion, and often people confuse one with the other. We have to be careful about this. And what becomes of what you call matter? The forces permeate all matter; they all dissolve into ether, from which they again come out; and the first to come out is *akâsa*. Whether you translate it as ether, or as anything else, this is the idea, that this *akâsa* is the primal form of matter. This *akâsa* vibrates under the action of *prâna*, and when the next *srishti* is coming up, as the vibration becomes quicker, the *akâsa* is lashed into all those wave forms which we call the suns, moons, and systems.

We read again, "Everything in this universe has been projected, *prâna* vibrating, (*ejati*.) You must remark the word *ejati*, because it comes from *ej*, to vibrate. *Nissritam*—projected, *yadidamkincha jagat*— whatever is this universe.

This is a part of the cosmological side. There are many details working into it. For instance, how the process takes place, how there is first ether, and how from the ether evolve other things, how that ether begins to vibrate, and how from that comes *vâyu* (air). But the one idea is here, that it is from the finer that the grosser has come. Gross matter is the last to emerge and is the most external, and this gross matter had the finer matter before it. Yet we see that the whole thing has been resolved into two, but there is not yet a final unity. There is the unity of force, *prâna*; there is the unity of matter, called *akâsa*. Is there any unity to be found behind them? Can they be melted into one. Our modern science is mute here, has not yet found its way out, and if it is finding its way out, just as it slowly found the same old *prâna* and the same ancient *akâsa*, it will also have to seek this unity along similar lines. The next unity is the omnipresent, impersonal being, known by its old mythological name as *Brahma*, the four-headed *Brahma*, and psychologically called *Mahat*. This is where the two unite. What is called your mind is only a bit of this *mahat* caught in the trap of the brain, and the sum total of all brains caught in the meshes of *mahat* is what you call *samashti* (the aggregate, the universal). Analysis had to go further; it was not yet complete. In this view we were each one of us, as it were, a microcosm, and the world taken altogether the macrocosm. But whatever is in the *vyashti* (the particular), we may safely conjecture that a similar thing is also in the universal. We may feel reasonably sure that if we had the power to analyze our own minds we should find in them what we find outside. What is this mind, is the question. In modern times, in Western countries, as physical science is making rapid progress, as physiology is step by step conquering stronghold after stronghold of old beliefs, people do not know where to stand, because to their great despair modern physiology has identified the mind with the brain at every step. But that we in India have known always. It was the first proposition the Hindu boy should learn, that the mind is matter, only finer. The body is gross, and behind the body is what we call the *sûkshma sharira*, the fine body or mind. This is also material, only finer; but it is not the *Atman*. I will not translate this word to you in English, because the idea does not exist in Europe, it is untranslatable.

The modern attempt of German philosophers is to translate the word *âtman* by the word "self," but until that word is universally accepted it is impossible to use it. So, call it self or anything, it is our *âtman*. This *âtman* is the real man behind. It is the *âtman* that uses the material mind as its instrument, its *antahkarana* (internal instrument), as the psychological term for the mind is. And the mind by means of a series of internal organs works the visible organs of the body. What is this mind? It was comparatively only the other day that Western philosophers arrived at the knowledge that the eyes are not the real organs of vision, but that behind these are other organs, the *indriyas*, and if these are destroyed a man may have a thousand eyes, like Indra, but there will be no sight for him. Aye, your philosophy starts with this assumption, that by vision is not meant the external vision. The real vision belongs to the internal organs, the brain centres inside. You may call them what you like, but the *indriyas* are not the eyes, or the nose, or the ears. And the sum total of all these *indriyas* plus the *manas, buddhi, chitta, ahankara*, etc., is what is called the mind, and if the modern physiologist comes to tell you that the brain is what is called the mind and that the brain is formed of so many organs, you need not be afraid at all; tell him your philosophers knew it always, it is the very alpha of your religion.

Next we have to understand what is meant by this *manas, buddhi, chitta, ahankara,* etc. First of all let us consider the *chitta;* it is the "mind-stuff"—a part of the *mahat*—and is the generic name for the mind itself, including all its various states.

Suppose here is a lake on a summer evening, smooth and calm, without a ripple on its surface. Let us call this the *chitta*. And suppose some one throws a stone into this lake. What happens?

First there is the action, the blow given to the water, next the water rises and sends a reaction towards the stone, and that reaction takes the form of a wave. First the water vibrates a little, then immediately sends back a reaction in the form of a wave. This *chitta* let us compare to this lake, and the external objects are like these stones thrown into it. As soon as it comes in contact with any external object by means of these *indriyas*— the *indriyas* must be there to carry these external objects inside—there is a vibration, what is called the *manas*, indecisive. Next there is a reaction, the determinative faculty, *buddhi*, and along with this *buddhi* flashes the idea *aham* (egoism) and the external object. Suppose there is a mosquito sitting on my hand. This sensation is carried to my *chitta* and it vibrates a little, this is the psychological *manas*. Then there is reaction, and immediately comes the idea that I have a mosquito on my hand, and that I shall have to drive it off. Thus these stones are thrown into the lake, but in the case of the lake, every blow that comes to it is from the external world, while in the case of the lake of the mind the blows may either come from the external world, or the internal world. This whole series—chitta, manas, etc., form what is called the *antahkarana*. Along with it you ought to understand one thing more that will help us in understanding the Advaita system later on. It is this. All of you must have seen pearls, and most of you know how pearls are made. Some irritating grain of dust or sand enters into the body of the pearl oyster and sets up an irritation there, and the oyster's body reacts towards the irritation and covers the little grain with its own juice. That crystallizes and forms the pearl. So the whole universe is like that, the universe is the pearl which is being formed by us. What we get from the external world is simply the blow. Even to know that blow we have to react, and as soon as we react we project really a portion of our own mind towards the blow, and when we come to know of it, it is really our own mind as it has been shaped by the blow. Therefore it is clear even to those who wish to believe in a hard and fast realism of an external world, (and they cannot but admit it in these days of physiology,) that, supposing that we represent the external world by "X" what we really know is "X" plus mind, and this mind element is so great that it has covered the whole of that "X" which has remained unknown and unknowable throughout, therefore if there be an external world it is always unknown and unknowable. What we know of it is as moulded, formed, fashioned by our own mind. So with the internal world. The same applies to our own soul, the *âtman*. In order to know the *âtman* we shall have to know it through the mind, and therefore what little we know of this *âtman* is simply the *âtman* plus the mind. That is to say, the *âtman* covered over, fashioned, and moulded by the mind, and nothing more. We shall revert to this a little later, but we will remember it here.

The next thing to understand is this. The statement was made that this body is merely the name of one continuous stream of matter. Every moment we are adding material to it, and every moment material is being thrown off by it, like unto a continually flowing river in which vast masses of water are always changing place; yet we take up the whole in imagination, and call it the same river. What do we call the river? Every moment the water is changing, the shore is changing, every moment the trees and plants, the leaves, and the foliage are changing; what is the river? It is the name of this series of changes. So with the mind.

There is the Buddhistic side, the great *Kshanika Vijnâna Vada* doctrine, most difficult to understand, but most rigorously and logically worked out; and this also arose in India in opposition to some part of the Vedânta. It had to be answered, and we will see how, later on, it could only be answered by the Advaita and by nothing else. We shall also see how, in spite of people's curious notions about Advaita, people's fright about Advaita, it is the salvation of the world, because therein alone is to be found the reason of things. Dualism and other "isms" are very good as means of worship, very satisfying to the mind; it may be that they have helped the mind onward; but if man wants to be rational and religious at the same time, Advaita is the one system in the world for him.

We will regard the mind as a similar river, continually emptying itself at one end, and filling itself at the other end. Where is that unity which we call the *âtman?* The idea is that, in spite of this continuous change in the body, and in spite of this continuous change in the mind, there is in us something that is unchangeable. When rays of light coming from different quarters fall upon a screen, or a wall, or upon something that is not changeable, then and then alone it is possible for them to form one complete whole. Where is this background in the human mind, falling upon which, as it were, the various ideas will come to unity and become one complete whole? This certainly cannot be the mind itself, seeing that it also changes.

Therefore there must be something which is neither the body nor the mind, something which changes not, something permanent, upon which all our sensations, all our ideas fall to form a unity and a complete whole, and this is the real soul, the *âtman* of man. And seeing that everything material, even if you call it fine matter, or mind, must be changeful; seeing that what you call gross matter, the external world, must be more changeful in comparison to that; this unchangeable something cannot be of material substance; it must be spiritual; that is to say, it is not matter; it is indestructible, unchangeable.

Next will come another question—apart from those old arguments which only rise in the external world, the arguments from design—who created this external world, who created matter, etc.? The idea here is to know truth only from the inner nature of man, and the question arises just in the same way as it arose about the soul. Taking for granted that there is an unchangeable soul in each man, which is neither the mind, nor the body, there is still a unity of idea among these souls, a unity of feeling, of sympathy. How is it possible that my soul can act upon your soul, where is the medium through which it can work, where is the medium through which it can act? How is it I can feel anything about your soul? What is it that is in touch both with your soul and with my soul? Herein arises a metaphysical necessity for admitting another soul, for it must be a soul which acts in contact with all the different souls; one Soul which covers and interpenetrates all the infinite number of souls in the world, in and through which they live, in and through which they sympathize and love and work for one another. And this universal Soul is *Paramâtman*, the Lord God of the universe. Again, it follows that because the soul is not composed of matter, because it is spiritual, it cannot obey the laws of matter, it cannot be judged by the laws of matter. It is therefore deathless and changeless. "This Self the fire cannot burn, nor instruments pierce, the sword cannot cut it asunder, the air cannot dry it up, nor can water melt it; unconquerable, deathless, and birthless is this Self of man." What is this Self doing then? We have known that according to the *Gîtâ* and according to Vedânta, this individual Self is also *vibhu* (all pervading), is, according to *Kapila*, omnipresent. Of course there are sects in India which regard this Self as *anu* (infinitely small), but what they mean is *anu* in manifestation; its real nature is *vibhu*.

There comes another idea, startling perhaps, yet a characteristically Indian idea, and if there is any idea that is common to all our sects it is this. Therefore I beg you to pay attention to this one idea and to remember it, for this is the very foundation of everything that we have in India. The idea is this. You have heard of the doctrine of physical evolution preached in the Western world, by the German and English savants. It tells us that the bodies of the different animals differ only in degree, not in kind. The differences that we see are but varying expressions of the same series, but from the lowest worm to the highest and most saintly man it is but one chain of expression, the one changing into the other, going up and up, higher and higher, until it attains perfection. We had that idea also. Declares our Yogi Patanjali, "*Jâtyantara parinâmah*," "one species (the jâti is species) changes into another species," (evolution); *parinâmah* means one thing changing into another, just as one species changes into another. Where do we differ from the Europeans? Patanjali says:

"*Prakrityâpûrât*"—"By the infilling of nature." The European says it is competition, natural and sexual selection, etc., that forces one body to take the form of another. But here is another idea, a still better analysis, going deeper into the thing, and saying "By the infilling of nature." What is meant by this infilling of nature? We admit that the *amoeba* goes higher and higher until it becomes a Buddha; we admit this, but we are, at the same time, equally certain that you cannot get any amount of work out of a machine until you put it on the other side. The sum total of the energy remains the same whatever the form it may take. If you want a mass of energy at one end you have got to put it in at the other end, it may be in another form, but the amount must be the same. Therefore, if a Buddha is the one end of the change, the very *amoeba* must have been "the Buddha also. If the Buddha is the evolved *amoeba*, the *amoeba* was the involved Buddha. If this universe is the manifestation of an almost infinite amount of energy, when this universe was in a state of *pralaya* (rest), it must have represented the same amount of involved energy. It cannot have been otherwise. As such it follows that every soul is infinite. From the lowest worm that crawls under our feet to the noblest and greatest saints, all possess this infinite power, infinite purity, and infinite everything. The apparent difference is in the degree of manifestation. The worm is manifesting only a little bit of that energy; you have manifested more, another god-man has manifested still more; that is all the difference. But that infinite power is there all the same. Says Patanjali; "*Tatah kshetrikavat*"—"Just as the peasant irrigating his field." He has a little canal that comes into his field and brings water from a reservoir somewhere, and perhaps he has a little lock that prevents the water from rushing into his field. When he wants water he has simply to open the lock and in rushes the water by its own power. The power has not to be added, it is already there in the reservoir. So, every one of us, every being has as his own background such a reservoir of strength, infinite power, infinite purity, infinite bliss, and infinite existence, only these locks, these bodies are hindering us from fully expressing what we really are. And as these bodies become more and more finely organized, as the *tamasa guna* (dullness) becomes the *rajasa guna* (activity) and as the *rajasa guna* becomes *sattva guna* (purity), more and more of this power and purity will become manifest; and it is for this reason that our people have been so careful about their eating and drinking. It may be that the original ideas have been lost, just as with our child-marriage, which, though not belonging to the subject, I may take as an example. If I have another opportunity I will talk more fully about it, for the ideas behind child-marriage are the only ideas through which there can be a real civilization. There cannot be anything else. If a man, or a woman, is allowed the freedom to take up any man or woman, as wife or husband, if individual pleasure, or satisfaction of animal instincts, were to be allowed to run loose in society, the result must be evil, evil children, wicked and demoniacal. Aye, man in every country is, on the one hand, producing these evil children, and on the other hand multiplying the police force to keep down their brutal instincts.

The question is not how to destroy evil that way, but how to prevent the very birth of evil, and as long as you live in society, your marriage certainly affects every member of it; therefore society has the right to dictate whom you shall marry, and whom you shall not. And great ideas of this kind have been behind the system of child-marriage here, what they call the astrological *jati* of the bride and bridegroom. And in passing I may remark that according to Manu a child who is born of lust is not an *Aryan*. The child whose very conception and whose death is according to the rules or Vedas, such is an *Aryan*. Yes, and less of these *Aryan* children are being produced in every country, and the result is the mass of evil which we call *Kali Yuga* (Black Age). But we have lost these ideals, we cannot carry these ideas to the fullest length now. It is perfectly true that we have made almost a caricature of some of them. It is lamentably true that fathers and mothers are not what they were in the old times, neither is society so educated as it used to be, neither has society that love for individuals that it used to have. But however faulty the working out may be, the principle is sound; and if its application has become defective, if one method has failed, take up the principle and work it out better; why kill the principle? The same applies to the food question, the work and details are bad, very bad indeed, but that does not affect the principle. The principle is eternal and must be kept. Work it out afresh, and make a reform application.

This great idea of the *âtman* is the one in India which every one of our sects has got to believe; only, as we will find, the dualists preach that this *âtman* by evil works becomes *sankocha*, that is, all its powers and its nature become contracted, and by good works its nature again expands. The Advaitist, on the other hand, says that the *âtman* never expands or contracts, but only seems to do so; it appears to have become contracted.

That is the only difference; but all have the one idea that the *âtman* has all power already; that nothing will come to it from outside, that nothing will drop into it from the skies. Mark you, your Vedas are not inspired, but expired; they come not from somewhere outside, but are eternal laws living in every soul. The Vedas are in the soul of the ant, in the soul of the god. The ant has only to evolve and get the body of a sage or a *Rishi*, and the Vedas will come out, eternal laws expressing themselves. This is the one great idea to understand, that our power is already ours, our salvation is already within us. Say either that it has become contracted, or say that it has been covered with the evil of *mâyâ*, it matters little; the idea is there; you must believe in that, believe in the possibilities of everybody, that even in the lowest man there is the same possibility as in the Buddha. This is doctrine of the *âtman*.

But now comes a tremendous fight. Here are the Buddhists, who equally analyze the body into a material stream, and as equally analyze the mind into another. About this *âtman*, however, they state that it is unnecessary; that we need not assume the *âtman* at all. What use of a substance and qualities inhering in the substance? Why not say *gunas*, qualities, and qualities alone? It is illogical to assume two causes where one will explain the whole thing. And the fight went on, and all the theories which held the doctrine of substance were thrown to the ground by the Buddhists. There was a break up all along the line of those who held to the doctrine of substance and qualities, that you have a soul, and I have a soul, and every one has a soul separate from the mind and body—and each one individual. So far we have seen that the idea of dualism is all right, for there is the body, there is then the fine mind, there is this *âtman*, and in and through all the *âtmans* is that *Paramâtman*, God. The difficulty is here, that this *âtman* and *Paramâtman* are both so-called substance, in which the mind and body inhere like so many qualities. Nobody has ever seen substance, none can ever conceive it; what is the use of thinking of this substance? Why not say that whatever exists is this succession of mental currents and nothing more. They do not inhere in each other, they do not form a unit, one is chasing the other, like waves in the ocean, never complete, never forming one unit whole. Man is a succession of waves, and when one goes away it generates another, and so on, and the cessation of these waveforms is what is called *Nirvâna*. You see that dualism is mute before this, it is impossible that it can bring up any argument, and the dualistic God also cannot be retained here. The idea of a God that is omnipresent, and yet is a person who creates without hands, and moves without feet, and who has created the universe as a *kumbhakara* (potter) creates a *ghata* (pot), the Buddhist declares is childish, and that if this be God he is going to deny and not worship Him. This universe is full of misery; if it be the work of a God, we are going to fight Him. And secondly, this God is illogical and impossible, as all of you are aware. We need not go into the defects of the design theory, nor into all the arguments against the idea of a personal God. Truth and nothing but truth can prevail. The Advaitist watchword is: *Satayameva jayati*—"Truth alone triumphs, and not untruth." Through truth alone the way to *Devayanam* lies. Everybody marches forward under that banner; but it is not meant to crush the weak man's position.

You come with your dualistic idea of God to pick a quarrel with a poor man who is worshipping an image, and you think you are wonderfully rational. You can confound him, but if he turns round and shatters your own personal God, and calls that an imaginary ideal, where are you? You fall back on faith, or raise up the cry of atheism, the old cry of weak man—whosoever defeats him is an atheist. If you are to be rational, be rational all along the line; and if not, allow others the same privilege which you ask for yourselves. How can you prove the existence of this God? On the other hand, it can be almost disproved. There is not a shadow of proof as to

His existence, and there are very strong arguments to the contrary. How will you prove His existence, with your God, and his *gunas*, and an infinite number of souls which are substance and each soul an individual? In what are you an individual? You are not as a body, for you know to-day better even than the Buddhists of old knew that what may have been matter in the sun has just now become matter in you, and shortly will go out and become matter in the plants, where is your individuality, you Mr. So and So? You have one thought to-night and another to-morrow. You do not think the same way that you thought when a child, and old men do not think as they did when they were young. Where is your individuality? Do not say it is in consciousness, this *ahankara*, because this only covers a small part of your existence. While I am talking to you all my organs are working and I am not conscious of it. If consciousness is the proof of existence they do not exist then, because I am not conscious of them. Where are you then with your personal God theories? How can you prove such a God? Again, the Buddhists will stand up and declare, not only is it illogical, but immoral, for it teaches man to be a coward and to seek assistance outside, and nobody can give him such help. Here is the universe, man made it, why, then, depend on an imaginary being outside, whom nobody ever saw or felt, or got help from? Why then do you make cowards of yourselves, and teach your children that the highest state of man is to be a dog, to go crawling before this imaginary being, saying that you are weak and impure, and that you are everything vile in this universe? On the other hand, the Buddhists may urge not only that you are telling a lie, but that you are bringing a tremendous amount of evil upon your children, for, mark you, this world is one of hypnotization. Whatever you tell yourself that you believe. Almost the first words the great Buddha uttered were: "What you think, that you are; what you will think, that you will be." If this be true—and who can deny it—do not teach yourselves that you are nothing, and that you cannot do anything unless you are helped by somebody who does not live here, who sits above the damp clouds. The result will be that you will be more and more weakened every day; and by constantly repeating: "We are very impure; Lord, make us pure," you will hypnotize yourselves into all sorts of vices.

The Buddhists say that ninety per cent. of the vices that are found in every society arise from this idea of inferiority and become as a dog before God; this awful idea of the human being that the end and aim of this expression of life, this wonderful expression of life, is to become like a worm of the dust. Says the Buddhist to the Vaishnavist, if your ideal, your aim and goal is to go to a place called *Vaikunta*, where God lives, and there stand before Him with folded hands all through eternity, it is better to commit suicide. The Buddhist may even urge that it is better to believe in annihilation to escape this.

I am putting these ideas before you as a Buddhist just for the time being, because nowadays all these Advaitic ideas are said to make you immoral, and I am trying to tell you how the other side looks. Let us face both sides boldly and bravely. We have seen first of all that the Buddhists claim that the idea of personal God creating the world cannot be proved; is there any child that can believe this to-day? Because a *kumbhakara* creates a *ghata*, therefore a God created the world. If this be so, then your *kumbhakara* is a god also, and if anyone tells you that he acts without head and hands you may take him to a lunatic asylum. Has your God, the Creator of the world, your personal God, to whom you cry all your life, ever helped you, and what help have you received is the next challenge from modern science?

They will prove that any help you have had could have been obtained by your own exertion, and better still, you need not have spent your energy in that crying, you could have done it all without weeping or crying at all. We have seen that along with this idea of a personal God comes tyranny and priestcraft.

Tyranny and priestcraft have prevailed wherever this idea existed, and until the lie is knocked on the head, say the Buddhists, tyranny will not cease. So long as man thinks he has to cower before a supernatural being, so long there will be priests to claim rights and privileges and to make men cower before them, while these poor men will continue to ask some priest to stand as interceder for them.

You may knock the Brahmin on the head, but mark me that those who do so will stand in his place, and will be worse; because these ancient Brahmins have a certain amount of generosity in them, and upstarts are always the worst tyrants. If a beggar gets wealth, he thinks the whole world is a bit of straw. So priests there will be, as long as this personal God idea continues, and it will be impossible to think of any great morality in society. Priestcraft and tyranny will go hand in hand as long as the need of mediation is felt by mankind. It is the idea of a thunderer, who kills everyone who does not obey him. Next the Buddhist says, you have been so rational up to this point that you say that everything is the result of the law of *Karma*. You believe in an infinity of souls and the belief in the law of *Karma* is perfectly logical no doubt. There cannot be a cause without an effect, the present must have had its cause in the past, and will have its effect in the future. The Hindu says the *karma* is *jada* (non-intelligent) and not *chaitanya* (intelligent), therefore some *chaitanya* is necessary to bring this cause to fruition. Is it that *chaitanya* is necessary to bring the plant to fruition? If I add water and plant the seed, no *chaitanya* is necessary. You may say there was some original *chaitanya*, but the souls themselves were the *chaitanya*, none else is necessary. If human souls have it too, what necessity is there for a God, as say the Jains, who, unlike the Buddhists, believe in souls and do not believe in God. Where are you logical, where are you moral? And when you try to maintain that Advaita will make for immorality, just read a little of what has been done in India by dualistic sects, and what has been brought before law courts. If there have been ten thousand Advaitist blackguards, there will be twenty thousand Dvaitist blackguards. Generally speaking, there will be more Dvaitist blackguards, because it takes a better type of mind to understand Advaita, and they can scarcely be frightened into anything. What stands for you then? There is no escape from the arguments of the Buddhist. You may quote the Vedas, but he does not believe in them. He will say: "My *Tripetakas* say otherwise, and they are without beginning or end, not even written by Buddha, for Buddha says he is only reciting them, they are eternal." And he adds that yours are wrong and his are the true Vedas, yours are manufactured by the Brahmin priests, therefore out with them. How do you escape?

Here is the way out. Take up the first objection, the metaphysical one, that substance and qualities are different.

Says the Advaitist they are not. There is no difference between substance and qualities. You know the old illustration, how the rope is taken for the snake, and when you see the snake you do not see the rope at all, the rope has vanished. Dividing the thing into substance and quality is a metaphysical something in the brains of philosophers, never can it have an objective reality. You see substance if you are an ordinary man, and qualities if you are a great *yogi*, but you never see both at the same time. So, Buddhists, your quarrel about substance and qualities has been but a quibble which does not exist in fact. But, if substance is qualified, there can only be one. If you take qualities from the soul, and show that these qualities are in the mind, really superimposed on the soul, then there can never be two souls, for it is qualification that makes the difference between one soul and another. How do you know that one soul is different from another? Owing to certain differentiating marks, certain qualities. And where qualities do not exist, how can there be differentiations? Therefore there are not two souls, there is but One, and your *Paramâtman* is unnecessary, it is this very soul. That one is called *Paramâtman*, that very one is also called *jivâtman*, and so on, and you dualists, such as *Sânkhya* and others, who say that the soul is omnipresent, *vibhu*, tell me, how can there be two Infinites? There can be only one. What else? This one is the one Infinite *Atman*, everything else is Its manifestation. There the Buddhist stops, but there it does not end.

The Advaitist position is not merely a weak one of criticism. The Advaitist criticises others when they come too near him, just throws them away, that is all, but he propounds his own position. He is the only one that criticises, and does not stop with criticism and showing books. You say the universe is a thing of continuous motion. In *vyashti* everything is moving, you are moving, the table is moving, motion everywhere, *samsâra:* continuous motion, this is *jagat* (the universe). Therefore there cannot be individuality in this *jagat*, because individuality means that which does not change; there cannot be any changeful individuality, it is a contradiction in terms. There is no such thing as individuality in this little world of ours, the *jagat*. Thought and feeling, mind and body, plants and animals and so on, are in a continuous state of flux. But suppose you take the universe as a unit whole; can it change or move? Certainly not. Motion is possible only in comparison with something which is a little less in motion, or entirely motionless. The universe as a whole, therefore, is motionless, unchangeable. You are, therefore, an individual then and then alone, when you are the whole of it, when you realize: "I am the universe." That is why the Vedantist says that so long as there are two, fear does not cease. It is only when one does not see another, does not feel another that fear ceases; then alone death vanishes, then alone *samsâra* disappears. Advaita teaches us therefore that man is individual in being universal, and not in being particular. You are immortal only when you are the whole. You are fearless and deathless when you are the universe, and then that which you call the universe is the same as that which you call God. It is the same undivided existence which is taken to be many by people having the same state of mind as we have, looking upon this universe as we see it, suns, and moons, and so on. People who have made a little better *karma* and have another state of mind, when they die look upon it as *svarga* (Heaven), and see Indras and so forth. People still higher will see the very same thing as *Brahma Loka*, and the perfect ones will neither see the earth nor the heavens, nor any *loka* at all. This universe will have vanished, and *Brahman* will be in its stead.

Can we know this *Brahman?* I have told you of the painting of the infinite in the *Samhita*. Here we shall find another side taken, the infinite internal. That was the infinite of the muscles. Here we shall have the infinite of thought. There the attempt was made to paint the infinite in positive language here that language failed, and the attempt has been made to paint it in negative language. Here is this universe, and even admitting that it is *Brahman*, can we know it? No! No! You must understand this one thing very clearly. Again and again this doubt will come to you, if this be *Brahman*, how can we know it? "By what, O Maitreyi, can the knower be known; how can the knower be known?" The eyes see everything; can they see themselves? They cannot, because the very fact of knowledge is a degradation. Children of *Aryas* you must remember this, for herein lies a great error. All the Western temptations that come to you, have their metaphysical basis in that one claim—that there is nothing higher than sense knowledge. In the East, we say in our Vedas that this knowledge is lower than the thing itself, because it is always a limitation. When you want to know a thing, it immediately becomes limited by your mind. They cite that instance of the oyster making pearls to show how knowledge is limitation, gathering a thing, bringing it into consciousness, and not knowing it as a whole. This is true about all knowledge, and can it be less so about the infinite? Can you thus limit Him who is the Substance of all knowledge, Him who is the *Sâkshi*, the Witness, without whom you cannot have any knowledge, Him who has no qualities, who is the Witness of the whole universe, the Witness in our souls? How can you know Him? By what means can you encompass Him? Everything, the whole universe, is a false attempt to do so. As it were this infinite *Atman* is trying to see his own face, and all from the lowest animal to the highest of gods, are like so many mirrors to reflect himself in, and he is taking up still others, finding them insufficient, and so on, until in the human body he comes to know that it is finite of the finite, that all is finite; that there cannot be any expression of the infinite in the finite. Then comes the retrograde march, and this is what is called renunciation, *vairâgyam*. Back from the senses, back: do not go to the senses, is the watchword of *vairâgyam*. This is the watchword of all morality, this is the watchword of all well-being, for you must remember that the universe begins in *tapasya*, in renunciation; and as you go back and back all the forms are being manifested before you, and they are left aside one after the other until you remain what you really are. This is *moksha* or liberation.

This idea we have to understand—"How to know the knower;" the knower cannot be known, because if it be known, it will not be the knower. If you look at your eyes in a mirror, the reflection is no more your eyes, but something else, a reflection only. Then if this

Soul, this universal, infinite being which you are, is only a witness, what good is it? It cannot live, and move about, and enjoy the world, as we do. People cannot understand how the witness can enjoy. Oh, you Hindus have become quiescent, and good for nothing, through this doctrine that you are witnesses. First of all it is only the witness that *can* enjoy. The more and more you are the witness of anything in life the more you enjoy it. And this is *ânandam* (bliss), and therefore infinite bliss can only be yours when you have become the witness of this universe, then alone you are a *mukta* (free soul.) It is the witness alone that can work without any desire, without any idea of going to heaven, without any fear of blame, without any desire for praise. The witness alone enjoys, and none else.

Coming to the moral aspect, there is one thing between the metaphysical and the moral aspect of Advaitism, it is the theory of *Mâyâ*. Every one of these points in the Advaita system requires years to understand and months to tell.

Therefore you will excuse me if I only just touch upon them *en passant*. This theory of *mâyâ* has been the most difficult thing to understand in all ages. Let me tell you in a few words that it is more than a theory, it is the combination of the three ideas *Desa-kâla-nimitta*—Space, time, and causation, which have been further reduced to *nama-rupa*—name and form. Suppose there is a wave in the ocean. The wave is distinct from the ocean only in its form and name, and this form and this name cannot have any separate existence from the wave, they exist only with the wave. The wave may subside, but the same amount of water remains, even if the name and form that were on the wave vanish forever. So this *mâyâ* is what makes the difference between me and you, between all animals and man, between men and gods. In fact it is this *mâyâ* that causes the *Atman* to be caught, as it were, in so many millions of beings, and these are distinguishable only through name and form. If you let name and form go, all this variety vanishes forever, and you are what you really are. This is *mâyâ*. It is again no theory, but a statement of facts.

When the realist states that this world exists, what he means is that this table has an independent existence of its own, that it does not depend on the existence of anything else in the universe, and if the rest of the universe were destroyed and annihilated this table would remain just as it is now. A little knowledge shows you this cannot be. Everything here in the sense-world is dependent and inter-dependent, relative and correlative, the existence of one depending on the other. There are three steps, therefore, in our knowledge of things; the first is that each thing is individual and separate from every other; the next step is to find that there is relation and correlation between all things; and the third is that there is only one thing which we see as many. The first idea of God with the ignorant is that God is somewhere outside of the universe; that is to say, the conception of God is extremely human, He does just what a man does only on a higher scale. And we have seen how that idea of God is proved in a few words to be unreasonable and insufficient. And next is the idea of a power that we see manifested everywhere. This is the real personal God we get in the *Chandi* (a book of praise of the Divine Mother), but, mark me, not the God whom you make the reservoir of all good qualities only. You cannot have two Gods, God and Satan, you must have only one, and dare to call Him good and bad, but have only one, and take the logical consequences.

"Thus we salute Thee, O Divine Mother, who lives in every being as peace, who lives in all beings as purity." At the same time we must take the whole consequence of it. "All this bliss, O Gargi, wherever there is bliss, there is a portion of the Divine."

You may use it how you like. You may try to give a poor man a hundred rupees, another man may forge your name, but the sunlight will be the same for both. This is the second stage, and the third is that God is neither outside nature, nor inside nature, but God and nature and soul and universe are all convertible terms. You never see two things, it is your metaphysical words that have deluded you. You assume that you are a body and have a soul, and that you are both together. How can that be? Try in your own mind. If there is a *yogi* among you, he knows himself as *chaitanya*, for him the body has vanished. An ordinary man thinks of himself as a body; the idea of spirit has vanished; but because the metaphysical ideas exist that man has a body and a soul and all these things, you think they are all simultaneously there. One thing at a time. Do not talk of God when you see matter, you see the effect and the effect alone, and the cause you cannot see, and the moment you can see the cause the effect will have vanished. Where then is this world, and who has taken it off?

"One that is formless and limitless, beyond all compare, beyond all qualities, O sage, O learned man, such a *Brahman* will shine in your heart in *samâdhi*" (the superconscious state.)

"Where all the changes of nature cease forever, thought beyond all thoughts, whom the Vedas declare, who is the essence in what we call our existence, such a *Brahman* will manifest himself in you in *samâdhi*."

"Beyond all birth and death, the Infinite One, incomparable, like the whole universe deluged in water in *mahâpralaya* ("the great dissolution")—water above, water beneath, water on all sides, and on the face of that water not a wave, not a ripple, silent and calm, all visions have died out, all fights and quarrels and wars of fools and saints have ceased forever, such a *Brahman* will shine in your hearts in *samâdhi*." That also comes, and when that comes the world has vanished.

We have seen then, that this *Brahman*, this Reality is unknown and unknowable, not in the sense of the agnostic, but because to know Him would be blasphemy, because you are He already. We have also seen that this *Brahman* is not this table and yet is this table. Take off the name and form, and whatever is reality is He. He is the reality in everything. "Thou art the woman, thou art the man, thou the young man walking in the pride of youth, thou the old man tottering on his stick, thou art all in all, in everything, and I am Thou, I am Thou."

That is the theme of Advaitism. A few words more. Herein we find the explanation of the essence of things. We have seen how here alone we can take a firm stand against all the onrush of logic and scientific knowledge. Here at last reason has a firm foundation. At the same time the Indian Vedantist does not curse the preceding steps. He looks back and he blesses them, for he knows that they were true, only wrongly perceived and wrongly stated. They were seen through the glass of *mâyâ*, distorted it may be, yet truth and nothing but truth. The same God whom the ignorant man saw outside nature, the same whom the little-knowing man saw as interpenetrating the universe, and the same whom the sage realizes as his own self, as the whole universe itself, all are one and the same being, the same entity seen from different points of view, seen through different glasses of *mâyâ*, perceived by different minds. All the difference is caused by that. Not only so, but one view must lead to the other. What is the difference between science and common knowledge? Go out into one of these streets and if something is happening, ask one of *gonwars* (boors) what it is. It is ten to one that he will tell you that a ghost is causing the phenomenon. He is always going after ghosts and spirits outside, because it is the nature of ignorance to seek for causes outside of effects. If a stone falls it has been thrown by a devil or a ghost, says the ignorant man, but the scientific man says it is the law of nature, the law of gravitation.

What is the fight between science and religion everywhere?

Religions are encumbered with a mass of explanations which are outside, one angel is in charge of the sun, another of the moon, and so on *ad infinitum*; every change is caused by a spirit, the one point of agreement being that they are all outside the thing itself; while science means that the cause of a thing is to be sought in the nature of the thing itself. As step by step science is progressing, it has taken the explanation of natural phenomena out of the hands of spirits and angels. Because Advaitism has done likewise, it is the most scientific religion. This universe has not been created by any extra-cosmic God, nor is it the work of any outside genius. It is self-created, self-manifesting, self-dissolved, one infinite existence, the *Brahman*. "*Tat tvam asi Svetaketo*"—"O Svetaketu, That thou art." Thus you see that this, and this alone, can be the scientific religion, and with all the prattle about science that is going on daily at the present time in modern half-educated India, with all the talk about rationalism and reason that I hear every day, I expect that whole sects will come over and dare to be Advaitists, and dare to preach it to the world in the words of Buddha, "for the good of many, for the happiness of many." If you do not, I take you for cowards. If you are cowards, if fear is your excuse, allow the same liberty unto others, do not try to overthrow the poor idol-worshipper, do not call him a devil, do not go about preaching to every man who does not agree entirely with you; know first that you are cowards yourselves, and if society frightens you, if your own superstitions of the past frighten you so much, how much more will these superstitions frighten and bind down those who are ignorant? That is the Advaitist position. Have mercy on others. Would to God that the whole world were Advaitists to-morrow, not only in theory, but in realization; but if that cannot be, let us do the next best thing. Let us take our less enlightened brothers by the hand, lead them gently step by step just as they can go, and know that every step in all religious growth in India has been progressive. It is not from bad to good, but from good to better.

Something more must be said about the moral relation. Our boys blithely talk nowadays, they learn from somebody—Lord knows from whom—that Advaita will make people immoral, because if we are all one and all God, we need not be moral at all. In the first place, that is the argument of the brute, who can only be kept down by the whip. If you are such a brute, commit suicide first, rather than be the kind of human being that has to be kept down by the whip. If the whip goes away, you will be a demon! You ought all to be killed just here, if such is the case; there is no help for you; you must always be living under this whip and rod, and there is no salvation, no escape for you. In the second place, Advaita and Advaita alone explains morality. Every religion preaches that the essence of all morality is to do good unto others. And why? Be unselfish. And why? Some god has said it? He is not for me. Some texts have told it? Let them all tell it; that is nothing to me; let them all tell it. And if they do, what is it? Each one for himself, and somebody for the hindermost, that is all the morality in the world, at least with many. What is the reason why I should be moral? You cannot explain it except when you come to know. "He who sees every one in himself, and himself in every one, thus seeing the same God living in all in the same manner, he (the sage) no more kills the self by the self." Know through Advaita that whomever you hurt, you hurt yourself; they are all you. Whether you know it or not, through all hands you work, through all feet you move, you are the king enjoying in the palace, you are the beggar leading that miserable existence in the street; you are the ignorant as well as the learned, you are the man who is weak, and you are the strong; know this and be sympathetic. And that is why we must not hurt others. That is why I do not even care whether I have got to starve, because there will be millions of mouths eating at the same time, and they are all mine. Therefore I should not care what becomes of me and mine, for the whole universe is mine, I am enjoying all the bliss at the same time; and who can kill me, or the universe? Herein Advaita alone explains morality. The others teach it, but cannot give you its reason. So much for explanation.

What is the gain? Strength is the gain. Take off that veil of hypnotism which you have cast upon the world, send not out thoughts and words of weakness unto humanity. Know that all sins and all evil can be summed up in that one word weakness. It is weakness that is the motive power in all evil doing; it is weakness that is the source of all selfishness, it is weakness that makes men injure each other, it is weakness that makes them manifest as they are not really. Let them all know what they are; let them tell day and night what they are. Let them suck it with their mothers' milk, this idea of strength. Let them ever repeat *"Soham, Soham,"* "I am He, I am He." And then let them think of it, and lastly let them deeply meditate upon it, and out of that heart will proceed works such as the world has never seen. What has to be done? This Advaitism is said by some to be impracticable; that is to say, it is not yet manifesting itself on the material plane. To a certain extent this is true, for, remember the saying of the Vedas—"*Om*, this is the great secret; *Om*, this is the greatest possession; he who knows the secret of this *Om*, whatever he desires that he gets."

Therefore first know the secret of this "*Om*," that you are the "*Om*"; know the secret of this "*Tat tvam asi*," and then, and then alone, whatever you want shall come to you. If you want to be great materially, believe that you are so. I may be a little bubble, and you may be a wave mountain-high, but know that for both of us the infinite ocean is the background, the infinite *Brahman* is our magazine of power and strength, and we can draw as much as we like, both of us,

I the bubble and you the mountain-high wave. Believe therefore in yourselves. The secret of Advaita is—Believe in yourselves first, and then believe in anything else. In the history of the world, you will find that only those nations that have believed in themselves have become great and strong. In the history of each nation, you will always find that only those individuals who have believed in themselves have become great and strong. Here, in India, came an Englishman, who was only a clerk, and for want of funds and other reasons he twice tried to blow out his brains, and when he failed he believed that he was born to do great things, and that man became Lord Clive, the founder of the Empire. If he had believed the *padris* and gone crawling all his life—"Oh Lord, I am weak and I am low"—where would he have been? In a lunatic asylum. They have made weaklings of you with these evil teachings. I have seen all the world over the bad effects of these weak teachings of humility, destroying the human race.

This is on the practical side. Believe, therefore, in yourselves, and if you want material wealth work it out; it will come to you. If you want to be intellectual let it work out on the intellectual plane and intellectual giants you shall be. And if you want to attain to freedom let it work out on the spiritual plane, and gods you shall be. "Enter into *Nirvana*, the blissful." The defect is here; so far the Advaita has only been tried on the spiritual plane, and nowhere else, now the time has come when you must make it practical. It shall no more be a secret, it shall no more live with monks in caves and forests, and in the Himalayas; it must come down to the daily, everyday life of the people; it shall be worked out in the palace of the king, in the cave of the recluse, it shall be worked out in the cottage of the poor, by the beggar in the street, everywhere, anywhere it can be worked out. Therefore do not fear if you are a woman or a *Sudra*, or anything, for this religion is so great, says Lord Krishna, that even the least done brings a great amount of good. Therefore children of the Âryans, do not sit idle, awake and arise, and stop not until the goal is reached. The time has come when this Advaita is to be worked out practically. Let us bring it down from heaven unto earth; this is the present dispensation. Aye, the voices of our forefathers of old are telling us to stop—stop here my children. Let these great teachings come down lower and lower until they have permeated the world, till they have entered into every pore of society, till they have become the common property of everybody, till they have become part and parcel of our lives, till they have entered into our veins and tingle with every drop of blood there.

You may be astonished to hear it, but as practical Vedantists the Americans are better than we are. I used to stand on the sea-front of New York, and look at the emigrants coming from different countries, crushed, down-trodden, hopeless, with a little bundle of clothes as their only possession, their clothes in rags, unable to look a man in the face; if they saw a policeman they were afraid and tried to get to the other side of the footpath. And, mark you, in six months those very men were walking erect, well clothed, looked everybody in the face; and what makes this wonderful difference? Suppose a man comes from Armenia, or from any other place where he was crushed down beyond all recognition, where everybody told him he was a born slave, born to remain in a low state all his life, and where at the least move on his part he was trodden upon. There everything cried out to him, "Slave; you are a slave; remain such. Helpless you were born, helpless remain." Even the very air murmured round him, "There is no hope for you, hopeless and a slave remain;" while stronger men crushed the life out of him. And when that same man landed in New York he went about, and found a new life; he found that there was a place in the world where he was a man among men. Perhaps he went to Washington, shook hands with the President of the United States, and perhaps there he saw men coming from distant villages, peasants, and ill clad, all shaking hands with the President. Then the veil of *mâyâ* slipped away from him. He who had been hypnotized into slavery and weakness, is once more awake, and he rises up and finds himself a man in the world of men.

In this country of ours, the very birthplace of Vedânta, our masses have been hypnotized for ages into that very state. To touch them is pollution. To sit with them is pollution. Hopeless they were born; hopeless they must remain; and the result is that they have been sinking, sinking, sinking, and have come to the last stage to which a human being can come. For what other country is there in the world where man has to sleep with the cattle? And for this blame nobody else, do not commit the mistake of the ignorant. The effect is here and the cause is here too. We are to blame. Stand up, be bold, and take the blame on your shoulders. Do not go about throwing mud at others; for all the pangs you suffer you are the sole and only cause.

Young men of Lahore, understand this, that this great sin, hereditary and national, is on your shoulders. There is no hope for us. You may make thousands of societies, twenty thousand political assemblages, fifty thousand institutions. These will be of no use until there is that sympathy, that love, that heart, which thinks of all, until Buddha's heart comes once more into India, until the words of Lord Krishna are brought to their practical use there is no hope for us. You go on imitating the Europeans and their societies and their assemblages, but let me tell you a story, a fact that I saw with my own eyes. A company of Burmans was taken over to London by some persons from India, who turned out to be Eurasians. They exhibited these people in London, took all the money, and then took these Burmans over to the Continent, and left them there for good or ill. These poor people did not know one word of any European language, but the English Consul in Austria sent them over to London. They were helpless in London, not knowing any one. But an English lady heard of them, took these foreigners from Burmah into her own house, gave them her own clothes, her bed, and everything, and then sent the news to the newspapers. And, mark you, the next day the whole nation was, as it were, aroused. Money poured in and these people were helped out, and sent back to Burmah. On this sort of sympathy are based all English political and other institutions, it is the rock foundation of love, for themselves at least. They may not love the world; they may be enemies all round, but in that country, it goes without saying, there is this great love for their own people, for truth and justice and charity to the stranger at the door. I would be the most ungrateful man, if I did not continually tell you how wonderfully and how hospitably I was received in every country in the West. Where is the heart here to build upon?

No sooner do we start a little joint-stock company then we cheat each other, and the whole thing comes down with a crash. You talk of imitating the English, and building as big a nation as they have. But where are the foundations? Ours are only sand, and therefore the building comes down with a crash in no time. Young men of Lahore, raise once more that wonderful banner of Advaita, for on no other ground can you have that all-embracing love, until you see that the same Lord is present in the same manner everywhere; unfurl that banner of love. "Arise, awake and stop not till the goal is reached." Arise, arise once more, for nothing can be done without renunciation. If you want to help others, your own little self must go. In the words of the Christians, you cannot serve God and mammon at the same time. Have *vairâgyam*—your ancestors gave up the world to do great things. At the present time there are men who give up the world to help their own salvation. Throw away everything, even your own salvation, and go and help others. Aye, you are always talking bold words, but here is practical Vedânta before you. Give up this little life of yours. What matters if you die of starvation, you and I and thousands like us, so long as this nation lives? The nation is sinking, the curse of unnumbered millions is on our heads; to whom we have been giving ditch-water to drink when they have been dying of thirst, while the perennial river of water was flowing past; the unnumbered millions whom we have allowed to starve in sight of plenty; the unnumbered millions to whom we have talked of Advaita and whom we have hated with all our strength; the unnumbered millions to whom we have talked theoretically that all are one, and that all are the same Lord, without even an ounce of practice. O my friends, must it only be in the mind and never in practice?

Wipe off this blot. Arise and awake. What matters it if this little life goes; every one has to die, the saint or the sinner, the rich or the poor. The body never remains for any one. Arise and awake and be perfectly sincere. What we want is character, that steadiness and character that make a man cling to a thing like grim death. "Let the sages blame or let them praise, let *Lakshmi* come to-day, let her go away, let death come just now, or in a hundred years; he indeed is the sage who does not make one false step from the path of right."

Arise and awake, for the time is passing and all our energies will be frittered away in vain talking. Arise and awake, let minor things and quarrels over little details, and fights over little doctrines be thrown aside, for here is the greatest of all works, here are the sinking millions. Mark, when the Mohammedans first came into India, there were sixty millions of Hindus here; to-day there are less than twenty millions. Every day they will become less and less till the whole disappear. Let them disappear, but with them will disappear the marvellous ideas of which with all their defects and all their misrepresentations they have stood as representatives. And with them will disappear this sublime Advaita, the crown jewel of all spiritual thought. Therefore, arise, awake, with your hands stretched out to protect the spirituality of the world. And first of all, work it out for your own country. What we want is not so much spirituality, as the bringing down of a little of Advaita into the material world, first bread and then religion. We stuff them too much with religion, when the poor fellows have been starving. No dogmas will satisfy the cravings of hunger. There are two curses here, first our weakness, second our hatred, our dried-up hearts. You may talk doctrines by the thousand, you may have sects by the hundreds of thousands; but it is nothing until you have the heart to feel, feel for them as your Veda teaches you; till you find that they are parts of your own bodies, till you realize that you and they, the poor and the rich, the saint and the sinner, all are parts of one Infinite whole which you call *Brahman*.

Gentlemen, thus I have tried to place before you only a few of the most brilliant points of the Advaita system, and to show that the time has come when it should be carried out into practice, not only in this country, but everywhere. Modern science and its sledgehammer blows are pulverizing the porcelain foundations of all dualistic religions everywhere. Not only here are the dualists torturing texts till they will extend no longer, for texts are not india-rubber; it is not only here that they are trying to get into the nooks and corners to protect themselves, it is still more so in Europe and America. And even there something of this idea will have to go from India. It has already reached there. It will have to increase and increase, and to save their civilizations too. For, in the West, the old order of things is vanishing, giving way to a new order of things, which is the worship of gold, the worship of Mammon. Even the old crude system of religion was better than the modern system— namely, competition and gold. No nation, however strong, can stand on such foundations, and the history of the world tells us that all those which had similar foundations are dead and gone. In the first place we have to stop the incoming of such a wave in India. Therefore preach the Advaita to every one, so that religion may withstand the shock of modern science. Not only so, you will have to help others, your thought must reach out to Europe and America. But above all let me once more remind you that there is need of practical work, and the first part of this is to go down to the sinking millions of India. Take them by the hand, remembering the words of Lord Krishna: "Even in this life they have conquered heaven whose minds are firmly fixed in this sameness, for God is pure and the same to all; therefore such are said to be living in God."

VEDÂNTA PHILOSOPHY: JNÂNA YOGA. PART II. SEVEN LECTURES

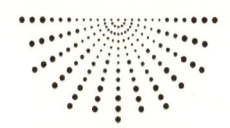

EDITOR'S PREFACE

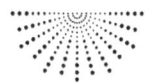

The lectures given in this volume were originally delivered by Swâmi Vivekânanda in New York in the beginning of 1896, and were received with the greatest enthusiasm.

Their purely philosophical character, however, made it doubtful as to whether they would appeal to the general public, and for that reason they were not brought out in book form at once.

The great success of the London lectures on Jnâna Yoga, which were published several years ago and which have already gone through two editions, now encourages the belief that this series will meet with an equally favorable reception. The conception of Jnâna according to Vedânta is a bold and daring one, and reaches the highest possible ideal, for it teaches the absolute unity of all existence. As will be easily understood by the students of the former volume, Jnâna Yoga is purely monistic on the highest spiritual plane. Speaking about this phase of Vedânta, Prof. Max Müller writes: "None of our philosophers, not excepting Heraclitus, Plato, Kant, or Hegel has ventured to erect such a spire, never frightened by storms or lightnings. Stone follows on stone in regular succession after once the first step has been made, after once it has been clearly seen that in the beginning there can have been but One, as there will be but

One in the end, whether we call It Âtman or Brahman." This may be a difficult thought for many to grasp at the outset, but it is worth careful study, and once understood will be a never-failing light to guide the enquiring soul to the crowning truth of all philosophy.

This universe of ours, the universe of the senses, the rational, the intellectual, is bounded on both sides by the illimitable, the unknowable, the ever unknown. Herein is the search, herein are the inquiries, here are the facts, from this comes the light which is known to the world as religion. Essentially, however, religion belongs to the supersensuous and not to the sense plane. It is beyond all reasoning and is not on the plane of intellect. It is a vision, an inspiration, a plunge into the unknown and unknowable, making the unknowable more than known, for it can never be "known." This search has been in the human mind, as I believe, from the very beginning of humanity. There cannot have been human reasoning and intellect in any period of the world's history without this struggle, this search beyond. In our little universe, this human mind, we see a thought arise. Whence it arises we do not know, and when it disappears, where it goes we know not either. The macrocosm and the microcosm are, as it were, in the same groove, passing through the same stages, vibrating in the same key.

In these lectures I shall try to bring before you the Hindu theory that religions do not come from without, but from within. It is my belief that religious thought is in man's very constitution, so much so that it is impossible for him to give up religion until he can give up his mind and body, until he can give up thought and life. As long as a man thinks, this struggle must go on, and so long man must have some form of religion. Thus we see various forms of religion in the world. It is a bewildering study, but it is not, as many of us think, a vain speculation. Amidst this chaos there is harmony, throughout these discordant sounds there is a note of concord, and he who is prepared to listen to it will catch the tone.

The great question of all questions at the present time is this: Taking for granted that the known and the knowable are bounded on both sides by the unknowable and the infinitely unknown, why struggle for that infinite unknown? Why shall we not be content with the known? Why shall we not rest satisfied with eating, drinking, and doing a little good to society? This idea is in the air. From the most learned professor to the prattling baby, we are told to do good to the world, that is all of religion, and that it is useless to trouble ourselves about questions of the beyond. So much is this the case that it has become a truism. But fortunately we *must* question the beyond. This present, this expressed, is only one part of that unexpressed. The sense universe is, as it were, only one portion, one bit of that infinite spiritual universe projected into the plane of sense consciousness. How can this little bit of projection be explained, be understood, without knowing that which is beyond? It is said of Socrates that one day while lecturing at Athens, he met a Brahmin who had travelled into Greece, and Socrates told the Brahmin that the greatest study for mankind is man. The Brahmin sharply retorted: "How can you know man until you know God?" This God, this eternally unknowable, or absolute, or infinite, or without name,—you may call Him by what name you like,—is the rational, the only explanation, the *raison d'etre* of that which is known and knowable, this present life. Take anything before you, the most material thing; take one of the most material sciences, as chemistry or physics, astronomy or biology, study it, push the study forward and forward, and the gross forms will begin to melt and become finer and finer, until they come to a point where you are bound to make a tremendous leap from these material things into the immaterial. The gross melts into the fine, physics into metaphysics, in every department of knowledge.

Thus man finds himself driven to a study of the beyond. Life will be a desert, human life will be vain if we cannot know the beyond. It is very well to say: Be contented with the things of the present; the cows and the dogs are, and all animals, and that is what makes them animals. So if man rests content with the present and gives up all search into the beyond, mankind will have to go back to the animal plane again. It is religion, the inquiry into the beyond, that makes the difference between man and an animal. Well has it been said that man is the only animal that naturally looks upwards; every other animal naturally looks prone. That looking upward and going upward and seeking perfection are what is called salvation, and the sooner a man begins to go higher, the sooner he raises himself towards this idea of truth as salvation. It does not consist in the amount of money in your pocket, or the dress you wear, or the house you live in, but in the wealth of spiritual thought in your brain. That is what makes for human progress, that is the source of all material and intellectual progress, the motive power behind, the enthusiasm that pushes mankind forward.

Religion does not live in bread, does not dwell in a house. Again and again you hear this objection advanced, "What good can religion do? Can it take away the poverty of the poor"? Supposing it cannot, would that prove the untruth of religion? Suppose a baby stands up among you when you are trying to demonstrate an astronomical theorem, and says: "Does it bring gingerbread?" "No, it does not," you answer. "Then," says the baby, "it is useless." Babies judge the whole universe from their own standpoint, that of producing gingerbread, and so are the babies of the world. We must not judge of higher things from a low standpoint. Everything must be judged by its own standard and the infinite must be judged by an infinite standard. Religion permeates the whole of man's life, not only the present, but the past, present, and future. It is therefore the eternal relation between the eternal soul and the eternal God. Is it logical to measure its value by its action upon five minutes of human life?

Certainly not. These are all negative arguments.

Now comes the question, can religion really accomplish anything? It can. It brings to man eternal life. It has made man what he is and will make of this human animal a god. That is what religion can do. Take religion from human society and what will remain? Nothing but a forest of brutes. Sense-happiness is not the goal of humanity; wisdom (Jnânam) is the goal of all life. We find that man enjoys his intellect more than an animal enjoys its senses, and we see that man enjoys his spiritual nature even more than his rational nature. So the highest wisdom must be this spiritual knowledge. With this knowledge will come bliss. All these things of this world are but the shadows, the manifestations in the third or fourth degree of the real Knowledge and Bliss.

One question more: What is the goal? Nowadays it is asserted that man is infinitely progressing, forward and forward, and there is no goal of perfection to attain to. Ever approaching, never attaining, whatever that may mean and however wonderful it may be, it is absurd on the face of it. Is there any motion in a straight line? A straight line infinitely projected becomes a circle, it returns to the starting point. You must end where you begin, and as you began in God, you must go back to God. What remains? Detail work. Through eternity you have to do the detail work.

Yet another question. Are we to discover new truths of religion as we go on? Yea and nay. In the first place we cannot know anything more of religion, it has all been known. In all the religions of the world you will find it claimed that there is a unity within us. Being one with divinity, there cannot be any further progress in that sense. Knowledge means finding this unity. I see you as men and women, and this is variety. It becomes scientific knowledge when I group you together and call you human beings. Take the science of chemistry, for instance. Chemists are seeking to resolve all known substances into their original elements and if possible to find the one element from which all these were derived. The time may come when they will find one element that is the source of all other elements. Reaching that, they can go no farther; the science of chemistry will have become perfect. So it is with the science of religion. If we can discover this perfect unity, there cannot be any farther progress.

The next question is can such a unity be found? In India the attempt has been made from the earliest times to reach a science of religion and philosophy, for the Hindus do not separate these as is customary in Western countries. We regard religion and philosophy as but two aspects of one thing which must equally be grounded in reason and scientific truth. In the lectures that are to follow I shall try to explain to you first the system of the *Sânkhya* philosophy, one of the most ancient in India, or in fact in the world. Its great exponent Kapila is the father of all Hindu psychology and the ancient system that he taught is still the foundation of all accepted systems of philosophy in India to-day,—which are known as the *Dârsanas*.

They all adopt his psychology, however widely they differ in other respects.

Next I shall endeavor to show you how Vedânta, as the logical outcome of the *Sânkhya*, pushes its conclusions yet farther. While its cosmology agrees with that taught by Kapila, the Vedânta is not satisfied to end in dualism, but continues its search for the final unity which is alike the goal of science and religion. To make clear the manner in which the task is accomplished will be the effort of the later lectures in this course.

I. THE SÂNKHYA COSMOLOGY.

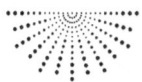

Here are two words, the microcosm and the macrocosm, the internal and the external. We get truths from both of these by means of experience; there is internal experience and external experience. The truths gathered from internal experience are psychology, metaphysics and religion; from external experience the physical sciences. Now a perfect truth should be in harmony with experience in both these worlds.

The microcosm must bear testimony to the macrocosm, and the macrocosm to the microcosm; physical truth must have its counterpart in the internal world, and the internal world must have its verification in the outside. Yet as a rule we find that many of these truths are constantly conflicting. At one period of the world's history the "internals" became supreme, and they began to fight the "externals;" at the present time the "externals," the physicists, have become supreme, and they have put down many claims of the psychologists and metaphysicians. So far as my little knowledge goes, I find that the really essential parts of psychology are in perfect accordance with the essential parts of modern physical knowledge.

It is not given to every individual to be great in every respect; it is not given to the same race, or nation, to be equally strong in the research of all the fields of knowledge. The modern European nations are very strong in their researches into external physical knowledge, but the ancient Europeans were weak in their researches into the internal part of man. On the other hand, the Orientals have not been very strong in their researches in the external physical world, but have excelled in their researches into the internal, and therefore we find that some of the Oriental theories are not in accordance with Occidental physics, neither is Occidental psychology in harmony with Oriental teachings on this subject. The Oriental physicists have been criticised by Occidental scientists. At the same time each rests on truth, and, as we stated before, real truth in any field of knowledge will not contradict itself, the truths internal are in harmony with the truths external.

We know the present theories of the Cosmos according to the modern astronomers and physicists, and at the same time we know how wofully they hurt the old school of theologians, and how every new scientific discovery that is made is as a bomb thrown into their house, and how they have attempted in every age to put down all these researches. In the first place, let us go over the psychological and scientific ideas of the Orientals as to cosmology and all that pertains to it, and you will find how wonderfully it is in accordance with all the latest discoveries of modern science, and when there is anything lacking you will find that it is on the side of modern science. We all use the word Nature, and the old Hindu philosophers called it by two different names, *Prakriti*, which is almost the same as the English word "nature," and by the more scientific name, *Avyaktam* ("undifferentiated"), from which everything proceeds, out of which come atoms and molecules, matter and force, and mind and intellect. It is startling to find that the philosophers and metaphysicians of India ages ago stated that mind is but matter in a finer form, for what are our present materialists striving to do but to show that mind is as much a product of nature as the body? And so is thought; and we shall find by and by that the intellect also comes from the same nature which is called *avyaktam*, the undifferentiated.

The ancient teachers define *avyaktam* as the "equilibrium of the three forces," one of which is called *Sattva*, the second *Rajas* and the third *Tamas*. *Tamas*, the lowest force, is that of attraction, a little higher is *Rajas*, that of repulsion, and the highest is the control of these two, *Sattva*, so that when the two forces, attraction and repulsion, are held in perfect control, or balance, by the *Sattva*, there is no creation, no movement; but as soon as this equilibrium is lost, the balance is disturbed and one of these forces gets stronger than the other. Then change and motion begin and all this evolution goes on. This state of things is going on cyclically, periodically; that is to say, there is a period of disturbance of the balance, when all these forces begin to combine and recombine, and this universe is projected; and there is also a period when everything has a tendency to revert to the primal state of equilibrium, and the time comes when a total absence of all manifestation is reached. Again, after a period, the whole thing is disturbed, projected outward, again it slowly comes out in the form of waves; for all motion in this universe is in the form of waves, successive rise and fall.

Some of these old philosophers taught that the whole universe quiets down for a period; others maintained that this quieting down applies only to systems. That is to say, that while our system here, this solar system, will quiet down and go back into that undifferentiated state, there are millions of other systems going the other way. I should rather follow the second opinion, that this quieting down is not simultaneous over the whole universe, but that in different parts different things are going on. But the principle remains the same, that all that we see, that Nature herself is progressing in successive rises and falls. The one stage, going back to the balance, to the perfect equilibrium, is called the end of a cycle. The whole *Kalpa*, the evolution and the involution, has been compared by theistic writers in India to the inbreathing and outbreathing of God; God, as it were, breathes out the universe, and it returns into Him again. When it quiets down, what becomes of the universe? It still exists, only in finer form, as it is called in Sanskrit, in the "causal state" (*Kârana Sarira*). Causation, time and space are still there, only they are potential. This return to an undifferentiated condition constitutes involution. Involution and evolution are eternally going on, so that when we speak of a beginning, we refer only to the beginning of a cycle.

The most extraneous part of the universe is what in modern times we call gross matter, The ancient Hindus called it the *Bhutas*, the external elements. There is one element which according to them is eternal; every other element is produced out of this one, and this eternal element is called *Âkâsa*. It is somewhat similar to the modern idea of ether, though not exactly the same. This is the primal element out of which everything proceeds, and along with this element there was something called *Prâna*: we shall see what it is as we go on. This *prâna* and this *âkâsa* eternally exist, and they combine and recombine and form all manifestation. Then at the end of the cycle everything subsides and goes back to the unmanifested form of *âkâsa* and *prâna*. There is in the Rig Veda, the oldest scriptures in existence, a beautiful passage describing creation, and it is most poetical—"When there was neither ought nor nought, when darkness was rolling over darkness, what existed?" and the answer is given, "It (the Eternal One) then existed without motion." *Prâna* and *âkâsa* were latent in that Eternal One, but there was no phenomenal manifestation. This state is called *Avyaktam*, which literally means "without vibration," or unmanifested. At the beginning of a new cycle of evolution, this *avyaktam* begins to vibrate and blow after blow is given by *prâna* to the *âkâsa*. This causes condensation and gradually, through the forces of attraction and repulsion, atoms are formed. These in turn condense into molecules and finally into the different elements of Nature.

We generally find these things very curiously translated; people do not go to the ancient philosophers or to their commentators for their translation and have not learning enough to understand for themselves. They translate the elements as "air," "fire," and so on. If they would go to the commentators they would find that they do not mean anything of the sort. The *âkâsa*, made to vibrate by the repeated blows of *prâna*, produces *vâyu* or the vibratory state of the *âkâsa*, which in turn produces gaseous matter. The vibrations growing more and more rapid generate heat, which in Sanskrit is called *tejas*. Gradually it is cooled off and the gaseous substance becomes solid, *prithivi*. We had first *âkâsa*, then came heat, then it became liquified, and when still more condensed appeared as solid matter. It goes back to the unmanifested condition in exactly the reverse way. The solids will be converted into liquid and the liquid into a mass of heat, that will slowly go back into the gaseous state, disintegration of atoms will begin, finally equilibrium of all forces will be reached, vibration will stop and the cycle of evolution which in Sanskrit is called *Kalpa* is at an end. We know from modern astronomy that this earth and sun of ours are undergoing the same transitions, this solid earth will melt down and become liquid once more, and will eventually go back to the gaseous state.

Prâna cannot work alone without the help of *âkâsa*. All that we know is that motion or vibration and every movement that we see is a modification of this *prâna*, and everything that we know in the form of matter, either as form or as resistance, is a modification of this *âkâsa*. This *prâna* cannot exist alone, or act without a medium, but in every state of it, whether as pure *prâna*, or when it changes into other forces of nature, say gravitation or centrifugal attraction, it can never be separate from *âkâsa*. You have never seen force without matter or matter without force; what we call force and matter being simply the gross manifestations of these same things, which, when superfine, we call *prâna* and *âkâsa*. *Prâna* you can call in English the life, or vital energy, but you must not restrict it to the life of man, nor should you identify it with the spirit, *Âtman*. Creation is without beginning and without end; it cannot have either, it is an eternal on-going.

The next question that comes is rather a fine one. Some European philosophers have asserted that this world exists because "I" exist, and if "I" do not exist, the world will not exist. Sometimes it is expressed in this way; they say, if all the people in the world were to die, and there were no more human beings, and no animals with powers of perception and intelligence, all manifestations would disappear. It seems paradoxical, but gradually we shall see clearly that this can be proved. But these European philosophers do not know the psychology of it, although they know the principle; modern philosophy has got only a glimpse of it.

First we will take another proposition of these old psychologists which is rather startling, that the grossest elements are the *bhutas*, but that all gross things are the results of fine ones. Everything that is gross is composed of a combination of minute things, so the *bhutas* must be composed of certain fine particles, called in Sanskrit the *tanmâtras*. I smell a flower; to smell that, something must come in contact with my nose; the flower is there and I do not see it move towards me; but without something coming in contact with my nose I cannot smell the flower. That which comes from the flower and into contact with my nose are the *tanmâtras*, fine molecules of that flower, so fine that no diminution can be perceived in the flower. So with heat, light, sight, and everything. These *tanmâtras* can again be subdivided into atoms. Different philosophers have different theories, and we know these are only theories, so we leave them out of discussion. Sufficient for us that everything gross is composed of things that are very, very minute. We first get the gross elements, which we feel externally, and composing them are the fine elements, which our organs touch, which come in contact with the nerves of the nose, eyes and ears.

That ethereal wave which touches my eyes, I cannot see, yet I know it must come in contact with my optic nerve before I can see the light. So with hearing, we can never see the particles that come in contact with our ears, but we know that they must be there. What is the cause of these *tanmâtras*? A very startling and curious answer is given by our psychologists,— self-consciousness. That is the cause of these fine materials, and the cause of the organs. What are these organs? Here is first the eye, but the eye does not see. If the eyes did see, when a man is dead, and his eyes are still perfect, they would still be able to see. There is some change somewhere; something has gone out of the man, and that something, which really sees, of which the eye is the instrument, is called the organ. So this nose is an instrument, and there is an organ corresponding to it. Modern physiology can tell you what that is, a nerve centre in the brain. The eyes, ears, etc., are simply the external instruments. It may be said that the organs, *Indriyas*, as they are called in Sanskrit, are the real seats of perception.

What is the use of having one organ for the nose, and one for the eyes, and so on? Why will not one serve the purpose? To make it clear to you,—I am talking, and you are listening, and you do not see what is going on around you because the mind has attached itself to the organ of hearing, and has detached itself from the sight organ. If there were only one organ the mind would hear and see at the same time, it would see and hear and smell at the same time, and it would be impossible for it not to do all three at the same time. Therefore it is necessary that there should be separate organs for all these centres. This has been borne out by modern physiology. It is certainly possible for us to see and hear at the same time, but that is because the mind attaches itself partially to both centres, which are the organs. What are the instruments? We see that these are really made of the gross materials. Here they are,—eyes, nose, and ears, etc. What are the organs? They are also made of materials, because they are centres. Just as this body is composed of gross material for transforming *prâna* into different gross forces, so these finer organs behind, are composed of the fine elements, for the manufacture of *prâna* into the finer forces of perception and all kindred things. All these organs or *indriyas* combined, plus the internal instrument or *antahkarana*, are called the finer body of man,—the *linga* (or *sûkshma*) *sarira*.

It has a real form, because everything material must have a form. Behind the *indriyas* is what is called the *manas*, the *chitta* in *vritti*, what might be called the vibratory state of the mind, the unsettled state. If you throw a stone into a calm lake, first there will be vibration, and then resistance. For a moment the water will vibrate and then it will react on the stone. So, when any impression comes on the *chitta*, or "mind stuff," it vibrates a little. This state of the mind is called the *manas*. Then comes the reaction, the will. There is another thing behind this will which accompanies all the acts of the mind, which is called egoism, the *ahamkâra*, the self-consciousness, which says "I am," and behind that is what is called *Buddhi*, the intellect, the highest form of nature's existence. Behind the intellect is the true Self of man, the *Purusha*, the pure, the perfect, who is alone the seer, and for whom is all this change. The Purusha is looking on at all these changes; he himself is never impure; but by implication, what the Vedantists call *adhyâsam*, by reflection, he appears to be impure. It is like a red flower held before a piece of crystal; the crystal will look red; or a blue flower and the crystal will look blue; and yet the crystal itself is colorless. We will take for granted that there are many selves; each self is pure and perfect, but it is all these various divisions of gross matter and fine matter that are imposing on the self, and making it variously colored. Why is nature doing all this? Nature is undergoing all these changes for the improvement of the soul; all this creation is for the benefit of the soul, so that it may be free. This immense book which we call the universe is stretched before man so that he may read, and come out, as an omniscient and omnipotent being. I must here tell you that some of our best psychologists do not believe in a personal God in the sense in which you believe in Him. The real father of our psychologists, Kapila, denies the existence of God as a Creator. His idea is that a personal God is quite unnecessary; Nature itself is sufficient to work out all that is good. What is called the "Design" theory he repudiated, and said a more childish theory was never advanced. But he admits a peculiar kind of God; he says we are all struggling to get free, and when man becomes free he can, as it were, melt away into Nature for the time being, only to come out at the beginning of the next cycle and be its ruler; come out an omniscient and omnipotent being. In that sense he can be called God; you and I and the humblest beings will be gods in different cycles. Kapila says such a God will be temporal, but an eternal God, eternally omnipotent and eternally ruler of the universe, cannot be. If there were such a God, there would be this difficulty: he must either be bound or free. A God who is perfectly free would not create; there would be no necessity. If he were bound, he would not create because he could not, he would be weak himself. So, in either case, there cannot be an omnipotent or omniscient eternal ruler. So wherever the word God is mentioned in our Scriptures, Kapila says it means those perfected souls who have become free. The *Sânkhya* system does not believe in the unity of all souls. Vedânta believes that all individual souls are united in one cosmic Being called *Brahman*, but Kapila, the founder of the *Sânkhya*, was dualistic. His analysis of the universe so far as it goes is really marvellous. He was the father of Hindu evolutionists, and all the later philosophical systems are simply outcomes of his thought.

According to this system all souls will regain their freedom and their natural rights, which are omnipotence and omniscience. Here the question may be asked, whence is this bondage of the souls? The *Sânkhya* says it is without beginning, but if it be without beginning it must also be without end, and we shall never be free. Kapila explains that this "without beginning" means not in a constant line. Nature is without beginning and without end, but not in the same sense as is the soul, because Nature has no individuality, just as a river flowing by us is every moment getting a fresh body of water, and the sum total of all these bodies of water is the river, so the river is not a constant quantity. Similarly everything in Nature is constantly changing, but the soul never changes. Therefore as Nature is always changing, it is possible for the soul to come out of its bondage. One theory of the *Sânkhya* is peculiar to this psychology. The whole of the universe is built upon the same plan as one single man, or one little being; so, just as I have a mind, there is also a cosmic mind. When this macrocosm evolves there must be first intelligence, then egoism, then the *tanmâtras* and the organs, and then the gross elements. The whole universe according to Kapila is one body, all that we see are the grosser bodies, and behind these are the finer bodies, and behind them, a universal egoism, and behind that a universal Intelligence, but all this is *in* Nature, all this is manifestation of Nature, not outside of Nature. Each one of us is a part of that cosmic consciousness. There is a sum-total of intelligence out of which we draw what we require, so there is a sum-total of mental force in the universe out of which we are drawing eternally, but the seed for the body must come from the parents. The theory includes heredity and reincarnation too. The material is given to the soul out of which to manufacture a body, but that material is given by hereditary transmission from the parents.

We come now to that proposition that in this process there is an involution and an evolution. All is evolved out of that indiscreet Nature; and then is involved again and becomes *Avyaktam*. It is impossible, according to the *Sânkhyas*, for any material thing to exist, which has not as its material some portion of consciousness. Consciousness is the material out of which all manifestation is made. The elucidation of this comes in our next lecture, but I will show how it can be proved. I do not know this table as it is, but it makes an impression; it comes to the eyes, then to the *indriyas*, and then to the mind; the mind then reacts, and that reaction is what I call the table. It is just the same as throwing a stone into a lake; the lake throws a wave against the stone; this wave is what we know. The waves coming out are all we know. In the same way the fashion of this wall is in my mind; what is external nobody knows; when I want to know it, it has to become that material which I furnish; I, with my own mind, have furnished the material for my eyes, and the something which is outside is only the occasion, the suggestion, and upon that suggestion I project my mind, and it takes the form of what I see. The question is, how do we all see the same things? Because we all have a part of this cosmic mind.

Those who have mind will see the thing, and those who have not will not see it. This goes to show that since this universe has existed there has never been a want of mind, of that one cosmic mind. Every human being, every animal, is also furnished out of that cosmic mind, because it is always present and furnishing material for their formation.

II. PRAKRITI AND PURUSHA.

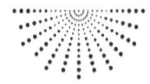

We will take up the categories we have been discussing and come to the particulars. If we remember we started with *Prakriti*, or Nature. This Nature is called by the *Sânkhya* philosophers indiscrete or inseparate, which is defined as perfect balance of the materials in it; and it naturally follows that in perfect balance there cannot be any motion. All that we see, feel, and hear is simply a compound of motion and matter. In the primal state, before this manifestation, where there was no motion, perfect balance, this *Prakriti* was indestructible, because decomposition comes only with limitation. Again, according to the *Sânkhya*, atoms are not the primal state. This universe does not come out of atoms, they may be the secondary, or tertiary state. The original matter may compound into atoms, which in turn compound into greater and greater things, and as far as modern investigations go, they rather point towards that. For instance, in the modern theory of ether, if you say ether is also atomic, that will not solve the proposition at all. To make it clearer, say that air is composed of atoms, and we know that ether is everywhere, interpenetrating, omnipresent, and these atoms are floating, as it were, in ether. If ether again be composed of atoms, there will still be some space between two atoms of ether. What fills up that?

And again there will be another space between the atoms of that which fills up this space. If you propose that there is another ether still finer you must still have something to fill that space, and so it will be *regressus in infinitum*, what the *Sânkhya* philosophers call *anavasthâ*,—never reaching a final conclusion. So the atomic theory cannot be final. According to the *Sânkhyas* this Nature is omnipresent, one omnipresent mass of Nature in which are the causes of everything that exists. What is meant by cause? Cause is the more subtle state of the manifested state, the unmanifested state of that which becomes manifested. What do you mean by destruction? It is reverting to the cause,—the materials out of which a body is composed go back into their original state. Beyond this idea of destruction, any idea such as annihilation, is on the face of it absurd. According to modern physical sciences, it can be demonstrated that all destruction means that which Kapila called ages ago "reverting to the causal state." Going back to the finer form is all that is meant by destruction. You know how it can he demonstrated in a laboratory that matter is indestructible. Those of you who have studied chemistry will know that if you burn a candle and put a caustic pencil inside a glass tube beneath the candle, when the candle has burned away, if you take the caustic pencil out of the tube and weigh it, you will find that the pencil will weigh exactly its previous weight, plus the weight of the candle,—the candle became finer and finer, and went on to the caustic. So that in this present stage of our knowledge, if any man claims that anything becomes annihilated, he is only making himself absurd. It is only uneducated people who would advance such a proposition, and it is curious that modern knowledge coincides with what those old philosophers taught. The ancients proceeded in their inquiry by taking up mind as the basis; they analyzed the mental part of this universe and came to certain conclusions, while modern science is analyzing the physical part, and it also comes to the same conclusions. Both analyses must lead to the same truth.

You must remember that the first manifestation of this *Prakriti* in the cosmos is what the *Sânkhyas* called *Mahat*. We may call it universal intelligence, the great principle; that is the literal meaning. The first manifestation of *Prakriti* is this intelligence; I would not translate it by self-consciousness, because that would be wrong. Consciousness is only a part of this intelligence, which is universal. It covers all the grounds of consciousness, sub-consciousness and super-consciousness. In Nature, for instance, certain changes are going on before your eyes which you see and understand, but there are other changes so much finer that no human perception can catch them. They are from the same cause, the same *Mahat* is making these changes. There are other changes, beyond the reach of our mind or reasoning, all this series of changes is in this *Mahat*. You will understand it better when I come to the individual. Out of this *Mahat* comes the universal egoism, and these are both material. There is no difference between matter and mind save in degree. It is the same substance in finer or grosser form; one changes into the other, and this will exactly coincide with the modern physiological research, and it will save you from a great deal of fighting and struggling to believe that you have a mind separate from the brain, and all such impossible things. This substance called *Mahat* changes into the material egoism, the fine state of matter, and that egoism changes into two varieties. In one variety it changes into the organs. Organs are of two kinds—organs of sensation and organs of reaction. They are not the eyes or nose, but something finer, what you call brain centres, and nerve centres. This egoism becomes changed, and out of this material are manufactured these centres and these nerves. Out of the same substance, the egoism, is manufactured a yet finer form, the *tanmâtras*, fine particles of matter, those for instance which strike your nose and cause you to smell. You cannot perceive these fine particles, you can only know that they are there. These *tanmâtras* are manufactured out of that egoism, and out of these *tanmâtras*, or subtle matter, is manufactured the gross matter, air, water, earth, and all the things that we see and feel. I want to impress this on your mind. It is very hard to grasp it, because, in Western countries, the ideas are so queer about mind and matter. It is hard to take these impressions out of our brains. I myself had a tremendous difficulty, being educated in Western philosophy in my childhood. These are all cosmic things. Think of this universal extension of matter, unbroken, one substance, undifferentiated, which is the first state of everything, and which begins to change just as milk becomes curd, and it is changed into another substance called *Mahat*, which in one state manifests as intelligence and in another state as egoism. It is the same substance, and it changes into the grosser matter called egoism; thus is the whole universe itself built, as it were, layer after layer; first undifferentiated Nature (*Avyaktam*), and that changes into universal intelligence (*Mahat*), and that again is changed into universal egoism (*Ahamkâra*), and that changes into universal sensible matter. That matter changes into universal sense-organs, again changes into universal fine particles, and these in turn combine and become this gross universe. This is the cosmic plan, according to the *Sânkhyas*, and what is in the cosmos or macrocosm, must be in the individual or microcosm.

Take an individual man. He has first a part of undifferentiated nature in him, and that material nature in him becomes changed into *mahat*, a small particle of the universal intelligence, and that small particle of the universal intelligence in him becomes changed into egoism—a particle of the universal egoism. This egoism in turn becomes changed into the sense-organs, and out of these sense-organs come the *tanmâtras*, and out of them he combines and manufactures his world, as a body. I want this to be clear, because it is the first stepping stone to Vedânta, and it is absolutely necessary for you to know, because this is the philosophy of the whole world. There is no philosophy in the world that is not indebted to Kapila, the founder of this *Sânkhya* system. Pythagoras came to India and studied his philosophy and carried some of these ideas to the Greeks. Later it formed the Alexandrian school, and still later formed the basis of Gnostic philosophy. It became divided into two parts; one went to Europe and Alexandria, and the other remained in India, and became the basis of all Hindu philosophy, for out of it the system of Vyâsa was developed. This was the first rational system that the world saw, this system of Kapila. Every meta-physician in the world must pay homage to him. I want to impress on your mind that as the great father of philosophy, we are bound to listen to him, and respect what he said. This wonderful man, most ancient of philosophers, is mentioned even in the Vedas. How wonderful his perceptions were! If there is any proof required of the power of the Yogis to perceive things beyond the range of the ordinary senses, such men are the proofs. How could they perceive them? They had no microscopes, or telescopes. How fine their perception was, how perfect their analysis and how wonderful!

To revert again to the microcosm, man. As we have seen, he is built on exactly the same plan. First the nature is "indiscrete" or perfectly balanced, then it becomes disturbed, and action sets in and the first change produced by that action is what is called *mahat*,— intelligence. Now you see this intelligence in man is just a particle of the cosmic intelligence,—the *Mahat*. Out of it comes self-consciousness, and from this the sensory and the motor nerves, and the finer particles out of which the gross body is manufactured. I will here remark that there is one difference between Schopenhauer and Vedânta. Schopenhauer says the desire, or will, is the cause of everything. It is the will to exist that makes us manifest, but the Advaitists deny this. They say it is the intelligence. There cannot be a single particle of will which is not a reaction. So many things are beyond will. It is only a manufactured something out of the ego, and the ego is a product of something still higher, the intelligence, and that is a modification of "indiscrete" Nature, or *Prakriti*.

It is very important to understand this *mahat* in man,—the intelligence. This intelligence itself is modified into what we call egoism, and this intelligence is the cause of all these motions in the body. This covers all the grounds of sub-consciousness, consciousness and super-consciousness. What are these three states? The sub-conscious state we find in animals, what we call instinct. This is nearly infallible, but very limited. Instinct almost never fails. An animal instinctively knows a poisonous herb from an edible one, but its instinct is limited to one or two things; it works like a machine. Then comes the higher state of knowledge, which is fallible, makes mistakes often, but has a larger scope, although it is slow, and this you call reason. It is much larger than instinct, but there are more dangers of mistake in reasoning than in instinct. There is a still higher state of the mind, the super-conscious, which belongs only to the Yogis, men who have cultivated it. This is as infallible as instinct, and still more unlimited than reason. It is the highest state. We must remember that in man this *mahat* is the real cause of all that is here, that which is manifesting itself in various ways, covers the whole ground of sub-conscious, conscious and super-conscious states, the three states in which knowledge exists. So in the Cosmos, this universal Intelligence, *Mahat*, exists as instinct, as reason, and as super-reason.

Now comes a delicate question, which is always being asked. If a perfect God created the universe, why is there imperfection in it? What we call the universe is what we see, and that is only this little plane of consciousness or reason, and beyond that we do not see at all. Now the very question is an impossible one. If I take up only a bit out of a mass and look at it, it seems to be imperfect. Naturally. The universe seems imperfect because we make it so. How? What is reason? What is knowledge? Knowledge is finding associations. You go into the street and see a man, and know it is a man. You have seen many men, and each one has made an impression on your mind, and when you now see this man, you calmly refer to your store of impressions, see many pictures of men there, and you put this new one with the rest, pigeon-hole it and are satisfied. When a new impression comes and it has associations in your mind, you are satisfied, and this state of association is called knowledge. Knowledge is, therefore, pigeon-holing one experience with the already existing fund of experience, and this is one of the great proofs that you cannot have any knowledge until you have already a fund in existence. If you are without experience, or if, as some European philosophers think, the mind is a *tabula rasa*, it cannot get any knowledge, because the very fact of knowledge is the recognition of the new by comparison with already existing impressions. There must be a store ready to which to refer a new impression. Suppose a child is born into this world without such a fund, it would be impossible for him to get any knowledge. Therefore the child must have been in a state in which he had a fund, and so knowledge is eternally going on. Show me any way of getting out of this. It is mathematical experience. This is very much like the Spencerian and other philosophies. They have seen so far that there cannot be any knowledge without a fund of past knowledge. They have drawn out the idea that the child is born with knowledge. They say that the cause has entered the effect. It comes in a subtle form in order to be developed. These philosophers say that these impressions with which the child comes, are not from the child's own past, but were in his forefathers'; that it is hereditary transmission. Very soon they are going to find this theory untenable, and some of them are now giving hard blows to these ideas of heredity. Heredity is very good, but incomplete. It only explains the physical side. How do you explain the influence of environment? Many causes produce one effect. Environment is one of the modifying causes. On the other hand we in turn make our own environment, because as our past was, so we find our present. In other words, we are what we are here and now, because of what we have been in the past.

You understand what is meant by knowledge. Knowledge is pigeon-holing a new impression with old impressions— recognizing a new impression. What is meant by recognition? Finding its association with the similar impressions that we already have. Nothing further is meant by knowledge. If that be the case, it must be that we have to see the whole series of similars. Is it not? Suppose you take a pebble; to find the association, you have to see the whole series of pebbles similar to it. But with the universe we cannot do that, because in our reasoning we can only go after one perception of our universe, and neither see on this side nor on that side, and we cannot refer it to its association. Therefore the universe seems unintelligible, because knowledge and reason are always finding associations.

This bit of the universe cut off by our consciousness is a startling new thing, and we have not been able to find its associations. Therefore we are struggling with it, and thinking it is so horrible, so wicked, and bad;—sometimes we think it is good, but generally we think it is imperfect. The universe will be known only when we find the associations. We shall recognize them when we go beyond the universe and consciousness, and then the universe will stand explained. Until we do that all our fruitless striving will never explain the universe, because knowledge is the finding of similars, and this conscious plane gives us only a partial view. So with our idea of the universal *Mahat*, or what in our ordinary everyday language we call

God. All that we have of God is only one perception, just as of the universe we see only one portion, and all the rest is cut off and covered by our human limitation. "I, the Universal, so great am I that even this universe is a part of me." That is why we see God as imperfect, and we can never understand Him, because it is impossible. The only way to understand is to go beyond reason, beyond consciousness. "When thou goest beyond the heard and hearing, the thought and thinking, then alone wilt thou come to truth." (Bhagavad Gita II. 52.) "Go thou beyond the Scriptures, because they teach only up to Nature, up to the three qualities." (Gita II. 45.) When we go beyond them we find the harmony, not before.

So far it is clear that this macrocosm and microcosm are built on exactly the same plan, and in this microcosm we know only one very small part. We know neither the sub-conscious, nor the super-conscious. We know only the conscious. If a man says "I am a sinner," he is foolish, because he does not know himself. He is the most ignorant of men about himself; one part only he knows, because the fact of knowledge covers only one part of the "mind-ground" he is in. So with this universe; it is possible to know only one part through reasoning, but Nature comprises the whole of it, the sub-conscious, the conscious and the super-conscious, the individual *mahat* and the universal *Mahat* with all their subsequent modifications, and these lie beyond reason.

What makes nature change? We see that Up to this point everything, all *Prakriti*, is *jadâ* (insentient). It is working under law; it is all compound and insentient. Mind, intelligence, and will, all are insentient. But they are all reflecting the sentiency, the *Chit* (Intelligence) of some Being who is beyond all this, and whom the Sànkhya philosophers call *Purusha*. This *Purusha* is the unwitting cause of all these changes in Nature—in the universe. That is to say, this *Purusha*, taking Him in the universal sense, is the God of the universe. It is claimed that the will of the Lord created the universe. This is very good as a common daily expression, but that is all. How could it be will? Will is the third or fourth manifestation in Nature. Many things exist before it, and what created *them*? Will is a compound, and everything that is a compound is a production out of Nature. Will itself cannot create Nature. It is not a simple. So to say that the will of the Lord created the universe is illogical. Our will only covers a little portion of self-consciousness, and moves our brain, they say. If it did you could stop the action of the brain, but you cannot. It is not the will. Who moves the heart? It is not the will, because if it were you could stop it or not at your will. It is neither will that is working your body, nor that is working the universe. But it is something of which will itself is one of the manifestations. This body is being moved by the power of which will is only a manifestation in one part. So in the universe there is will, but that is only one part of the universe. The whole of the universe is not guided by will, that is why we do not find the explanation in will. Suppose I take it for granted that the will is moving the body, and then I begin to fret and fume. It is my fault, because I had no right to take it for granted that it was will. In the same way, if I take the universe and think it is will that moves it and then find things that do not coincide, it is my fault. This *Purusha* is not will, neither can it be intelligence, because intelligence itself is a compound. There cannot be any intelligence without some sort of matter. In man, this matter takes the form which we call brain. Wherever there is intelligence there must be matter in some form or other. But that intelligence itself is a compound. What then is this *Purusha*? It is neither intelligence nor *buddhi* (will), but yet it is the cause of both these; it is His presence that sets them all vibrating and combining. *Purusha* may be likened to some of these substances which by their mere presence promote chemical reaction, as in the case of cyanide of potassium which is added when gold is being smelted. The cyanide of potassium remains separate and unaffected, but its presence is absolutely necessary to the success of the process. So with the *Purusha*. It does not mix with Nature: it is not Intelligence, or *Mahat*, or any one of these, but the Self, the Pure, the Perfect. "I am the Witness, and through My witnessing, Nature is producing all that is sentient and all that is insentient." (Gita IX. 10.)

What is this sentiency in Nature? The basis of sentiency is in the *Purusha*, is the nature of the *Purusha*. It is that which cannot be spoken, but which is the material of all that we call knowledge. This *Purusha* is not consciousness, because consciousness is a compound, but whatever is light and goodness in this consciousness belongs to It. Sentiency is in the *Purusha*, but the *Purusha* is not intelligent, not knowing, it is knowledge itself. The *Chit* in the *Purusha*, plus *Prakriti*, is what is known to us as intelligence and consciousness. Whatever is pleasure and happiness and light in the universe belongs to the *Purusha*, but it is a compound because it is that *Purusha* plus Nature. "Wherever there is any happiness, wherever there is any bliss, there is one spark of that immortality, which is *Purusha*." This *Purusha* is the great attraction of the universe, untouched by, and unconnected with the universe, yet it attracts the whole universe. You see a man going after gold, because therein is a spark of the *Purusha*, even though he knows it not. When a man desires children, or a woman a husband, what is the attracting power? That spark of *Purusha* behind the child or wife, behind everything. It is there, only overlaid with matter. Nothing else can attract. "In this world of insentiency that *Purusha* alone is sentient." This is the *Purusha* of the *Sânkhyas*. As such it necessarily follows that this *Purusha* must be omnipresent. That which is not omnipresent must be limited. All limitations are caused; that which is caused must have beginning and end. If the *Purusha* is limited it will die, will not be final, will not be free, but will have been caused. Therefore if not limited, it is omnipresent. According to Kapila there are many *Purushas*, not one. An infinite number of them, you are one, I am one, each is one; an infinite number of circles, each one infinite, running through this universe. The *Purusha* is neither born nor dies. It is neither mind nor matter, and the reflex from it is all that we know. We are sure if it be omnipresent it knows neither death nor birth. Nature is casting her shadow upon it, the shadow of birth and death, but it is by its own nature eternal. So far we have found the theory of Kapila wonderful.

Next we will have to take up the proofs against it. So far the analysis is perfect, the psychology cannot be controverted. There is no objection to it. We will ask of Kapila the question: Who created Nature? and his answer will be that Nature (*Prakriti*) is uncreate. He also says that the *Purusha* is omnipresent and that of these *Purushas* there is an infinite number. We shall have to controvert this last proposition, and find a better solution, and by so doing we shall come to the ground taken by Vedânta. Our first doubt will be how there can be these two infinites. Then our argument will be that it is not a perfect generalization, and that therefore we have not found a perfect solution. And then we shall see how the Vedantists find their way out of all these difficulties and reach a perfect solution. Yet all the glory really belongs to Kapila. It is very easy to give a finish to a building that is nearly complete.

III. SÂNKHYA AND ADVAITA.

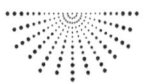

I will give you first a *resumé* of the *Sânkhya* philosophy, through which we have been going, because in this lecture we want to find where its defects are, and where Vedânta comes in as supplementary to these defects. You must remember that according to the *Sânkhya* philosophy, Nature is causing all these manifestations which we call thought and intellect, reason, love, hatred, touch, taste; that everything is from Nature. This Nature consists of three sorts of elements, one called *Sattva*, another *Rajas*, and the third *Tamas*. These are not qualities, but the materials out of which the whole universe is being evolved, and at the beginning of a cycle they remain in equilibrium. When creation comes this equilibrium is disturbed and these elements begin to combine and recombine, and manifest as the universe. The first manifestation of this is what the *Sânkhya* calls the *Mahat* (universal Intelligence), and out of that comes consciousness. And out of consciousness is evolved *Manas* (universal Mind). Out of this consciousness are also evolved the organs of the senses, and the *tanmâtras*,— sound particles, touch particles, taste particles, and so forth. All fine particles are evolved from this consciousness, and out of these fine particles come the gross particles which we call matter. After the *tanmâtras* (those particles which cannot be seen, or measured) come the gross particles which we can feel and sense. The *chitta* "mind-stuff") in its three-fold functions of intellect, consciousness and mind, is working and manufacturing the forces called *prânas*. These *prânas* have nothing to do with breath, you must at once get rid of that idea. Breath is one effect of the Prana (universal Energy). By these *prânas* are meant the nervous forces that are governing and moving the whole body, which are manifesting themselves as thought, and as the various functions of the body. The foremost and the most obvious manifestation of these *prânas* is the breathing motion. If it were caused by air, a dead man would breathe. The *prâna* acts upon the air, and not air upon it. These *prânas* are the vital forces which manipulate the whole body, and they in turn are manipulated by the mind and the *indriyas* (the two kinds of organs). So far so good. The psychology is very clear and most precise, and just think of the age of it, the oldest rational thought in the world! Wherever there is any philosophy or rational thought, it owes something to Kapila. Wherever there is any attempt at psychology, or philosophy, there is some indebtedness to the great father of this thought, to this man Kapila.

So far we see that this psychology is wonderful, but we shall have to differ with it on some points, as we go on. We find that the principal idea on which Kapila works is evolution. He makes one thing evolve out of another, because his very definition of causation is "the effect is the cause reproduced in another form," and because the whole universe, so far as we see it, is progressive and evolving. This whole universe must have evolved out of some material, out of *Prakriti* or Nature. Therefore this Nature cannot be essentially different from its cause, only when it takes form it becomes limited. The material itself is without form. But according to Kapila, from undifferentiated nature down to the last stage of differentiation, none of these is the same as *Purusha*, the "Enjoyer," or "Enlightener." Just as a lump of clay, so is a mass of mind, or the whole universe. By itself it has no light, but we find reason and intelligence in it, therefore there must be some Existence behind it, behind the whole of Nature, whose light is percolating through it and appearing as *Mahat* and consciousness and all these various things, and this

Existence is what Kapila calls the *Purusha*, the *Âtman* or Self of the Vedantist. According to Kapila, the *Purusha* is a *simple* factor, not a compound. It is immaterial, the only one that is immaterial, whereas all the various manifestations are material.

The *Purusha* alone knows. Suppose I see a blackboard, first the external instruments will bring that sensation to the organ (to the *indriya* according to Kapila), from the organ it will go to the mind and make an impression; the mind will cover it up with another factor,—consciousness, and will present it to the *buddhi* (intelligence), but *buddhi* cannot act; it is the *Purusha* behind that acts. These are all its servants, bringing the sensation to It, and It gives the orders, and the *buddhi* reacts.

The *Purusha* is the Enjoyer, the Perceiver, the real One, the King on his throne, the Self of man, and It is immaterial. Because It is immaterial, it necessarily follows that It must be infinite, It cannot have any limitation whatever. So each one of these *purushas* is omnipresent, each is all-pervading, but can act only through fine and gross manifestations of matter. The mind, the self-consciousness, the organs and the vital forces compose what is called the fine body, or what in Christian philosophy is called the "spiritual body" of man. It is this body that comes to reward or punishment, that goes to the different heavens; that incarnates and reincarnates; because we see from the very beginning that the going and coming of the soul (*Purusha*) is impossible. Motion means going and coming, and that which goes from one place to another cannot be omnipresent. It is this *linga-sarira* (subtle body) which comes and goes. Thus far we see from Kapila's psychology that the soul is infinite, and that the soul is the only principle that is not an evolution of Nature. It is the only one that is outside of Nature, but It has apparently got bound by Nature. This Nature is around the *Purusha* and It has identified Itself with Nature. It thinks "I am the *linga-sarira*," It thinks "I am the gross matter, the gross body," and as such is enjoying pleasure and pain; but these do not really belong to the soul, they belong to this *linga-sarira*, and to the gross body. When certain nerves are hurt we feel pain. We recognize that immediately. If the nerves in our fingers were dead we could cut the fingers and not feel it. So pleasure and pain belong to the nerve-centres. Suppose my organ of sight is destroyed, I do not feel pleasure or pain from color, although my eyes are there. So it is obvious that pleasure and pain do not belong to the soul.

They belong to the mind and the body.

The soul has neither pleasure nor pain; it is the Witness of everything, the eternal Witness of things that are going on, but it takes no fruits from any work. "As the sun is the cause of sight in every eye, yet is not itself affected by the defects in any eye; as a piece of crystal appears red when red flowers are placed before it, so this *Purusha* appears to be affected by pleasure or pain from the reflection cast upon It by Nature, but it remains ever unchanged." The nearest way to describe Its state is that it is meditation. This meditative state is that in which you approach nearest to the *Purusha*. Thus we see why the meditative state is always called the highest state by the *Yogi*, neither a passive nor an active state, but the meditative state. This is the *Sânkhya* philosophy.

Next, the *Sânkhyas* say that this manifestation of Nature is for the soul, all the combinations are for something outside of Nature. So these combinations which we call Nature, these constant changes are going on for the enjoyment of the soul, for its liberation, that it may gain all this experience from the lowest to the highest, and when it has gained it, the soul finds that it never was in Nature. It was entirely separate, and it finds that it is indestructible, that it neither goes nor comes, that going to heaven and being born again were in Nature and not in the soul. So the soul becomes free. All of Nature is working for the enjoyment and experience of the soul. It is getting this experience in order to reach the goal, and that goal is freedom. These souls are many, according to the *Sânkhya* philosophy. There is an infinite number of souls. And the other conclusion is that there is no God, as the Creator of the universe. Nature herself is sufficient to produce all these forms. God is not necessary, say the *Sânkhyas*.

Now we shall have to contest these three positions of the *Sânkhyas*. First that intelligence or anything of that sort does not belong to the soul, but that it belongs entirely to Nature; the soul being simply qualitiless, colorless. The second point is that there is no God, but Vedânta will show that without a God there cannot be any explanation whatever. Thirdly, we shall have to contend that there cannot be many souls, that there cannot be an infinite number, that there is only One Soul in the universe, and that One is appearing as many.

We will take the first proposition, that intelligence and reason belong entirely to Nature, and not to the soul. The Vedânta says that the soul is in its essence Existence-Knowledge-Bliss; but we agree with the *Sânkhyas* that all that they call intelligence is a compound. For instance, let us look at our perceptions. We remember that the *chitta* (or the "mind-stuff") is what is combining all these things, and upon which all these impressions are made, and from which reactions come. Suppose there is something outside. I see the blackboard. How does the knowledge come? The blackboard itself is unknown, I can never know it. It is what the German philosophers call the "thing in itself." That blackboard, that "X," is acting on my mind, and the *chitta* reacts. The *chitta* is like a lake; throw a stone upon it, and as soon as the stone strikes it a reactionary wave comes towards the stone. This wave is what you really know. And this wave is not like the stone at all, it is a wave. So that blackboard, "X," is the stone which strikes the mind and the mind throws up a wave towards that object which strikes it, and this wave which is thrown towards it is what we call the blackboard. I see you.

You as reality are unknown and unknowable. You are "X" and you act upon my mind, and the mind throws a wave towards the point from which the action came, and that wave is what I call Mr. or Mrs. So-and-So.

There are two elements in this, one from inside and the other from outside, and the combination of these two, "X" plus mind, is our external universe. All knowledge is by reaction. In the case of a whale it has been determined by calculation how long after its tail is struck, its mind reacts upon the tail and the tail feels the pain. Take the case of the pearl oyster, in which the pearl is formed by the oyster throwing its own juice around the grain of sand that enters the shell and irritates him. There are two things which cause the pearl. First the oyster's own juice, and second the blow from outside.

So this table is "X" plus my mind. The very attempt to know it will be made by the mind; therefore the mind will give some of its own substance to enable it to understand, and when we understand it, it has become a compound thing,—"X" plus the mind. Similarly in internal perception; when we want to know ourselves. The real Self, which is within us, is also unknown and unknowable. Let us call it "Y." When I want to know myself as Mr. So-and-So it is "Y" plus the mind. That "Y" strikes a blow on the mind, and when I want to know myself I must throw a blow upon the mind also. So our whole world is "X" plus mind (the external world), and "Y" plus mind (the internal world). We shall see later how this Advaitist idea can be demonstrated mathematically.

"X" and "Y" are simply the algebraic unknown quantities. We have seen that all knowledge is a combination, and this world, the universe, is a combination, and intelligence is similarly a combination. If it is internal intelligence it is "Y" plus the mind, if an external object, it is "X" plus the mind. Knowledge is a combination of "Y" plus the mind and matter is a combination of "X" plus the mind. We first take the internal group. Intelligence which we see in Nature cannot be wholly in Nature, because intelligence itself is a compound of "Y" plus the mind.

"Y" comes from the Self. So the intelligence that we know is a compound of the power of the light of the soul plus nature.

Similarly, the existence which we know must be a compound of "X" plus the mind. We find therefore that in these three factors, I exist, I know and I am blessed, the idea that I have no want, which comes from time to time, is the central idea, the grand basic idea of our life, and when it becomes limited, and becomes a compound, we think it happiness and misery. These factors manifest as existence phenomenal, knowledge phenomenal, and love phenomenal. Every man exists, and every man must know, and every man is made for bliss. He cannot help it. So through all existence; animals and plants, from the lowest to the highest existence, all must love. You may not call it love; but they must all exist, must all know and must all love. So this existence which we know is a compound of "X" and the mind, and knowledge also is a compound of that "Y" inside plus mind, and that love also is a compound of that "Y" and mind. Therefore these three factors which come from inside and are combining themselves with the external things to manufacture phenomenal existence, knowledge and love, are called by the Vedantists "Existence Absolute, Knowledge Absolute, Bliss Absolute."

That Absolute Existence which is limitless, which is unmixed, uncombined, which knows no change, is the free soul, and that Real Existence, when it gets mixed up, muddled up, as it were, with the elements of Nature is what we call human existence. It is limited and manifests as plant life, animal life, human life, just as infinite space is apparently limited by the walls of this room, or by any other enclosure. That Knowledge Absolute means not the knowledge we know, not intelligence, not reason, not instinct, but that which when it becomes manifested we call by these names. When that Knowledge Absolute becomes limited we call it intuition, and when it becomes still more limited we call it reason, instinct, etc. That Knowledge Absolute is *Vijnâna*. The nearest translation of it is "all-knowingness." There is no combination in it. It is the nature of the soul. That Bliss Absolute when it becomes limited we call love, attraction for the gross body, or the fine bodies, or for ideas. These are but distorted manifestations of this blessedness which is not a quality of the soul, but the essence, the inherent nature of the soul. Absolute Existence, Absolute Knowledge, and Absolute Blessedness are not qualities of the soul, but its essence; there is no difference between them and the soul. And the three are one; we see the one thing in three different lights. They are beyond all knowledge and by their reflection Nature appears to be intelligent.

It is that eternal Knowledge Absolute of the Self percolating through the mind of man that becomes our reason and intelligence. It varies according to the medium through which it is shining. There is no difference as soul between me and the lowest animal, only his brain is a poorer medium through which the knowledge shines, and we call it instinct. In man the brain is much finer, so the manifestation is much clearer, and in the highest man it has become entirely clear, like a piece of glass. So with existence; this existence which we know, this limited bit of existence is simply a reflection of that Existence Absolute which is the nature of the soul. So with bliss; that which we call love or attraction is but the reflection of the eternal blessedness of the Self, because with these manifestations come limitations, but the unmanifested, the natural, essential existence of the soul is unlimited, to that blessedness there can be no limit. But in human love there are limitations. I may love you one day, I may cease to love you the next. My love increases one day, decreases the next, because it is only a limited manifestation.

The first thing therefore that we find against Kapila is that he conceives the soul to be a mere qualitiless, colorless, inactive something. Vedânta teaches that it is the essence of all Existence, Knowledge, and Bliss; infinitely higher than all knowledge that we know, infinitely more blessed than any human love that we can think of, infinitely existing. The soul never dies. Death and birth are simply unthinkable in connection with the Self, because it is Existence Absolute.

The second point where we will contend with Kapila is with regard to his idea of God. Just as this series of limited manifestations of Nature, beginning with the individual intellect and ending with the individual body, requires the Self behind as the ruler and governor on the throne, so in the Cosmos, we must enquire what the universal Intelligence, the universal Mind, the universal fine and gross materials have as their ruler and governor? How will that series become complete without one universal Self behind it as its ruler and governor? If we deny that there is a universal governor, we must deny there is a soul behind the lesser series, because the whole universe is a repetition of the same plan. When we know one lump of clay we know the nature of all clay. If we can analyze one human being, we shall have analyzed the whole universe, because it is all built on the same plan. Therefore if it be true that behind this individual series there stands one who is beyond all nature, who is not composed of materials, the *purusha*, the very same logic will apply to this universe, and this universe too will require such a Soul. The Universal Soul which is behind the modifications of Nature is called by Vedânta *Isvara*, the Supreme Ruler, God.

Now comes the more difficult point to fight. There can be but one Soul. To begin with, we can give the *Sânkhyas* a good blow by taking up their theories and proving that each soul must be omnipresent, because it is not composed of anything. Everything that is limited must be limited by something else. Here is the existence of the table. Its existence is circumscribed by many things, and we find that every limitation presupposes some limiting thing. If we think of space, we have to think of it as a little circle, but beyond that is more space. We cannot imagine a limited space in any other way. It can only be understood and perceived through the infinite. To perceive the finite, in every case we must apprehend the infinite; both stand or fall together. When you think of time, you have also to think of time beyond any particular period of time. The latter is limited time and the larger is unlimited time. Wherever you endeavor to perceive the finite, you will find it impossible to separate it from the infinite. If this be the case, we shall prove thereby that this Self must be infinite, omnipresent. Then comes a fine question. Can the omnipresent, the infinite be two? Suppose there are two infinites, one will limit the other. Suppose there are two infinites,—A and B; the infinite "A" limits the infinite "B," because the infinite "B" you can say is not the infinite "A," and the infinite "A" it can be said is not the infinite "B." Therefore there can be but one infinite. Secondly, the infinite cannot be divided. Infinity divided into any number of parts must still be infinity, for it cannot be separated from itself. Suppose there is an infinite ocean of water, could you take up one drop from there? If you could, that ocean would no longer be infinite, that drop would limit it. The infinite cannot be divided by any means.

But there are stronger proofs that the Self is One. Not only so, but that the whole universe is one. We will once more take up our "X" and "Y". We have shown how what we call the external world is "X" plus mind, and the internal world "Y" plus mind. "X" and "Y" are both unknown quantities, unknown and unknowable. What is the mind? The mind is the "time, space and causation." This idea is the nature of the mind. You can never think without time, you can never conceive of anything without space, and you can never imagine anything without causation. These three are the forms in which both "X" and "Y" are caught, and which become the mind. Beyond that there is nothing to the mind. Take off these three forms which of themselves do not exist,—what remains? It is all one; "X" and "Y" are one. It is only this mind, this form, that has limited them apparently, and made them differ as internal and external world. "X" and "Y" are both unknown and unknowable. We cannot attribute any quality to them. As such they are both the same.

That which is qualitiless and attributeless and absolute must be one. There cannot be two absolutes. When there are no qualities there can be only One. "X" and "Y" are both without qualities because they take qualities only in the mind, therefore this "X" and "Y" are one.

The whole universe is One. There is only One Self in the universe, only One Existence, and that One Existence, when it is passing through the forms of time, space and causation, is called *buddhi*, fine matter, gross matter, etc. All physical and mental forms, everything in the universe is that One, appearing in various ways. When a little bit of it gets into this network of time, space and causation, it apparently takes forms; remove the network and it is all One. This whole universe is all one, and is called in the Advaitist philosophy *Brahman*. *Brahman* appearing behind the universe is called God; appearing behind the little universe—the microcosm, is the soul. This very "Self" or Âtman therefore is God in man. There is only one *Purusha*, and He is called God, and when God and man are analyzed they are one. The universe is you yourself, the unbroken you; you are throughout this universe. "In all hands you work, through all mouths you eat, through all nostrils you breathe, through all minds you think." The whole universe is you; this universe is your body; you are the universe, both formed and unformed. You are the soul of the universe, its body also. You are God, you are the angels, you are man, you are the animals, you are the plants, you are the minerals, you are everything; all manifestation is you. Whatever exists is you—the *real* "You"— the one undivided Self—not the little, limited personality that you have been regarding as yourself.

The question now arises,—how have you, that Infinite Being, broken into parts, become Mr. So-and-So, and the animals and so on? The answer is that all this division is only apparent. We know that the infinite cannot be divided, therefore this idea that you are a part has no reality, and never will have: and this idea that you are Mr. So-and-So was never true at any time; it is but a dream. Know this and be free. That is the Advaitist conclusion. "I am neither the mind, nor the body, nor am I the organs; I am Existence-Knowledge-Bliss Absolute; I am He, I am He," This is knowledge, and everything besides this is ignorance. Everything that is, is but ignorance, the result of ignorance. Where is knowledge for me, for I am knowledge itself! Where is life for me, for I am life itself! Life is a secondary manifestation of my nature. I am sure I live, for I am life, the one Being, and nothing exists except through me, and in me, and as me. I am manifested through elements, but I am the one free. Who seeks freedom? Nobody seeks freedom. If you think that you are bound, you remain bound; you make your own bondage. If you realize that you are free, you are free this moment. This is knowledge, knowledge of freedom. Freedom is the goal of all Nature.

IV. THE FREE SOUL.

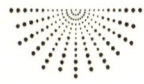

We have seen that the analysis of the *Sânkhyas* stops with the duality of existence, Nature and souls. There are an infinite number of souls, which, being simple, cannot die, and must therefore be separate from Nature. Nature in itself changes and manifests all these phenomena, and the soul, according to the *Sânkhyas* is inactive. It is a simple by itself, and Nature works out all these phenomena for the liberation of the soul, and liberation consists in the soul discriminating that it is not Nature. At the same time we have seen that the *Sânkhyas* were bound to admit that every soul was omnipresent. Being a simple the soul cannot be limited, because all limitation comes either through time, space, or causation. The soul being entirely beyond these cannot have any limitation. To have limitation one must be in space, which means the body, and that which is body must be in Nature. If the soul had form, it would be identified with Nature; therefore the soul is formless, and that which is formless cannot be said to exist here, there, or anywhere. It must be omnipresent. Beyond this the *Sânkhya* philosophy does not go.

The first argument of the Vedantists against this is that this analysis is not a perfect one. If this Nature be a simple, and the soul is also a simple, there will be two simples, and all the arguments that apply in the case of the soul to show that it is omnipresent, will apply in the case of Nature, and Nature too will be beyond all time, space, and causation, and as the result there will be no change or manifestation. Then will come the difficulty of having two simples, or two absolutes, which is impossible. What is the solution of the Vedantist? His solution is that, just as the *Sânkhyas* say, it requires some sentient being as the motive power behind, which makes the mind think and Nature work, because Nature in all its modifications, from gross matter up to *Mahat* (Intelligence) is simply insentient. Now, says the Vedantist, this sentient being which is behind the whole universe is what we call *God*, and consequently this universe is not different from Him. It is He Himself who has become this universe. He not only is the instrumental cause of this universe, but also the material cause. Cause is never different from effect, the effect is but the cause reproduced in another form. We see that every day. So this Being is the cause of Nature. All the forms and phases of Vedânta, either dualistic, or qualified-monistic, or monistic, first take this position,—that God is not only the instrumental but also the efficient cause of this universe, that everything which exists is He. The second step in Vedânta is that these souls are also a part of God, one spark of that Infinite Fire. "As from a mass of fire millions of small particles fly, even so from this Ancient One have come all these souls." So far so good, but it does not yet satisfy. What is meant by a part of the Infinite? The Infinite is indivisible; there cannot be parts of the Infinite. The Absolute cannot be divided. What is meant therefore that all these sparks are from Him? The Advaitist, the non-dualistic Vedantist, solves the problem by maintaining that there is really no part; that each soul is really not a part of the Infinite, but actually *is* the Infinite *Brahman*. Then how can there be so many? The sun reflected from millions of globules of water appears to be millions of suns, and in each globule is a miniature picture of the sun-form; so all these souls are but reflections and not real. They are not the real "I" which is the God of this universe, the one undivided Being of the universe. And all these little different beings, men and animals, etc., are but reflections, and not real. They are simply illusory reflections upon Nature. There is but one Infinite Being in the universe, and that Being appears as you and as I, but this appearance of division is after all delusion. He has not been divided, but only appears to be divided. This apparent division is caused by looking at Him through the network of time, space, and causation. When I look at God through the network of time, space, and causation, I see Him as the material world. When I look at Him from a little higher plane, yet through the same network, I see Him as an animal, a little higher as a man, a little higher as a god, but yet He is the One Infinite Being of the universe, and that Being we are. I am That, and you are That. Not parts of It, but the whole of It. "It is the Eternal Knower standing behind the whole phenomena; He Himself is the phenomena." He is both the subject and the object, He is the "I" and the "You." How is this? "How to know the knower?" The Knower cannot know himself. I see everything but cannot see myself. The Self, the Knower, the Lord of all, the Real Being, is the cause of all the vision that is in the universe, but it is impossible for Him to see Himself or know Himself, excepting through reflection. You cannot see your own face excepting in a mirror, and so the Self cannot see its own nature until it is reflected, and this whole universe therefore is the Self trying to realize Itself. This reflection is thrown back first from the protoplasm, then from plants and animals, and so on and on from better and better reflectors, until the best reflector,—the perfect man,—is reached. Just as a man who, wanting to see his face, looks first in a little pool of muddy water, and sees just an outline. Then he comes to clearer water, and sees a better image, then to a piece of shining metal, and sees a still better image, and at last to a looking-glass, and sees himself reflected as he is. Therefore the perfect man is the highest reflection of that Being, who is both subject and object. You now find why man instinctively worships everything, and how perfect men are instinctively worshipped as God in every country. You may talk as you like, but it is they who are bound to be worshipped. That is why men worship Incarnations, such as Christ or Buddha. They are the most perfect manifestations of the eternal Self. They are much higher than all the conceptions of God that you or I can make. A perfect man is much higher than such conceptions. In him the circle becomes complete;

the subject and the object become one. In him all delusions go away and in their place comes the realization that he has always been that perfect Being. How came this bondage then? How was it possible for this perfect Being to degenerate into the imperfect? How was it possible that the free became bound? The *Advaitist* says he was never bound, but was always free. Various clouds of various colors come before the sky. They remain there a minute and then pass away. It is the same eternal blue sky stretching there forever. The sky never changes; it is the cloud that is changing. So you are always perfect, eternally perfect. Nothing ever changes your nature, or ever will. All these ideas that I am imperfect, I am a man, or a woman, or a sinner, or I am the mind, I have thought, I will think, all are hallucinations; you never think, you never had a body; you never were imperfect. You are the blessed Lord of this universe, the one Almighty ruler of everything that is and ever will be, the one mighty ruler of these suns and stars and moons and earths and plants, and all the little bits of our universe. It is through you the sun shines, and the stars shed their lustre, and the earth becomes beautiful. It is through your blessedness that they all love and are attracted to each other. You are in all, and you are all. Whom to avoid, and whom to take? You are the all in all. When this knowledge comes delusion immediately vanishes.

I was once travelling in the desert in India. I travelled for over a month and always found the most beautiful landscapes before me, beautiful lakes and all that. One day I was very thirsty and I wanted to have a drink at one of these lakes, but when I approached that lake it vanished. Immediately with a blow came into my brain the idea that this was a mirage about which I had read all my life, and then I remembered and smiled at my folly, that for the last month all the beautiful landscapes and lakes I had been seeing were this mirage, but I could not distinguish them then. The next morning I again began my march; there was the lake and the landscape, but with it immediately came the idea, "This is a mirage." Once known it had lost its powers of illusion. So this illusion of the universe will break one day. The whole of this will vanish, melt away. This is realization. Philosophy is no joke or talk. It will be realized; this body will vanish, this earth and everything will vanish, this idea that I am the body, or the mind, will for some time vanish, or if the *Karma* is ended it will disappear never to come back; but if one part of the *Karma* remains,—as a potter's wheel after the potter has finished the pot, will sometimes go on from the past momentum—so this body, when this delusion has vanished altogether, will go on for some time. Again this world will come, men and women and animals will come, just as the mirage came the next day, but not with the same force, along with it will come the idea that I know its nature now, and it will cause no bondage, no more pain, nor grief, nor misery. Whenever anything miserable will come, the mind will be able to say, "I know you as hallucination." When a man has reached that state he is called *jivan mukta*, "living free," free even while living. The aim and end in this life for the *Jnâna Yogi* is to become this *jivan mukta*, living freedom. He is *jivan mukta* who can live in this world without being attached. He is like the lotus leaves in water, which are never wet by the water. He is the highest of human beings, nay, the highest of all beings, for he has realized his identity with the Absolute, he has realized that he is one with God. So long as you think you have the least difference from God, fear will seize you, but when you have known that you are He, that there is no difference, entirely no difference, that you are He, all of Him, and the whole of Him, all fear ceases.

"There who sees whom? Who worships whom? Who talks to whom? Who hears whom? Where one sees another, where one talks to another, where one hears another, it is in law. Where none sees none, where none speaks to none that is the highest, that is the great, that is the *Brahman*." Being That, you are always That. What will become of the world then? What good shall we do to the world? Such questions do not arise.

"What becomes of my gingerbread if I become old?" says the baby. "What becomes of my marbles if I grow, so I will not grow," says the boy. "What will become of my dolls if I grow old?" says the little child. It is the same question in connection with this world; it has no existence in the past, present, or future. If we have known the *Âtman* as It is, if we have known that there is nothing else but this *Âtman*, that everything else is but a dream, with no existence in reality, then this world with its poverties, its miseries, its wickedness and its goodness will cease to disturb us. If they do not exist, for whom and for what shall we take trouble? This is what the *Jnâna Yogis* teach. Therefore, dare to be free, dare to go as far as your thought leads, and dare to carry that out in your life. It is very hard to come to *jnânam*. It is for the bravest and most daring, who dare to smash all idols, not only intellectual, but in the senses. This body is not I; it must go. All sorts of curious things may come out of this. A man stands up and says I am not the body, therefore my headache must be cured, but where is the headache if not in his body? Let a thousand headaches and a thousand bodies come and go. What is that to me? "I have neither birth nor death; father nor mother I never had; friends and foes I have none, because they are all I; I am my own friend and I am my own enemy; I am Existence-Knowledge-Bliss Absolute; I am He, I am He." If in a thousand bodies I am suffering from fever and other ills, in millions of bodies I am healthy. If in a thousand bodies I am starving, in other thousand bodies I am feasting. If in thousands of bodies I am suffering misery, in thousands of bodies I am happy. Who shall blame whom, who praise whom? Whom to seek, whom to avoid? I seek none, nor avoid any, for I am all the universe, I praise myself, I blame myself, I suffer for myself, I am happy at my own will, I am free. This is the *Jnâni*, brave and daring. Let the whole universe tumble down; he smiles and says it never existed. It was all an hallucination; we see the universe tumble down; where was it? Where has it gone?

Before going into the practical part, we will take up one more intellectual question. So far the logic is tremendously rigorous. If man reasons, there is no place for him to stand until he comes to this, that there is but One Existence, that everything else is nothing. There is no other way left for rational mankind but to take this view. But how is it that what is infinite, ever perfect, ever blessed, Existence-Knowledge-Bliss Absolute has come under these delusions? It is the same question that has been asked all the world over. In the vulgar form the question becomes "How did sin come into this world?" This is the most vulgar and sensuous form of the question, and the other is the more philosophic form, but the answer is the same. The same question has been asked in various grades and fashions, but in its lower forms it finds no solution, because the stories of apples and serpents and women do not give the explanation. In that state, the question is childish and so is the answer. But the question has assumed very high proportions now. "How this illusion came?" And the answer is as fine. The answer is that we cannot expect any answer to an impossible question. The very question is impossible in terms. You have no right to ask that question. Why? What is perfection? That which is beyond time, space and causation. That is perfect. Then you ask how the perfect became imperfect. In logical language the question may be put in this form—"How did that which is beyond causation become caused?" You contradict yourself. You first admit it is beyond causation, and then ask what causes it. This question can only be asked within the limits of causation. As far as time and space and causation extend, so far can this question be asked. But beyond that it will be nonsense to ask it, because the question is illogical. Within time, space and causation it can never be answered, and what answer may lie beyond these limits can only be known when we have transcended them, therefore the wise will let this question rest. When a man is ill, he devotes himself to curing his disease, without insisting that he must first learn how he came to have it.

There is another form of this question, a little lower, but more practical and illustrative. What produced this delusion? Can any reality produce delusion? Certainly not. We see that one delusion produces another, and so on. It is delusion always that produces delusion. It is disease that produces disease, and not health that produces disease. The wave is the same thing as the water, the effect is the cause in another form. The effect is delusion, and therefore the cause must be delusion. What produced this delusion? Another delusion. And so on without beginning. The only question that remains for you to ask is, does not this break your monism, because you get two existences in the universe, one yourself, and the other the delusion? The answer is,—delusion cannot be called an existence. Thousands of dreams come into your life, but do not form any part of your life. Dreams come and go; they have no existence; to call delusion existence will be sophistry. Therefore there is only one individual existence in the universe, ever free, and ever blessed, and that is what you are. This is the last conclusion reached by the *Advaitists*. It may then be asked, what becomes of all these various forms of worship? They will remain; they are simply groping in the dark for light, and through this groping light will come. We have just seen that the Self cannot see Itself. Our knowledge is within the network of *Mâyâ* (unreality), and beyond that is freedom; within the network there is slavery, it is all under law. Beyond that there is no law. So far as the universe is concerned, existence is ruled by law, and beyond that is freedom. As long as you are in the network of time, space and causation, to say you are free is nonsense, because in that network all is under rigorous law, sequence and consequence. Every thought that you think is caused, every feeling has been caused; to say that the will is free is sheer nonsense. It is only when the infinite existence comes, as it were, into this network of *Mâyâ* that it takes the form of will. Will is a portion of that being caught in the network of *Mâyâ*, and therefore "free-will" is a misnomer. It means nothing,—sheer nonsense. So is all this talk about freedom. There is no freedom in *Mâyâ*.

Every one is as much bound in thought, word, deed, and mind, as a piece of stone or this table. That I talk to you now is as rigorously in causation as that you listen to me. There is no freedom until you go beyond *Mâyâ*. That is the real freedom of the soul. Men, however sharp and intellectual, however clearly they see the force of the logic that nothing here can be free, are all compelled to think they are free; they cannot help. No work can go on until we begin to say we are free. It means that the freedom we talk about is the glimpse of the blue sky through the clouds, and that the real freedom—the blue sky itself,—is behind. True freedom cannot exist in the midst of this delusion, this hallucination, this nonsense of the world, this universe of the senses, body and mind. All these dreams, without beginning or end, uncontrolled and uncontrollable, ill-adjusted, broken, inharmonious, form our idea of this universe. In a dream, when you see a giant with twenty heads chasing you, and you are flying from him, you do not think it is inharmonious; you think it is proper and right. So is this law. All that you call law is simply chance without meaning. In this dream state you call it law. Within *Mâyâ*, so far as this law of time, space and causation exists, there is no freedom, and all these various forms of worship are within this *Mâyâ*. The idea of God and the ideas of brute and of man are within this *Mâyâ*, and as such equally hallucinations; all of them are dreams. But you must take care not to argue like some extraordinary men of whom we hear at the present time. They say the idea of God is a delusion, but the idea of this world is true. Both ideas stand or fall by the same logic. He alone has the right to be an atheist who denies this world, as well as the other. The same argument is for both. The same mass of delusion extends from God to the lowest animal, from a blade of grass to the Creator. They stand or fall by the same logic. The same person who sees falsity in the idea of God ought also to see it in the idea of his own body, or his own mind. When God vanishes, then also vanish the body and mind, and when both vanish, that which is the Real Existence remains forever. "There the eyes cannot go, nor the speech, nor the mind. We cannot see it, neither know it." And we now understand that so far as speech and thought and knowledge, and intellect go, it is all within this *Mâyâ*, within bondage. Beyond that is Reality. There neither thought, nor mind, nor speech, can reach.

So far it is intellectually all right, but then comes the practice. The real work in these classes is the practice. Are any practices necessary to realize this one-ness? Most decidedly. It is not that you become this *Brahman*. You are already that. It is not that you are going to become God or perfect; you are already perfect, and whenever you think you are not, it is a delusion. This delusion which says that you are Mr. So-and-So, or Mrs. So-and-So, can be got rid of by another delusion, and that is practice. Fire will eat fire, and you can use one delusion to conquer another delusion. One cloud will come and brush away another cloud, and then both will go away. What are these practices then? We must always bear in mind that we are not going to be free, but are free already. Every idea that we are bound is a delusion. Every idea that we are happy or unhappy, is a tremendous delusion; and another delusion will come,—that we have got to work and worship and struggle to be free,—and this will chase out the first delusion, and then both will stop. The fox is considered very unholy by the Mohammedans, also by the Hindus. Also, if a dog touches any bit of food it has to be thrown out, it cannot be eaten by any man. In a certain Mohammedan house a fox entered and took a little bit of food from the table, ate it up and fled. The man was a poor man, and had prepared a very nice feast for himself, and that feast was made unholy, and he could not eat it. So he went to a *Mulla*, a priest, and said: "This has happened to me; a fox came and took a mouthful out of my meal; what can be done? I had prepared a feast and wanted so much to eat it, and now comes this fox and destroys the whole affair." The *Mulla* thought for a minute, and then found only one solution and said: "The only way is for you to get a dog, and make him eat a bit out of the same plate, because dog and fox are eternally quarrelling. The food that was left by the fox will go into your stomach, and that not eaten by the dog will go there, and both will be purified." We are very much in the same Predicament. This is an hallucination that we are imperfect, and we take up another, that we have to practice to become perfect. Then one will chase the other, as we can use one thorn to extract another and then throw both away. There are people for whom it is sufficient knowledge to hear, "Thou art That." With a flash this universe goes away and the real nature shines, but others have to struggle hard to get rid of this idea of bondage.

  The first question is, who are fit to become *Jnâna Yogis*? Those who are equipped with these requisites. First, renunciation of all fruits of work and of all enjoyments in this life or another life. If you are the creator of this universe whatever you desire you will have, because you will create it for yourself. It is only a question of time. Some get it immediately; with others the past *samskâras* (impressions) stand in the way of getting their desires. We give the first place to desires for enjoyment, either in this or another life. Deny there is any life at all, because life is only another name for death. Deny that you are a living being. Who cares for life? Life is one of these hallucinations and death is its counterpart. Joy is one part of these hallucinations, and misery the other part, and so on. What have you to do with life or death? These are all creations of the mind. This is called giving up desires of enjoyment either in this life or another.

Then comes controlling the mind, calming it so that it will not break into waves and have all sorts of desires; holding the mind steady, not allowing it to get into waves from external or internal causes, controlling the mind perfectly just by the power of will. The *Jnâna Yogi* does not take any one of these physical helps, or mental helps, simply philosophic reasoning, knowledge and his own will, these are the instrumentality he believes in. Next comes *Titikshâ*, forbearance, bearing all miseries without murmuring, without complaining. When an injury comes, do not mind it. If a tiger comes, stand there. Who flies? There are men who practice *titikshâ*, and succeed in it. There are men who sleep on the banks of the Ganges in the mid-summer sun of India, and in winter float in the waters of the Ganges for a whole day; they do not care. Men sit in the snow of the Himâlayas, and do not care to wear any garment. What is heat? What is cold? Let things come and go, what is that to me, I am not the body. It is hard to believe this in these Western countries, but it is better to know that it is done. Just as your people are brave to jump at the mouth of a cannon, or into the midst of the battlefield, so our people are brave to think and act out their philosophy. They give up their lives for it.

"I am Existence-Knowledge-Bliss Absolute; I am He; I am He." Just as the Western ideal is to keep up luxury in practical life, so ours is to keep up the highest form of spirituality, to demonstrate that religion is not merely frothy words, but can be carried out, every bit of it, in this life. This is *titikshâ*, to bear everything, not to complain of anything. I myself have seen men who say "I am the soul; what is the universe to me? Neither pleasure, nor pain, nor virtue, nor vice, nor heat, nor cold are anything to me." That is *titikshâ*; not running after the enjoyments of the body. What is religion? To pray: "give me this and that"? Foolish ideas of religion! Those who believe them have no true idea of God and soul. My Master used to say the vulture rises high and high until he becomes a speck, but his eye is always in the piece of rotten carrion on the earth. After all, what is the result of your ideas of religion? To cleanse the streets, and have more bread and clothes. Who cares for bread and clothes? Millions come and go every minute. Who cares? Why care for the joys and vicissitudes of this little world? Go beyond that if you dare; go beyond law, let the whole universe vanish, and stand alone. "I am Existence-Absolute, Knowledge-Absolute, Bliss-Absolute; I am He; I am He."

V. ONE EXISTENCE APPEARING AS MANY.

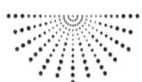

We have seen how *Vairâgyam*, or renunciation, is the turning point in all these various *Yogas*. The *Karmi* (worker) renounces the fruits of his work. The *Bhakta* (devotee) renounces all little loves for the almighty and omnipresent love. The *Yogi* renounces his experiences, because his philosophy is that the whole Nature, although it is for the experience of the soul, at last brings him to know that he is not in Nature, but eternally separate from Nature. The *Jnâni* (philosopher) renounces everything, because his philosophy is that Nature never existed, neither in the past, present nor future. We have also seen how the question of utility cannot be asked in these higher themes; it is very absurd to ask utility, and even if it be asked, after a proper analysis what do we find in this question of utility? The ideal of happiness, that which brings man greater happiness is of greater utility to him than those things which do not improve his material conditions or bring him such great happiness. All the sciences are for this one end, to bring happiness to humanity and that which brings the larger amount of happiness, mankind takes and gives up that which brings a lesser amount of happiness. We have seen how happiness is either in the body, or in the mind, or in the *Âtman*. With animals, and in the lowest of human beings, who are very much like animals, happiness is all in the body. No man can eat with the same pleasure as a famished dog, or a wolf; so, in the dog and the wolf the happiness is gone entirely into the body. In men we find a higher plane of happiness, that of thought, and in the *Jnâni* there is the highest plane of happiness in the Self, the *Âtman*. So to the philosopher this knowledge of the Self is of the highest utility, because it gives him the highest happiness possible. Sense gratifications or physical things cannot be of the highest utility to him because he does not find in them the same pleasure that he finds in knowledge itself; and after that, knowledge is the one goal, and is really the highest happiness that we know. All who work in ignorance are, as it were, the draught animals of the *devas*. The word *deva* is here used in the sense of a wise man. All the people that work, and toil, and labor like machines do not really enjoy life, but it is the wise man who enjoys. A rich man buys a picture at a cost of a hundred thousand dollars perhaps, but it is the man who understands art that enjoys it; and if a man is without knowledge of art it is useless to him, he is only the owner. All over the world, it is the wise man who enjoys the happiness of the world. The ignorant man never enjoys; he has to work for others unconsciously.

Thus far we have seen the theories of these Advaitist philosophers, how there is but one *Âtman*; there cannot be two. We have seen how in the whole of this universe there is but One Existence, and that One Existence when seen through the senses is called the world, the world of matter. When It is seen through the mind It is called the world of thoughts and ideas, and when It is seen as it is, then It is the One Infinite Being. You must bear this in mind; it is not that there is a soul in man, although I had to take that for granted in order to explain it at first, but that there is only One Existence, and that one the *Âtman*, the Self, and when this is perceived through the senses, through sense imageries, It is called the body. When It is perceived through thought, It is called the mind. When It is perceived in Its own nature, It is the *Âtman*, the One Only Existence. So, it is not that there are three things in one, the body and the mind and the Self, although that was a convenient way of putting it in the course of explanation; but all is that *Âtman*, and that one Being is sometimes called the body, sometimes the mind, and sometimes the Self, according to different vision. There is but one Being which the ignorant call the world. When a man goes higher in knowledge he calls the very same Being the world of thought. Again when knowledge itself comes, all illusions vanish, and man finds it is all nothing but *Âtman.* I am that One Existence. This is the last conclusion. There are neither three nor two in the universe; it is all One. That One, under the illusion of *Mâyâ* is seen as many, just as a rope is seen as a snake. It is the very rope that is seen as a snake. There are not two things there, a rope separate and a snake separate. No man sees two things there. Dualism and non-dualism are very good philosophic terms, but in perfect perception we never perceive the real and the false at the same time. We are all born monists, we cannot help it. We always perceive the one. When we perceive the rope, we do not perceive the snake at all, and when we see the snake, we do not see the rope at all; it has vanished. When you see illusion, you do not see real men. Suppose one of your friends is coming from a distance in the street; you know him very well, but through the haze and mist that is before you, you think it is another man. When you see your friend as another man, you do not see your friend at all, he has vanished. You are perceiving only one. Suppose your friend is Mr. A., but when you perceive Mr. A. as Mr. B. you do not see Mr. A. at all. In each case you perceive only one. When you see yourself as a body, you are body and nothing else, and that is the perception of the vast majority of mankind. They may talk of soul and mind, and all these things, but what they perceive is the physical form, the touch, taste, vision, and so on. Again, with certain men, in certain states of consciousness, they perceive themselves as thought. You know, of course, the story told of Sir Humphrey Davy, who was making experiments before his class with laughing-gas, and suddenly one of the tubes broke, and the gas escaping, he breathed it in. For some moments he remained like a statue. Afterwards he told his class that when he was in that state, he actually perceived that the whole world is made up of ideas. The gas, for a time, made him forget the consciousness of the body, and that very thing which he was seeing as the body, he began to perceive as ideas. When the consciousness rises still higher, when this little puny consciousness is gone forever, that which is the Reality behind shines, and we see it as the One Existence-Knowledge-Bliss, the one *Âtman*, the Universal. "One that is only knowledge itself, One that is bliss itself, beyond all compare, beyond all limit, ever free, never bound, infinite as the sky, unchangeable as the sky. Such an One will manifest Himself in your heart in meditation."

How does the Advaitist theory explain all these various phases of heavens and hells and all these various ideas we find in all religions? When a man dies it is said that he goes to heaven or hell, goes here or there, or that when a man dies he is born again in another body, either in heaven or in another world, or somewhere. These are all hallucinations. Nobody is ever born or dies, really speaking. There is neither heaven nor hell, nor this world; all three never really existed. Tell a child a lot of ghost stories, and let him go out into the street in the evening. There is a little stump of a tree. What does the child see? A ghost, with hands stretched out, ready to grab him. Suppose a man comes from the corner of the street, wanting to meet his sweetheart; he sees that stump of the tree as the girl. A police-man coming from the street corner sees the stump as a thief. The thief sees it as a policeman. It is the same stump of a tree that was seen in various ways. The stump is the reality, and the visions of the stump are the projections of the various minds. There is one Being, this Self; It neither comes nor goes.

When a man is ignorant, he wants to go to heaven or some place, and all his life he has been thinking and thinking of this, and when this earth dream vanishes he sees this world as a heaven, with *devas* and angels flying about, and all such things. If a man all his life desires to meet his forefathers he gets them all, from Adam downwards, because he creates them. If a man is still more ignorant and has always been frightened by fanatics with ideas of hell, when he dies he will see this very world as hell, with all sorts of punishments. All that is meant by dying or being born is simply changes in the plane of vision. Neither do you move, nor does that move upon which you project your vision. You are the permanent, the unchangeable. How can you go and come? It is impossible; you are omnipresent. The sky never moves, but the clouds move over the surface of the sky, and we may think that the sky itself moves. Just as you go into a railway train, and you think the land is moving. It is not so, but it is the train which is moving. You are where you are; this dream, these various clouds move. One dream follows another without connection. There is no such thing as law or connection in this world, but we are thinking that there is a great deal of connection. All of you have probably read "Alice in Wonderland." It is the most wonderful book for children written in this century. When I read it I was delighted, it was always in my head to write that sort of a book for children. What pleased me most in it was what you think most incongruous, that there is no connection there. One idea comes and jumps into another, without any connection. When you were children you thought that the most wonderful connection. So this man brought back his thoughts of childhood, perfectly connected to him as a child, and composed this book for children. And all these books which men write, trying to make children swallow their own ideas as men are nonsense. We too are grown up children, that is all. The world is the same unconnected thing,—"Alice in Wonderland,"—with no connection whatever. When we see things happen a number of times in a certain sequence, we call it cause and effect, and say that the thing will happen again. When this dream changes another dream will seem quite as connected as this. When we dream, the things we see all seem to be connected; during the dream we never think they are incongruous; it is only when we wake that we see the want of connection. When we wake from this dream of the world and compare it with the Reality, it will be found all incongruous nonsense, a mass of incongruity passing before us, we do not know whence or whither, but we know it will end; and this is called *Mâyâ*, and is like masses of fleeting, fleecy clouds. They represent all this changing existence, and the sun itself, the unchanging, is you. When you look at that unchanging Existence from the outside, you call it God, and when you look at it from the inside you call it yourself. It is but one. There is no God separate from you, no God higher than you, the real "you." All the gods are little beings to you, all the ideas of God and Father in heaven are but your reflection. God

Himself is your image. "God created man after His own image." That is wrong. Man creates God after his own image. That is right. Throughout the universe we are creating gods after our own image. We create the god, and fall down at his feet and worship; and when this dream comes, we love it!

This is a good point to understand,—that the sum and substance of this morning's lecture is that there is but One Existence, and that One Existence seen through different constitutions appears either as the earth, or heaven, or hell, or God, or ghosts, or men or demons, or world, or all these things. But among these many "He who sees that One in this ocean of death, he who sees that One Life in this floating universe, who realizes that One who never changes, unto him belongs eternal peace; unto none else, unto none else." This One Existence has to be realized. How, is the next question. How is it to be realized? How is this dream to be broken, how shall we wake up from this dream that we are little men and women, and all such things? We are the Infinite Being of the universe, and have become materialized into these little beings, men and women, depending upon the sweet word of one man, or the angry word of another man and so forth. What a terrible dependence, what a terrible slavery! I who am beyond all pleasure and pain, whose reflection is the whole universe, little bits of whose life are the suns and moons and stars,— I am held down as a terrible slave. If you pinch my body I feel pain. If one says a kind word I begin to rejoice. See my condition,—slave of the body, slave of the mind, slave of the world, slave of a good word, slave of a bad word, slave of passion, slave of happiness, slave of life, slave of death, slave of everything. This slavery has to be broken. How?

"This *Âtman* has first to be heard, then reasoned upon and then meditated upon." This is the method of the Advaita *Jnâni*. The truth has to be heard, then reflected upon and then to be constantly asserted. Think always—"I am *Brahman*"; every other thought must be cast aside as weakening. Cast aside every thought that says that you are men or women. Let body go, and mind go, and gods go, and ghosts go. Let everything go but that One Existence. "Where one hears another, where one sees another, that is but small; where one does not hear another, where one does not see another, that is infinite." That is the highest, when the subject and the object become one. When I am the listener and I am the speaker, when I am the teacher and I am the taught, when I am the creator and I am the created,— then alone fear ceases; there is not another to make us afraid. There is nothing but myself, what can frighten me? This is to be heard day after day. Get rid of all other thoughts. Everything else must be thrown aside, and this is to be repeated continually, poured through the ears until it reaches the heart, until every nerve and muscle, every drop of blood tingles with the idea that I am He, I am He. Even at the gate of death say "I am He." There was a man in India, a *Sannyâsin*, who used to repeat "*Shivoham*" ("I am Bliss Eternal"), and a tiger jumped on him one day and dragged him away and killed him, and as long as he was living the sound came "*Shivoham, Shivoham.*" Even at the gate of death, in the greatest danger, in the thick of the battle-field, at the bottom of the ocean, on the tops of the highest mountains, in the thickest of the forest, tell yourself "I am He, I am He." Day and night say "I am He." It is the greatest strength; it is religion.

"The weak will never reach the *Âtman.*" Never say: "O Lord, I am a miserable sinner." Who shall help you? You are the help of the universe. What in this universe can help you? Where is the man, or the god, or the demon to help you? What can prevail over you? You are the god of the universe; where can you seek for help? Never help came from anywhere but from yourself. In your ignorance, every prayer that you made and that was answered, you thought was answered by some Being, but you answered the prayer yourself, unknowingly. The help came from yourself, and you fondly imagined that some one was sending help to you. There is no help for you outside of yourself; you are the creator of the universe. Like the silkworm you have built a cocoon around yourself. Who will save you? Cut your own cocoon and come out as the beautiful butterfly, as the free soul.

Then alone you will see Truth. Ever tell yourself "I am He." These are words that will burn up the dross that is in the mind, words that will bring out the tremendous energy which is within you already, the infinite power which is sleeping in your heart. This is to be brought out by constantly hearing the truth and nothing else. Wherever there is thought of weakness, approach not the place. Avoid all weakness if you want to be *Jnâni*.

Before you begin to practise, clear your mind of all doubts. Fight and reason and argue, and when you have established it in your mind that this and this alone can be the truth and nothing else, do not argue any more; close your mouth. Hear not argumentation, neither argue yourself. What is the use of any more arguments? You have satisfied yourself, you have decided the question. What remains? The truth has now to be realized, therefore why waste valuable time in vain arguments?

The truth has now to be meditated upon and every idea that strengthens you must be taken up and every thought that weakens you must be rejected. The *Bhakta* meditates upon forms and images and all such things and upon God. This is the natural process, but a slower one. The *Yogi* meditates upon various centres in his body and manipulates powers in his mind. The *Jnâni* says the mind does not exist, neither the body. This idea of the body and of the mind must go, must be driven off; therefore it is foolish to think of them. It would be like trying to cure one ailment by bringing in another. His meditation therefore is the most difficult one, the negative; he denies everything, and what is left is the Self. This is the most analytical way. The *Jnâni* wants to tear away the universe from the Self by the sheer force of analysis. It is very easy to say, "I am a *Jnâni*," but very hard to really be one. "The way is long; it is, as it were, walking on the sharp edge of a razor, yet despair not. Awake, arise, and stop not until the goal is reached," say the Vedas.

So what is the meditation of the *Jnâni*? He wants to rise above every idea of body or mind, to drive away the idea that he is the body. For instance, when I say "I, Swâmi," immediately the idea of the body comes. What must I do then? I must give the mind a hard blow and say, "No, I am not the body, I am the Self." Who cares if disease comes or death in the most horrible form? I am not the body. Why make the body nice? To enjoy the illusion once more? To continue the slavery? Let it go, I am not the body. That is the way of the *Jnâni*. The *Bhakta* says: "The Lord has given me this body that I may safely cross the ocean of life and I must cherish it until the journey is accomplished."

The *Yogi* says: "I must be careful of the body so that I may go on steadily and finally attain liberation." The *Jnâni* feels that he cannot wait, he must reach the goal this very moment. He says: "I am free through eternity, I am never bound; I am the God of the universe through all eternity. Who shall make me perfect? I am perfect already." When a man is perfect he sees perfection in others. When he sees imperfection, it is his own mind projecting itself. How can he see imperfection if he has not got it in himself? So the *Jnâni* does not care for perfection or imperfection. None exists for him. As soon as he is free, he does not see good and evil. Who sees evil and good? He who has it in himself. Who sees the body? He who thinks he is the body. The moment you get rid of the idea that you are the body, you do not see the world at all. It vanishes forever. The *Jnâni* seeks to tear himself away from this bondage of matter by the force of intellectual conviction. This is the negative way,—the "*neti, neti*" ("not this, not this").

VI. UNITY OF THE SELF.

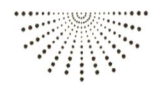

To illustrate the conclusion arrived at in our last lesson, I will read to you from one of the Upanishads, showing how these ideas were taught in India from the most ancient times.

Yajnavalkya was a great sage. You know the rule in India was that every man must give up the world when he became old. So *Yajnavalkya* said to his wife: "My beloved, here is all my money and my possessions, and I am going away." She replied:

"Sir, if I had this whole earth full of wealth would that give me immortality?" *Yajnavalkya* said: "No, that cannot be. Your life will be that of the rich, and that will be all, but wealth cannot give you immortality." She replied: "That through which I shall become immortal, what shall I do to gain that? If you know that, tell me." *Yajnavalkya* replied: "You have always been my beloved; you are more beloved now by this question. Come, take your seat, and I will tell you, and when you have heard, meditate upon it." He continued: "It is not for the sake of the husband that the wife loves the husband, but for the sake of the *Átman* (the Self) that she loves the husband, because she loves the Self. None loves the wife for the sake of the wife, but it is because he loves the Self that he loves the wife. None loves the children for the sake of the children, but because he loves the Self, therefore he loves the children. None loves wealth on account of the wealth, but because he loves the Self, therefore he loves wealth. None loves the Brahmin for the sake of the Brahmin, but because he loves the Self, he loves the Brahmin. So none loves the *Kshatriya* for the sake of the *Kshatriya*, but because he loves the Self. Neither does anyone love the world on account of the world, but because he loves the Self. None similarly loves the gods on account of the gods, but because he loves the Self. None loves anything for that thing's sake, but it is for the Self of that thing that he loves it. This Self therefore, is to be heard, is to be reasoned, and is to be meditated upon. Oh my *Maitreyi*, when that Self has been heard, when that Self has been seen, when that Self has been realized, then all these things become known."

What does this mean? Before us we find a curious philosophy. That the Self shines through all these various things which we call the world. The statement has been made that every love is selfishness in the lowest sense of the word; because I love myself, therefore I love another; it cannot be. There have been philosophers in modern times who have said that self is the only motive power in the world. That is true, and yet it is wrong. This self is but the shadow of that real Self which is behind. It appears wrong and evil because it is limited. That very love we have for the Self, which is the universe, appears to be evil, because it is seen through limitation. Even when a wife loves a husband, whether she knows it or not, she loves the husband for that Self. It is selfishness as it is manifested in the world, but that selfishness is really but a small part of that "Self-ness." Whenever one loves, one has to love in and through the Self.

This Self has to be known. Those that love the Self without knowing what It is, their love is selfishness. Those that love knowing what that Self is, their love is free, they are sages. None loves the Brahmin for the Brahmin, but because he loves the Self, which is appearing through the Brahmin. "Him the Brahmin gives up who sees the Brahmin as separate from the Self. Him the *Kshatriya* gives up who sees the *Kshatriya* as separate from the Self. The world gives him up who sees this world as separate from the Self. The gods give him up who believes the gods to be separate from the Self. All things give him up who knows them as separate from the Self. These Brahmins, these *Kshatriyas*, this world, these gods, whatever exists, everything is that Self. Thus *Yajnavalkya* explains what he means by that love. The difficulty comes when we particularize this love. Suppose I love a woman; as soon as that woman is particularized, is separated, from that *Âtman* (the Self), my love will not be eternal; it has become selfish and is likely to end in grief, but as soon as I see that woman as the *Âtman*, that Love becomes perfect, and will never suffer. So, as soon as you are attached to anything in the universe detaching it from the universe as a whole—from the *Âtman*—then comes a reaction. With everything that we love outside the Self, grief and misery will be the result. If we enjoy everything in the Self, and as the Self, no misery or reaction will come. This is perfect bliss.

How to come to this ideal? *Yajnavalkya* goes on to tell us the process by which to reach that state. The universe is infinite; how can we take every particular thing and look at it as the *Âtman*, without knowing the *Âtman*? "With a drum, when we are at a distance, we cannot conquer the sound by trying to control the sound waves, but as soon as we come to the drum, and put our hand on it, the sound is conquered. When the conch shell is being blown, we cannot conquer the sound, until we come near and get hold of the shell, and then it is conquered. When the vina is being played, as soon as we come to the vina, we can control the centre of the sound, whence the sound is proceeding. As when some one is burning damp fuel, all sorts of smoke and sparks of various kinds rise, even so from this great One has been breathed out history and knowledge; everything has come out of Him. He breathed out, as it were, all knowledge. As to all water the one goal is the ocean, as to all touch the hand is the one centre, as to all smell the nose is the one centre, as of all taste the tongue is the one centre, as of all form the eyes are the one centre, as of all sounds the ears are the one centre, as of all thought the mind is the one centre, as of all knowledge the heart is the one centre, as of all work the hands are the one centre, as of all speech the organ of speech is the one centre, as the concentrated salt is through and through the waters of the sea, yet not to be seen by the eyes; even so, oh *Maitreyi*, is this *Âtman* not to be seen by the eyes, yet He permeates this universe. He is everything. He is concentrated knowledge. The whole universe rises from Him, and again goes down unto Him. Reaching Him, we go beyond knowledge." We here get the idea that we have all come just like sparks from Him, and that when we know Him then we go back, and become one with Him again.

Maitreyi became frightened, just as everywhere people become frightened. She said: "Sir, here is exactly where you have thrown a confusion over me. You have frightened me by saying there will be no more gods; all individuality will be lost. When I reach that stage shall I know that *Âtman*, shall I reach the unconscious state and lose my individuality, or will the knowledge remain with me that I know Him? Will there be no one to recognize, no one to feel, no one to love, no one to hate? What will become of me?" "O *Maitreyi!*" replied her husband, "think not that I am speaking of an unconscious state, neither be frightened. This *Âtman* is indestructible, eternal in His essence; the stage where there are two is a lower one. Where there are two there one smells another, one sees another, one hears another, one welcomes another, one thinks of another, one knows another. But when the whole has become that *Âtman*, who is to be smelled by whom, who is to be seen by whom, who is to be heard by whom, who is to be welcomed by whom, who is to be known by whom? Who can know Him by whom everything is known? This *Âtman* can only be described as *"neti, neti"* (not this, not this). Incomprehensible, He cannot be comprehended by the intellect. Unchangeable, He never fades. Unattached, He never gets mixed up with Nature. Perfect, He is beyond all pleasure and pain. Who can know the Knower? By what means can we know Him? By no means; this is the conclusion of the sages, O *Maitreyi*! Going beyond all knowledge, is to attain Him and to attain immortality."

So far the idea is, that it is all One Infinite Being, that is the Real Individuality, when there is no more division, no more parts and parcels, no more such low and illusory ideas. And yet, in and through every part of this little individuality is shining that Infinite, the Real Individuality. Everything is a manifestation of the *Âtman*. How to reach to that? *Yajnavalkya* told us in the beginning that

—"This *Âtman* is first to be heard, then to be reasoned, then to be meditated upon." Thus far he has spoken about the Self, the *Âtman*, as being the essence of everything in this universe. Then reasoning on the Infinite nature of that Self and the finite nature of the human mind he comes to the conclusion that it is impossible for the finite mind to know the Knower of all—the Self. What is to be done then if we cannot know the Self? *Yajnavalkya* tells *Maitreyi* that It can be realized, although It cannot be known, and he enters upon a discourse as to how It is to be meditated upon. This universe is helpful to every being and every being is also helping this universe, for they are both part and parcel of each other, the development of the one helps the development of the other; but to the *Âtman*, the self-effulgent One, nothing can be helpful because It is perfect and infinite. All that is bliss, even in the lowest sense, is but the reflection of It. All that is good is the reflection of that *Âtman*, and when that reflection is less clear it is called evil. When the *Âtman* is less manifested it is called darkness—evil, and when it is more manifested it is called light—goodness. That is all. This good and evil are only a question of degree, the *Âtman* more manifested or less manifested. Just take the example of our own lives. How many things we see in our childhood which we think to be good, but which really are evil, and how many things seem to be evil which are good? How our ideas change! How an idea becomes higher and higher! What we thought very good at one time, we do not think so good now. Thus good and evil depend on the development of our minds, and do not exist objectively. The difference is only in the degree. All is a manifestation of that *Âtman*; It is being manifested in everything, only when the manifestation is very poor we call it evil, and when it is clearer we call it good. That *Âtman* Itself is beyond both good and evil. So everything that is in the universe is first to be meditated upon as all good, because it is a manifestation of that perfect One. He is neither evil nor good; He is perfect and the perfect can be only one. The good can be many, and the evil many, there will be degrees of variation between the good and the evil; but the perfect is only one, and that perfect One when seen through certain covering we call different degrees of good, and when seen through other covering we call evil. Our ideas of good and evil as two distinct things are mere superstition. There is only more good and less good and the less good we call evil. These mistaken ideas of good and evil have produced all sorts of dualistic delusions. They have gone deep into the hearts of human beings, terrorizing men and women in all ages. All the hatred with which we hate others is caused by these foolish ideas which we have imbibed since our childhood. Our judgment of humanity becomes entirely false; we make this beautiful earth a hell, but as soon as we can give up these false ideas of good and evil, it will become a heaven.

"This earth is blissful ('sweet' is the literal translation) to all beings, and all beings are sweet to this earth; they all help each other. And all this sweetness is the *Âtman*, that effulgent, immortal One." That one sweetness is manifesting itself in various ways. Wherever there is any love, any sweetness in any human being, either in a saint or a sinner, either in an angel or a murderer, either in the body or the mind or the senses, it is all He. How can there be anything but the One? Whatever is the lowest physical enjoyment is He, and the highest spiritual enjoyment is also He. There is no sweetness but He. Thus says *Yajnavalkya*. When you come to that state, and look upon all things with the same eyes; when you see in the drunkard's pleasure in drink only that sweetness, or in the saints' meditation only that sweetness, then you have got the truth, and then alone you will know what happiness means, what peace means, what love means. But as long as you make these vain distinctions, silly, childish, foolish superstitions, all sorts of misery will come. But that immortal One, the effulgent One, He is the background of the whole universe, it is all His sweetness. This body is a miniature universe, as it were; and through all the powers of the body, all the enjoyments of the mind, shines that effulgent One. That self-effulgent One who is in the body, He is the *Âtman*. "This world is so sweet to all beings, and every being is so sweet to it!" But the self-effulgent One, the Immortal is the bliss in this world. In us also, He is that bliss. He is the *Brahman*. "This air is so sweet to all beings, and all beings are so sweet to this air." But He who is that self-effulgent immortal Being in the air, He is also in this body. He is expressing Himself as the life of all beings.

"This sun is so sweet to all beings, and all beings are so sweet to this sun." He who is the self-effulgent Being in the sun, Him we reflect as smaller lights. What can there be but His reflection? He is in the body, and it is His reflection which makes us see the light. "This moon is so sweet to all beings, and all beings are so sweet to this moon." But that self-effulgent and immortal One who is the soul of that moon, He is in us expressing himself as mind. "This lightning is so sweet to all beings and all beings are sweet to this lightning," but the self-effulgent and immortal One is the soul of this lightning, and is also in us, because all is that *Brahman*. This *Brahman*, this *Âtman*, this Self, is the King of all beings. These ideas are very helpful to men; they are for meditation. For instance, meditate on the earth, think of the earth, at the same time knowing that we have in us that which is in the earth, that both are the same. Identify the body with the earth, and identify the soul with the Soul behind. Identify the air with the soul that is in the air and that is in you and so on. All these are one, manifested in different forms. To realize this unity is the end and aim of all meditation, and this is what *Yajnavalkya* was trying to explain to *Maitreyi*.

VII. THE HIGHEST IDEAL OF JNÂNA YOGA.

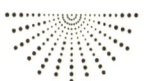

As this is the last of these classes it is better that I give a brief *resumé* of all that I have been trying to tell you. In the Vedas and Upanishads we find records of some of the very earliest religious ideas of the Hindus, ideas that long antedated the time of Kapila, ancient as this great sage is. He did not propound the *Sânkhya* philosophy as a new theory of his own. His task was to throw the light of his genius on the vast mass of religious theories that were existing in his time and bring out a rational and coherent system. He succeeded in giving India a psychology that is accepted to the present day by all the diverse and seemingly opposing philosophical systems to be found among the Hindus. His masterly analysis and his comprehensive statement of the processes of the human mind have not yet been surpassed by any later philosopher and he undoubtedly laid the foundation for the Advaita philosophy, which accepted his conclusions as far as they went and then pushed them a step farther, thus reaching a final unity beyond the duality that was the last word of the *Sânkhyas*.

Among the religious ideas that preceded the time of Kapila the first groups that we see coming up,—I mean among recognized religious ideas, and not the very low ones, which do not deserve the name of religion,—all include the idea of inspiration, and revealed book and so forth. In the earliest step, the idea of creation is very peculiar; it is that the whole universe is created out of zero, at the will of God; that all this universe did not exist, and out of nothingness all this has come. In the next stage we find this conclusion is questioned. The first step in Vedânta asks this question: How can existence be produced out of non-existence? If this universe is existent it must have come out of something, because it was easy for them to see that there is nothing coming out of nothing anywhere. All work that is going on by human hands requires materials. Naturally, therefore, the ancient Hindus rejected the first idea that this world was created out of nothing, and sought some material out of which this world was created. The whole history of religion, in fact, is this search for material. Out of what has all this been produced? Apart from the question of the efficient cause, or God, apart from the question whether God created the universe, the great question of all questions has been, out of what did God create it? All the philosophies are turning, as it were, on this question.

One solution is that nature and God and soul are eternal existences, as if three parallel lines are running eternally, of which nature and soul comprise what they call the dependent, and God the independent Being. Every soul, like every particle of matter, is perfectly dependent on the will of God. These and many other ideas we find already existing when the *Sânkhya* psychology was brought forward by Kapila. According to it, perception comes by the transmission of the suggestion, which causes perception first to the eyes, from the eyes to the organs, from the organs to the mind, the mind to the *buddhi* and from the *buddhi* to something which is a unit, which they call the *Âtman*. Coming to modern physiology we know that they have found centres for all the different sensations. First are found the lower centres, then a higher grade of centres, and these two will exactly correspond with the actions of the *buddhi* and the *manas* (mind), but not one centre has been found which controls all the other centres, so philosophy cannot answer what unifies all these centres. Where and how do the centres get unified? The centres in the brain are all different, and there is not one centre which controls all the others; therefore, so far as it goes, the *Sânkhya* psychology stands unchallenged upon this point. We must have this unification, something upon which the sensations will be reflected to form a complete whole. Until there is that something I cannot have any idea of you, or the picture, or anything else. If we had not that unifying something we would only see, then after a while hear, and then feel, and while we heard a man talking we should not see him at all, because all the centres are different.

This body is made of particles which we call matter, and it is dull and insentient. So is what is called the fine body. The fine body, according to the *Sânkhyas* is a little body, made of very fine particles, so fine that no microscope can see them. What is the use of it? It is the receptacle of what we call mind. Just as this gross body is the receptacle of the grosser forces, so the fine body is the receptacle of the finer forces, that which we call thought, in its various modifications. First is the body, which is gross matter, with gross force. Force cannot exist without matter. It can only manifest itself through matter, so the grosser forces work through the body and those very forces become finer; the very force which is working in a gross form works in a fine form and becomes thought. There is no real difference between them, simply one is the gross and the other the fine manifestation of the same thing. Neither is there any difference in substance between the fine body and the gross body. The fine body is also material, only very fine material.

Whence do all these forces come? According to the Vedânta philosophy there are two things in Nature, one of which they call *Âkâsa*, which is substance, or matter, infinitely fine, and the other they call *Prâna*. Whatever you see, or feel, or hear, as air or earth, or anything, is material. And everything is a form of this *âkâsa*. It becomes finer and finer, or grosser and grosser, and it changes under the action of *Prâna* (universal Energy). Like *âkâsa*, *prâna* is omnipresent, interpenetrating everything. *Âkâsa* is like the water, and everything else in the universe like blocks of ice, made out of that water and floating in it, and *prâna* is the power that changes the *âkâsa* into all these various forms. This body is the instrument made out of *âkâsa* for the manifestation of *prâna* in gross forms, as muscular motion, or walking, sitting, talking, and so on. The fine body also is made of *âkâsa*, a much finer form of *âkâsa*, for the manifestation of the same *prâna* in the finer form of thought. So, first there is this gross body, beyond that is the fine body, and beyond that is the *jiva* (soul), the real man. Just as these finger nails can be pared off a hundred times a year, and yet are still a part of our bodies, not different, so we have not two bodies. It is not that man has a fine and also a gross body; it is the one body, only it remains longer when it is a fine body, and the grosser it is the sooner it dissolves. Just as I can cut this nail a hundred times a year, so millions of times I can shed this body in one æon, but the fine body will remain. According to the dualists this *jiva*, or the real man, is very fine, minute.

So far we have seen that man is a being who has first a gross body which dissolves very quickly, then a fine body which remains through æons, and lastly a *jiva*. This *jiva*, according to the Vedânta philosophy, is eternal, just as God is eternal, and Nature is also eternal, but changefully eternal. The material of Nature, the *prâna* and the *âkâsa*, are eternal, but are changing into different forms eternally. Matter and force are eternal, but their combinations vary continually. The *jiva* is not manufactured, either of *âkâsa*, or of *prâna*; it is immaterial, and therefore will remain for ever. It is not the result of any combination of *prâna* and *âkâsa*, and whatever is not the result of combination will never be destroyed, because destruction is decomposition. That which is not a compound cannot be destroyed. The gross body is a compound of *âkâsa* and *prâna* in various forms and will be decomposed. The fine body will also be decomposed after a long time, but the *jiva* is a simple, and will never be destroyed. For the same reason, we cannot say it ever was born. Nothing simple can be born; the same argument applies. Only that which is a compound can be born.

The whole of this nature combined in these millions of forms is under the will of God. God is all pervading, omniscient, formless, everywhere, and He is directing this nature day and night. The whole of it is under His control. There is no independence of any being. It cannot be. He is the Ruler. This is the teaching of dualistic Vedânta.

Then the question comes, if God be the Ruler of this universe, why did He create such a wicked universe, why must we suffer so much? The answer is made that it is not God's fault. It is our own fault that we suffer. Whatever we sow that we reap. God does not do anything to punish us. If a man is born poor, or blind, or lame, he did something before he was born in that way, something that produced these results. The *jiva* has been existing for all time, was never created. It has been doing all sorts of things all the time. Whatever we do we suffer for. If we do good we shall have happiness, and if bad, unhappiness. This *jiva* is by its own nature pure, but ignorance covers its nature, says the dualist. As by evil deeds it has covered itself with ignorance, so by good deeds it can become conscious of its own nature again. Just as it is eternal, so its nature is pure. The nature of every being is pure. When through good deeds all its sins and misdeeds have been washed away, then the *jiva* becomes pure again, and when he becomes pure he goes after death by what is called *Devayana* (the path of the gods), to heaven, or the abode of the gods. If he has been only an ordinarily good man he goes to what is called the "Abode of the Fathers."

When the gross body falls, the organs of speech enter the mind.

You cannot think without words; wherever there are words there must be thought. The mind is resolved into the *prâna*, and the *prâna* resolves into the *jiva*. Then the *jiva* leaves the body and goes to that condition of reward or punishment which he has earned by his past life. *Devaloka* is the "place (or abode) of the gods." The word *deva* (god) means bright or shining one, and corresponds to what the Christians and Mohammedans call "angels." According to this teaching there are various heavenly spheres somewhat analogous to the various heavens described by Dante in the *Divine Comedy*. There are the heaven of the fathers (or *pitris*), *devaloka*, the lunar sphere, the electric sphere and highest of all the *Brahmaloka*, the heaven of *Brahma*. From all the lower heavens the *jiva* returns again to human birth, but he who attains to *Brahmaloka* lives there through all eternity. These are the highest men who have become perfectly unselfish, perfectly purified, who have given up all desires, do not want to do anything except to worship and love God. There is a second class, who do good works, but want some reward, want to go to heaven in return. When they die the *jiva* goes to the lunar sphere, where it enjoys and becomes a *deva* (god or angel). The gods, the *devas*, are not eternal, they have to die. In heaven they will all die. The only deathless place is *Brahmaloka*, where alone there is no birth and no death. In our mythology it is said there are also the demons, who sometimes give the gods chase. In all mythologies you read of these fights between the demons, or wicked angels, and the gods and sometimes the demons conquer the gods. In all mythologies also, you find that the *devas* were fond of the beautiful daughters of men. As a *deva*, the *jiva* only reaps results of past actions, but makes no new Karma. Only man makes Karma. Karma means actions that will produce effects, also those effects, or results of action. When a man dies and becomes a *deva* he has a period of pleasure, and during that time makes no fresh Karma; he simply enjoys the reward of his past good works. But when the good Karma is worked out then the other Karma begins to take effect.

In the Vedas there is no mention of hell. But afterwards the *Purânas*, the later books in our Scriptures, thought that no religion could become complete without a proper attachment of hells, and so they invented all sorts of hells, with as many, if not more, varieties of punishment than Dante saw in his *Inferno*, but our books are merciful enough to say that it is only for a period. Bad Karma is worked out in that state and then the souls come back to earth and get another chance. This human form is the great chance. It is called the *karmic* body, in which we decide our fate. We are running in a huge circle, and this is the point in the circle which determines the future. So a human body is considered the greatest body there is; man is greater than the gods. Even they return to human birth. So far with dualistic Vedânta.

Next comes a higher conception of Vedânta philosophy, which says that these ideas are crude. If you say there is a God who is an infinite Being, and a soul which is also infinite, and Nature which is also infinite, you can go on multiplying infinites indefinitely, but that is illogical, because each would limit the other and there would be no real infinite. God is both the material and the efficient cause of the universe; He projects this universe out of Himself. Does that mean that God has become these walls, and this table, that God has become the animal, the murderer and all the evils in the world? God is pure, how can He become all these degenerate things? He has not. God is unchangeable, all these changes are in Nature; just as I am a soul and have a body, this body is not different from me in a sense, yet I, the real "I," in fact am not this body. For instance, I am a child, I become a young man, an old man, but my soul has not changed. It remains the same soul. Similarly the whole universe comprises all Nature, and an infinite number of souls, or, as it were, the infinite body of God. He is interpenetrating the whole of it. He alone is unchangeable, but Nature changes and soul changes. In what way does Nature change? In its forms; it takes fresh forms. But the soul cannot change that way. The soul contracts and expands in knowledge. It contracts by evil deeds; those deeds which contract the natural knowledge and purity of the soul are called evil deeds. Those deeds, again, which bring out the natural glory of the soul, are called good deeds. All these souls were pure, but they have become contracted by their own acts. Still, through the mercy of God, and by doing good deeds, they will expand and become pure again. Every soul has the same chance, and, in the long run, must become pure and free itself from Nature. But this universe will not cease, because it is infinite. This is the second theory. The first is called dualistic Vedânta; the second teaches that there is God, soul, and Nature, that soul and Nature form the body of God, and that these three form one unit. Believers in this second theory are called qualified non-dualists (*Visishtadvaitins*).

The last and highest theory is pure monism, or as it is known in India, *Advaita*. It also teaches that God must be both the material and the efficient cause of this universe. As such, God has become the whole of this universe. This theory denies that God is the soul, and the universe is the body, and the body is changing. In that case what is the use of calling God the material cause of this universe? The material cause is the cause become effect; the effect is nothing but the cause in another form. Wherever you see effect, it is the cause reproduced. If the universe is the effect, and God the cause, this must be the reproduction of God. If it be claimed that the universe is the body of God and that that body becomes contracted and fine and becomes the cause, and out of that the universe is evolved, then the *advaitist* says it is God Himself who has become this universe. Now comes a very fine question. If God has become this universe, then everything is God. Certainly; everything is God. My body is God, and my mind is God, and my soul is God.

Then why are there so many *jivas*? Has God become divided into millions and millions of *jivas*? How can that infinite power and substance, the one Being of the universe become divided? It is impossible to divide infinity. How can the pure Being become this universe? If He has become the universe, He is changeful, and if He is changeful, He is in Nature, and whatever is in Nature is born and dies. If God is changeful, He must die some day. Remember that. Again, how much of God has become this universe? If you say "X," the algebraical unknown quantity, then God is God minus "X" now, and therefore not the same God as before this creation, because so much of Him has become this universe. The answer of the non-dualist is that this universe has no real existence, it exists in appearance only.

These *devas* and gods and angels and being born and dying, and all this infinite number of souls coming up and going down, all these things are mere dreams. All is the one Infinite. The one sun reflected on various drops of water appears to be many, millions of globules of water reflect so many millions of suns and in each globule will be a perfect image of the sun, yet there is only one sun, and so it is with all these *jivas*, they are but reflections of the one infinite Being. A dream cannot be without a reality, and that reality is the one infinite Existence. You, as body, mind, or soul, are a dream, but what you really are is Existence-Knowledge-Bliss Absolute. Thus says the *Advaitist*. All these births and rebirths, this coming and going are but parts of the dream. You are infinite. Where can you go? The sun, moon, and the whole universe are but a drop in your nature. How can you be born or die? The Self was never born, never will be born, never had father or mother, friends or foes, for it is Existence-Knowledge-Bliss Absolute.

What is the goal, according to this philosophy? That those who receive this knowledge are one with the universe; for them all heavens, even *Brahmaloka*, are destroyed, the whole dream vanishes, and they find themselves the eternal God of the universe. They attain their real individuality, infinitely beyond these little selves which we now think of so much importance. No individuality will be lost; an infinite and eternal Individuality will be realized. Pleasures in little things will cease. We are finding pleasure in this little body, in this little individuality. How much greater the pleasure when this whole universe is in our one body? If there be pleasure in these separate bodies, how much more when all bodies are one? The man who has realized this has attained to freedom, has gone beyond the dream and known himself in his real nature. This is the teaching of Advaita, the non-dualistic Vedânta.

These are the three steps which Vedânta philosophy has taken, and we cannot go beyond, because we cannot go beyond unity. When any science reaches a unity it cannot possibly go any farther. You cannot go beyond this idea of the Absolute, the One Idea of the universe, out of which everything else has evolved. All people cannot take up this *Advaita* philosophy; it is too hard. First of all, it is very difficult to understand it intellectually. It requires the sharpest of intellects, a bold understanding. Secondly, it does not suit the vast majority of people.

It is better to begin with the first of these three steps. Then by thinking of that and understanding it, the second one will open of itself. Just as a race travels, so individuals have to travel. The steps which the human race has taken to come to the highest pinnacle of religious thought, every individual will have to take. Only, while the human race took millions of years to reach from one step to another, individuals may live the whole life of the human race in a few years, or they may be able to do it more quickly, perhaps in six months. But each one of us will have to go through these steps. Those of you who are non-dualists can, no doubt, look back to the period of your lives when you were strong dualists. As soon as you think you are a body and a mind, you will have to accept the whole of this dream. If you have one piece you must take the whole. The man who says, here is this world but there is no God, is a fool, because if there be a world there will have to be a cause of the world, and that is what is called God. You cannot have an effect without knowing that there is a cause. God will only vanish when this world vanishes. When you have realized your one-ness with God, this world will no longer be for you. As long as this dream exists, however, we are bound to see ourselves as being born and dying, but as soon as the dream that we are bodies vanishes, so will vanish this dream that we are being born and dying, and so will vanish the other dream that there is a universe. That very thing which we now see as this universe will appear to us as God, and that very God who was so long external, will appear as the very Self of our own selves. The last word of *Advaita* is, *Tat tvam asi,*—"That thou art."

Copyright © 2021 by ALICIA EDITIONS
All rights reserved.
No part of this book may be reproduced in any form or by any electronic or mechanical means, including information storage and retrieval systems, without written permission from the author, except for the use of brief quotations in a book review.

www.ingramcontent.com/pod-product-compliance
Lightning Source LLC
LaVergne TN
LVHW040039080526
838202LV00045B/3410